Lipids: Update on Diagnosis and Management of Dyslipidemia

Editors

CONNIE B. NEWMAN
ALAN CHAIT

ENDOCRINOLOGY AND METABOLISM CLINICS OF NORTH AMERICA

www.endo.theclinics.com

Consulting Editor
ADRIANA G. IOACHIMESCU

September 2022 • Volume 51 • Number 3

ELSEVIER

1600 John F. Kennedy Boulevard • Suite 1800 • Philadelphia, Pennsylvania, 19103-2899

http://www.theclinics.com

ENDOCRINOLOGY AND METABOLISM CLINICS OF NORTH AMERICA Volume 51, Number 3
September 2022 ISSN 0889-8529, ISBN 13: 978-0-323-98695-3

Editor: Katerina Heidhausen
Developmental Editor: Jessica Cañaberal

Endocrinology and Metabolism Clinics of North America (ISSN 0889-8529) is published quarterly by Elsevier Inc., 360 Park Avenue South, New York, NY 10010-1710. Months of issue are March, June, September, and December. Periodicals postage paid at New York, NY and additional mailing offices. Subscription prices are USD 394.00 per year for US individuals, USD 1058.00 per year for US institutions, USD 100.00 per year for US students and residents, USD 467.00 per year for Canadian individuals, USD 1079.00 per year for Canadian institutions, USD 512.00 per year for international individuals, USD 1079.00 per year for international institutions, USD 100.00 per year for Canadian students/residents, and USD 245.00 per year for international students/residents. To receive student/resident rate, orders must be accompanied by name of affiliated institution, date of term, and the signature of program/residency coordinator on institution letterhead. Orders will be billed at individual rate until proof of status is received. Foreign air speed delivery is included in all *Clinics* subscription prices. All prices are subject to change without notice. **POSTMASTER:** Send address changes to *Endocrinology and Metabolism Clinics of North America*, Elsevier Health Sciences Division, Subscription Customer Service, 3251 Riverport Lane, Maryland Heights, MO 63043. **Customer Service: Telephone: 1-800-654-2452** (U.S. and Canada); **1-314-447-8871** (outside U.S. and Canada). **Fax: 1-314-447-8029. E-mail: journalscustomerservice-u-sa@elsevier.com (for print support); journalsonlinesupport-usa@elsevier.com (for online support)**.

Reprints. For copies of 100 or more, of articles in this publication, please contact the Commercial Rights Department, Elsevier Inc., 360 Park Avenue South, New York, NY 10010-1710; phone: +1-212-633-3874; fax: +1-212-633-3820; E-mail: reprints@elsevier.com.

Endocrinology and Metabolism Clinics of North America is covered in *MEDLINE/PubMed (Index Medicus), EMBASE/Excerpta Medica, Current Contents/Clinical Medicine, Current Contents/Life Sciences, Science Citation Index, ISI/BIOMED, BIOSIS,* and *Chemical Abstracts*.

Contributors

CONSULTING EDITOR

ADRIANA G. IOACHIMESCU, MD, PhD, FACE
Associate Professor of Medicine and Neurosurgery, Co-Director, The Emory Pituitary
Center, Emory University School of Medicine, Atlanta, Georgia, USA

EDITORS

CONNIE B. NEWMAN, MD
Adjunct Professor, Division of Endocrinology, Diabetes and Metabolism, Department of
Medicine, NYU Grossman School of Medicine, New York, New York, USA

ALAN CHAIT, MD
Professor Emeritus, Division of Metabolism, Endocrinology and Nutrition, Department of
Medicine, University of Washington, Seattle, Washington, USA

AUTHORS

ZAHRA ALIGABI, MS
Lipoprotein Metabolism Laboratory, Translational Vascular Medicine Branch, National
Heart, Lung, and Blood Institute, National Institutes of Health, Bethesda, Maryland, USA

MARCELLO ARCA, MD
Professor of Medicine, Department of Translational and Precision Medicine, University of
Rome, Sapienza, Italy

MAURIZIO AVERNA, MD
Professor of Medicine, University of Palermo, Italy

MICHAEL J. BLAHA, MD, MPH
Division of Cardiology, Department of Medicine, Ciccarone Center for the Prevention of
Cardiovascular Disease, Johns Hopkins School of Medicine, Baltimore, Maryland, USA

ALBERICO CATAPANO, MD, PhD
Professor of Pharmacology, Department of Pharmacological and Biomolecular Sciences,
Università degli Studi di Milano, Milan, Italy; IRCCS MultiMedica, Sesto San Giovanni, Italy

ALAN CHAIT, MD
Professor Emeritus, Division of Metabolism, Endocrinology and Nutrition, Department of
Medicine, University of Washington, Seattle, Washington, USA

HONG Y CHOI, PhD
Research Institute of the McGill University Health Centre, Montreal, Quebec, Canada

LAURA D'ERASMO, MD, PhD
Department of Translational and Precision Medicine, University of Rome, Sapienza, Italy

KENNETH R. FEINGOLD, MD
Emeritus Professor of Medicine, University of California, San Francisco, San Francisco, California, USA

EDWARD A. FISHER, MD, PhD
Professor, Division of Cardiology and Center for the Prevention of Cardiovascular Disease, NYU Grossman School of Medicine, New York, New York, USA

JACQUES GENEST, MD
Research Institute of the McGill University Health Centre, Montreal, Quebec, Canada

JANA GJINI, MS
Associate Research Technician, Division of Endocrinology, Diabetes and Metabolism, NYU Grossman School of Medicine, New York, New York, USA

IRA J. GOLDBERG, MD
Director, Division of Endocrinology, Diabetes and Metabolism, NYU Grossman School of Medicine, New York, New York, USA

RONALD B. GOLDBERG, MD
Professor of Medicine, Division of Endocrinology, Diabetes and Metabolism, Diabetes Research Institute, University of Miami Miller School of Medicine, Miami, Florida, USA

EARL GOLDSBOROUGH III, BS
Johns Hopkins School of Medicine, Baltimore, Maryland, USA

IULIA IATAN, PhD, MD
Research Institute of the McGill University Health Centre, Montreal, Quebec, Canada

WANN JIA LOH, MBBS, BSc
Department of Endocrinology, Changi General Hospital, Singapore

DIEGO LUCERO, PhD
Lipoprotein Metabolism Laboratory, Translational Vascular Medicine Branch, National Heart, Lung, and Blood Institute, National Institutes of Health, Bethesda, Maryland, USA

CONNIE B. NEWMAN, MD
Adjunct Professor, Division of Endocrinology, Diabetes and Metabolism, Department of Medicine, NYU Grossman School of Medicine, New York, New York, USA

NGOZI OSUJI, MD, MPH
Division of Cardiology, Department of Medicine, Ciccarone Center for the Prevention of Cardiovascular Disease, Johns Hopkins School of Medicine, Baltimore, Maryland, USA

AMISHA PATEL, MD
Department of Pediatrics, UT Southwestern Medical Center, Dallas, Texas, USA

NIVEDITA PATNI, MD
Division of Pediatric Endocrinology, Department of Pediatrics, UT Southwestern Medical Center, Dallas, Texas, USA

ALAN T. REMALEY, MD, PhD
Lipoprotein Metabolism Laboratory, Translational Vascular Medicine Branch, National Heart, Lung, and Blood Institute, National Institutes of Health, Bethesda, Maryland, USA

LISA R. TANNOCK, MD
Professor of Internal Medicine, Division of Endocrinology, Diabetes, and Metabolism, University of Kentucky, Department of Veterans Affairs, Lexington, Kentucky, USA

JONATHAN A. TOBERT, MD, PhD
Academic Visitor, Nuffield Department of Population Health, University of Oxford, Oxford, United Kingdom

SARAH TURECAMO, BA
Heart Disease Phenomics Laboratory, Epidemiology and Community Health Branch, National Heart, Lung, and Blood Institute, National Institutes of Health, Bethesda, Maryland, USA

GERALD F. WATTS, DSc, PhD, DM, FRACP, FRCP
School of Medicine, University of Western Australia, Crawley, Western Australia, Australia; Department of Cardiology and Internal Medicine, Royal Perth Hospital, Victoria Square, Perth, Western Australia, Australia

ANNA WOLSKA, PhD
Heart Disease Phenomics Laboratory, Epidemiology and Community Health Branch, National Heart, Lung, and Blood Institute, National Institutes of Health, Bethesda, Maryland, USA

ALBERTO ZAMBON, MD, PhD
Associate Professor of Medicine, Department of Medicine - DIMED, University of Padova, Padova, Italy

Contents

The exogenous lipoprotein pathway starts with the incorporation of dietary lipids into chylomicrons in the intestine. Chylomicron triglycerides are metabolized in muscle and adipose tissue and chylomicron remnants are formed, which are removed by the liver. The endogenous lipoprotein pathway begins in the liver with the formation of very low-density lipoprotein particles (VLDL). VLDL triglycerides are metabolized in muscle and adipose tissue forming intermediate-density lipoprotein (IDL), which may be taken up by the liver or further metabolized to low-density lipoprotein (LDL). Reverse cholesterol transport begins with the formation of nascent high-density lipoprotein (HDL) by the liver and intestine that acquire cholesterol from cells resulting in mature HDL. The HDL then transports the cholesterol to the liver either directly or indirectly by transferring the cholesterol to VLDL or LDL.

Based on decades of both basic science and epidemiologic research, there is overwhelming evidence for the causal relationship between high levels of cholesterol, especially low-density lipoprotein cholesterol and cardiovascular disease. Risk evaluation and monitoring the response to lipid-lowering therapies are heavily dependent on the accurate assessment of plasma lipoproteins in the clinical laboratory. This article provides an update of lipoprotein metabolism as it relates to atherosclerosis and how diagnostic measures of lipids and lipoproteins can serve as markers of cardiovascular risk, with a focus on recent advances in cardiovascular risk marker testing.

Assessment of atherosclerotic cardiovascular disease (ASCVD) risk is the cornerstone of primary ASCVD prevention, enabling targeted use of the most aggressive therapies in those most likely to benefit, while guiding a conservative approach in those who are low risk. ASCVD risk assessment begins with the use of a traditional 10-year risk calculator, with further refinement through the consideration of risk-enhancing factors (particularly

modifications with heart-healthy diet and moderate-vigorous activity are fundamental in the management of pediatric dyslipidemia. Pharmacotherapy has been evolving in children, and statins, bile acid sequestrants, ezetimibe and PCSK9 inhibitors, fibrates, niacin, and omega-3 fish oils are available for use in pediatric population.

Most endocrine disorders are chronic in nature, and thus even a minor effect to increase risk for cardiovascular disease can lead to a significant impact over prolonged duration. Although robust therapies exist for many endocrine disorders (eg suppression of excess hormone amounts, or replacement of hormone deficiencies), the therapies do not perfectly restore normal physiology. Thus, individuals with endocrine disorders are at potential increased cardiovascular disease risk, and maximizing strategies to reduce that risk are needed. This article reviews various endocrine conditions that can impact lipid levels and/or cardiovascular disease risk.

Elevated triglyceride and reduced high-density lipoprotein cholesterol (HDL-C) are common in type 2 diabetes, but increased atherogenic particles and dysfunctional HDL are demonstrable in both types 1 and 2 diabetes, contributing to a two-fold increase in atherosclerotic cardiovascular disease (ASCVD). ASCVD risk accelerates with diabetes duration and severity, aging, risk factors, and risk enhancers. Using statins or other LDL-C–lowering agents if needed in adults with intermediate or greater degrees of risk is recommended. Although hypertriglyceridemia enhances risk, most guidelines do not recommend fibrates or omega 3 fatty acid for risk reduction except for icosapent ethyl in patients with ASCVD.

Benefits of omega 3 fatty acids for cardiovascular and other diseases have been touted for more than 50 years. The one clear clinical benefit of these lipids is the reduction of circulating levels of triglycerides, making them a useful approach for the prevention of pancreatitis in severely hypertriglyceridemic patients. After a series of spectacularly failed clinical trials that were criticized for the choice of subjects and doses of omega 3 fatty acids used, Reduction of Cardiovascular Events with Icosapent Ethyl-Intervention Trial (REDUCE-IT) using a high dose of icosapent ethyl (IPE) reported a reduction in cardiovascular disease (CVD) events. However, this trial has generated controversy due to the use of mineral oil in the control group and the associated side effects of the IPA. This review will focus on the following topics: What are the epidemiologic data suggesting a benefit of omega 3 fatty acids? What might be the mechanisms for these benefits? Why have the clinical trials failed to resolve whether these fatty acids provide benefit? What choices should a clinician consider?

> Atherosclerotic cardiovascular disease (ASCVD) continues to represent a
> growing global health challenge. Despite guideline-recommended treat-
> ment of ASCVD risk, including antihypertensive, high-intensity statin ther-
> apy, and antiaggregant agents, high-risk patients, especially those with
> established ASCVD and patients with type 2 diabetes, continue to experi-
> ence cardiovascular events. Recent years have brought significant devel-
> opments in lipid and atherosclerosis research. Several lipid drugs owe
> their existence, in part, to human genetic evidence. Here, the authors
> briefly review the mechanisms, the effect on lipid parameters, and safety
> profiles of some of the most promising new lipid-lowering approaches
> that will be soon available in our daily clinical practice.

> This article reviews the safety of statins and non-statin medications for
> management of dyslipidemia. Statins have uncommon serious adverse ef-
> fects: myopathy/ rhabdomyolysis, which resolve with statin discontinua-
> tion, and diabetes, usually in people with risk factors for diabetes. The
> CVD benefit of statins far exceeds the risk of diabetes. Statin myalgia,
> without CK elevation, is likely caused by muscle symptoms with another
> etiology, or the nocebo effect. Notable adverse effects of non-statin med-
> icines include injection site reactions (alirocumab, evolocumab, inclisiran),
> increased uric acid and gout (bempedoic acid), atrial fibrillation/flutter
> (omega-3-fatty acids), and myopathy in combination with a statin
> (gemfibrozil).

> Combinations of lipid-lowering agents can often bring LDL cholesterol
> down to around 40 mg/dL (1 mmol/L). Randomized controlled trials indi-
> cate that this reduces the risk of atherosclerotic vascular events with min-
> imal adverse effects. This has raised the question of whether there is any
> concentration of LDL cholesterol below which further lowering is futile and/
> or a source of new adverse effects. This article examines several lines of
> evidence that lead to the conclusion that there is no known threshold
> below which lowering LDL cholesterol is harmful, but reduction of LDL
> cholesterol below 25 mg/dL may provide little if any further benefit.

ENDOCRINOLOGY AND METABOLISM CLINICS OF NORTH AMERICA

SERIES OF RELATED INTEREST

Medical Clinics
https://www.medical.theclinics.com
Primary Care: Clinics in Office Practice
https://www.primarycare.theclinics.com/

VISIT THE CLINICS ONLINE!
Access your subscription at:
www.theclinics.com

Foreword
Advances in Lipids

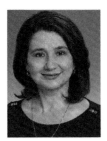

Adriana G. Ioachimescu, MD, PhD, FACE
Consulting Editor

The "Updates on Diagnosis and Management of Dyslipidemia" issue of the *Endocrinology and Metabolism Clinics of North America* reflects the significant progress in management of this multifaceted entity frequently encountered in the general population. The collection of articles offers a thorough review of the essential and novel aspects of lipid disorders, which will enhance the knowledge of medical students and trainees and will empower the health care practitioners who screen for and treat lipid disorders.

The guest editors are Connie B. Newman MD, Adjunct Professor at New York University Grossman School of Medicine, New York, New York and Alan Chait MD, Professor Emeritus, University of Washington, Seattle, Washington. Dr Newman and Dr Chait contributed to the Endocrine Society practice guidelines regarding management of lipid disorders in patients with endocrine conditions released in 2020.

An international group of distinguished researchers and clinical experts authored 13 articles that reflect our enhanced understanding of pathophysiology of lipid metabolism, the progress in lipid particle measurement and calculation, and steps toward personalized medicine to reduce the risk of atherosclerotic cardiovascular disease. In addition, an overview of the genetic diagnosis of hypercholesterolemia and hypertriglyceridemia and their consequences are provided, along with an update on the role of Lp(a) and HDL-cholesterol in atherosclerosis. Evidence-based information is presented regarding lipid disorders in children and adolescents, as well as in patients with diabetes mellitus, polycystic ovarian syndrome, thyroid dysfunction, and growth hormone abnormalities. Finally, treatment of dyslipidemia has made significant advances in the last decade. Our readers can find up-to-date information based on outcome trials with omega-3 fatty acid preparations, PCSK9 inhibitors, and statins. The status of emerging therapies currently under investigation and their potential role in the future of management of dyslipidemia are presented.

Endocrinol Metab Clin N Am 51 (2022) xiii–xiv
https://doi.org/10.1016/j.ecl.2022.03.001
0889-8529/22/© 2022 Published by Elsevier Inc.

endo.theclinics.com

I hope you will find this issue of the *Endocrinology and Metabolism Clinics of North America* a great resource for your practice and an interesting read. I would like to thank our guest editors and authors for their contribution and the Elsevier editorial staff for their continuous support.

Adriana G. Ioachimescu, MD, PhD, FACE
The Emory Pituitary Center Emory University School of Medicine, 1365 B Clifton Road, Northeast, B6209 Atlanta, GA 30322

E-mail address:
aioachi@emory.edu

Preface

Update on Lipids and Lipoproteins

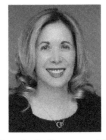
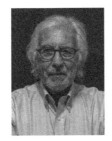

Connie B. Newman, MD   Alan Chait, MD

Editors

Significant progress in the field of lipids and lipoproteins has taken place in the last decade. This issue of *Endocrinology and Metabolism Clinics of North America* describes many of these advances. The measurement of lipids and lipoproteins for clinical use continues to evolve, especially in the estimation of low-density lipoprotein levels in the presence of hypertriglyceridemia or when levels have been dramatically reduced by drug therapy. Major advances have taken place in the genetic diagnosis of hypercholesterolemia and its management. There has been an increased understanding of the genetics of hypertriglyceridemia and its importance as a risk factor for atherosclerotic cardiovascular disease. There also has been an increased understanding of the pathogenesis of severe hypertriglyceridemia, its role in causing pancreatitis, and an approach to its management. New therapies that markedly reduce lipoprotein (a) (Lp(a)), are still somewhat underappreciated cardiovascular disease risk factor, are under investigation. However, clinical trials to determine whether lowering of Lp(a) will reduce clinical cardiovascular disease are in progress and had not been completed by the time this collection of articles was published. And although our understanding of the physiological role of high-density lipoprotein (HDL) and its role in atherosclerosis and other inflammatory states remains incomplete, clinical trials have failed to demonstrate the expected benefit of increasing HDL-cholesterol levels, raising questions about the importance of HDL as a true risk factor rather than a marker of cardiovascular disease. There have been updates in the evaluation and management of dyslipidemia in children and adolescents, and advances in the management of dyslipidemia in endocrine disorders and diabetes. Confusing information on the potential role of omega-3 fatty acids in the prevention of cardiovascular disease has become clearer in the recent past, including when to use specific omega-3 fatty acid preparations in the management of residual hypertriglyceridemia. Since lipids and lipoproteins were last featured in the *Endocrinology and Metabolism Clinics of*

Endocrinol Metab Clin N Am 51 (2022) xv–xvi
https://doi.org/10.1016/j.ecl.2022.02.013
0889-8529/22/© 2022 Published by Elsevier Inc.

North America, exciting new therapies for the management of dyslipidemia have become available, and several more are in development or are on the horizon. For example, a novel medication, a small interfering ribonucleic acid (RNA), FDA approved in December 2021 for hypercholesterolemia, markedly lowers low-density lipoprotein cholesterol (LDL-C) by significantly reducing the translation of proprotein convertase subtilisin/kexin type 9 (PCSK9) messenger RNA, and only requires 3 injections the first year, and 2 injections annually thereafter. In combination with statins, this medicine, and the others that inhibit PCSK9, can reduce LDL-C to very low levels (below 15–20 mg/dL). The last article summarizes the evidence for the efficacy and safety of low LDL-C.

To this end, we have assembled a group of outstanding leaders in the field to contribute to this issue of *Endocrinology and Metabolism Clinics of North America* to address these and several other topical issues, to provide a timely update to the current state of clinical disorders in this evolving area. We anticipate that the advances in diagnosis and treatment of dyslipidemia described in this issue will benefit our patients by further reducing their risk of atherosclerotic cardiovascular disease and pancreatitis.

Connie B. Newman, MD
Division of Endocrinology and Metabolism
Department of Medicine
New York University Grossman School of Medicine
435 East 30th Street
New York, NY 10016, USA

Alan Chait, MD
Division of Metabolism, Endocrinology and Nutrition
Department of Medicine
University of Washington
850 Republican Street, Mailstop 358062
Seattle, WA 98109, USA

E-mail addresses:
connie.newman@nyulangone.org (C.B. Newman)
achait@uw.edu (A. Chait)

Lipid and Lipoprotein Metabolism

Kenneth R. Feingold, MD

KEYWORDS

- Chylomicrons • VLDL • LDL • HDL • Lipoprotein (a) • Apolipoproteins
- Reverse cholesterol transport

KEY POINTS

- Chylomicrons are triglyceride-rich lipoproteins synthesized in the intestine. In the circulation, the triglycerides are removed by lipoprotein lipase (LPL) leading to the formation of chylomicron remnants which are taken up by the liver.
- Very low-density lipoprotein particles (VLDL) are triglyceride-rich lipoproteins synthesized in the liver. In the circulation, the triglycerides are removed by LPL leading to the formation of VLDL remnants (intermediate density lipoproteins) which may be taken up by the liver or further metabolized to low-density lipoprotein (LDL).
- The plasma level of LDL cholesterol is primarily determined by hepatic LDL receptor activity, which regulates both the production and clearance of LDL.
- High-density lipoprotein (HDL) are cholesterol and phospholipid-rich particles that mediate the transport of cholesterol and other compounds from peripheral tissues to the liver (ie, reverse cholesterol transport), which is one of the several potential mechanisms by which HDL may be anti-atherogenic.
- Chylomicron remnants, VLDL, VLDL remnants, LDL, and lipoprotein (a) are pro-atherogenic particles while HDL is anti-atherogenic.

INTRODUCTION

Lipids are insoluble in water and therefore cholesterol and triglycerides need to be transported in association with proteins (ie, lipoproteins) in the bloodstream. Lipoproteins play a crucial role in the transport of dietary lipids from the small intestine to the liver, muscle, and adipose tissue, in the transport of hepatic lipids to peripheral tissues, and the transport of cholesterol from peripheral tissues to the liver and intestine (ie, reverse cholesterol transport). Lipoproteins may have additional functions and studies have suggested that they may play a role in protection from disease.[1] For example, lipoproteins bind endotoxin (LPS) from gram-negative bacteria and lipoteichoic acid from gram-positive bacteria thereby reducing their toxic effects.[1] In addition, apolipoprotein L1, associated with HDL particles, has lytic activity against the

Department of Medicine, University of California-San Francisco, San Francisco, California, 94117, USA
E-mail address: Kenneth.feingold@ucsf.edu

Endocrinol Metab Clin N Am 51 (2022) 437–458
https://doi.org/10.1016/j.ecl.2022.02.008
0889-8529/22/© 2022 Elsevier Inc. All rights reserved.

endo.theclinics.com

parasite *Trypanosoma brucei* and lipoproteins can neutralize viruses.[2,3] Thus, while this article will focus on the transport properties of lipoproteins the reader should recognize that lipoproteins may have other important functions.

LIPOPROTEIN STRUCTURE

The surface of lipoproteins is a hydrophilic membrane consisting of phospholipids, free cholesterol, and apolipoproteins which surrounds a central hydrophobic core of nonpolar lipids, primarily cholesteryl esters and triglycerides (**Fig. 1**).[4] Lipoprotein particles are divided into 7 classes based on size, apolipoprotein composition, and lipid composition (**Fig. 2, Table 1**).

ANTI-ATHEROGENIC LIPOPROTEIN PARTICLES
High-Density Lipoprotein Particles

High-density lipoprotein particles are enriched in cholesterol and phospholipids and apolipoproteins A-I, A-II, A-IV, C-I, C-II, C-III, and E are associated with HDL particles.[5,6] The core structural protein is Apo A-I and each HDL particle may contain multiple Apo A-I proteins. In addition, using mass spectrometry proteins involved in proteinase inhibition, complement activation, and the acute-phase response have been found associated with HDL particles.[7] HDL particles may be classified based on density, size, charge, and apolipoprotein composition and are very heterogeneous (**Table 2**). HDL particles mediate the transport of cholesterol and other compounds from peripheral tissues to the liver (ie, reverse cholesterol transport), which is one of the several potential mechanisms by which HDL may be anti-atherogenic. In addition, HDL particles have

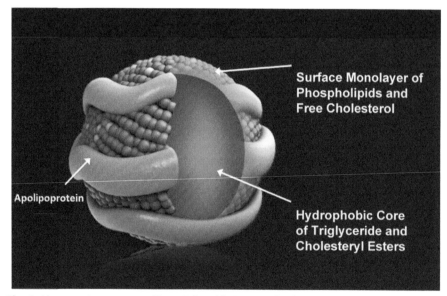

Fig. 1. Lipoprotein structure. (*From* Feingold KR. Introduction to Lipids and Lipoproteins. 2021 Jan 19. In: Feingold KR, Anawalt B, Boyce A, Chrousos G, de Herder WW, Dhatariya K, Dungan K, Hershman JM, Hofland J, Kalra S, Kaltsas G, Koch C, Kopp P, Korbonits M, Kovacs CS, Kuohung W, Laferrère B, Levy M, McGee EA, McLachlan R, Morley JE, New M, Purnell J, Sahay R, Singer F, Sperling MA, Stratakis CA, Trence DL, Wilson DP, editors. Endotext [Internet]. South Dartmouth (MA): MDText.com, Inc.; 2000–.)

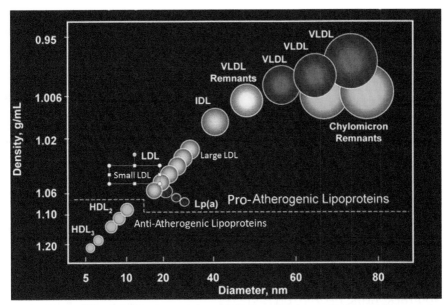

Fig. 2. Classes of lipoproteins. (*From* Feingold KR. Introduction to Lipids and Lipoproteins. 2021 Jan 19. In: Feingold KR, Anawalt B, Boyce A, Chrousos G, de Herder WW, Dhatariya K, Dungan K, Hershman JM, Hofland J, Kalra S, Kaltsas G, Koch C, Kopp P, Korbonits M, Kovacs CS, Kuohung W, Laferrère B, Levy M, McGee EA, McLachlan R, Morley JE, New M, Purnell J, Sahay R, Singer F, Sperling MA, Stratakis CA, Trence DL, Wilson DP, editors. Endotext [Internet]. South Dartmouth (MA): MDText.com, Inc.; 2000–.)

Table 1
Lipoprotein classes

Lipoprotein	Density (g/mL)	Size (nm)	Major Lipids	Major Apoproteins
Chylomicrons	<0.930	75–1200	Triglycerides	Apo B-48, Apo C, Apo E, Apo A-I, A-II, A-IV
Chylomicron Remnants	0.930–1.006	30–80	Triglycerides Cholesterol	Apo B-48, Apo E
VLDL	0.930–1.006	30–80	Triglycerides	Apo B-100, Apo E, Apo C
IDL VLDL remnants	1.006–1.019	25–35	Triglycerides Cholesterol	Apo B-100, Apo E, Apo C
LDL	1.019–1.063	18–25	Cholesterol	Apo B-100
HDL	1.063–1.210	5–12	Cholesterol Phospholipids	Apo A-I, Apo A-II, Apo C, Apo E
Lp (a)	1.055–1.085	∼30	Cholesterol	Apo B-100, Apo (a)

From Feingold KR. Introduction to Lipids and Lipoproteins. 2021 Jan 19. In: Feingold KR, Anawalt B, Boyce A, Chrousos G, de Herder WW, Dhatariya K, Dungan K, Hershman JM, Hofland J, Kalra S, Kaltsas G, Koch C, Kopp P, Korbonits M, Kovacs CS, Kuohung W, Laferrère B, Levy M, McGee EA, McLachlan R, Morley JE, New M, Purnell J, Sahay R, Singer F, Sperling MA, Stratakis CA, Trence DL, Wilson DP, editors. Endotext [Internet]. South Dartmouth (MA): MDText.com, Inc.; 2000–.

Table 2
Classification of HDL

Method of Classification	Types of HDL
Density gradient ultracentrifugation	HDL_2, HDL_3, very high-density HDL
Nuclear magnetic resonance	large, medium, and small
Gradient gel electrophoresis	HDL 2a, 2b, 3a, 3b, 3c
2-dimensional gel electrophoresis	pre-beta 1 and 2, alpha 1, 2, 3, 4
Apolipoprotein composition	A-I particles, A-I: A-II particles, A-I: E particles

From Feingold KR. Introduction to Lipids and Lipoproteins. 2021 Jan 19. In: Feingold KR, Anawalt B, Boyce A, Chrousos G, de Herder WW, Dhatariya K, Dungan K, Hershman JM, Hofland J, Kalra S, Kaltsas G, Koch C, Kopp P, Korbonits M, Kovacs CS, Kuohung W, Laferrère B, Levy M, McGee EA, McLachlan R, Morley JE, New M, Purnell J, Sahay R, Singer F, Sperling MA, Stratakis CA, Trence DL, Wilson DP, editors. Endotext [Internet]. South Dartmouth (MA): MDText.com, Inc.; 2000–.

anti-oxidant, anti-inflammatory, anti-thrombotic, and anti-apoptotic properties, which may also contribute to their ability to prevent atherosclerosis.

PRO-ATHEROGENIC LIPOPROTEIN PARTICLES
Chylomicron Particles

Chylomicrons are large triglyceride-rich particles secreted by the small intestine, which play a key role in the transport of dietary triglycerides and cholesterol to peripheral tissues and liver.[8] Each chylomicron particle contains one Apo B-48 molecule, which is the core structural protein. In addition, chylomicron particles also contain A-I, A-II, A-IV, A-V, B-48, C-II, C-III, and E. Chylomicrons vary in size depending on the amount of fat ingested with a high-fat meal leading to the formation of large chylomicron particles with an increased quantity of triglyceride, whereas in the fasting state or with the consumption of a low-fat meal the chylomicron particles are small carrying decreased quantities of triglyceride. Similarly, the amount of cholesterol transported in chylomicrons can also vary.

Chylomicron Remnant Particles

Chylomicron remnants are formed by the removal of triglyceride from chylomicrons by muscle and adipose tissue lipoprotein lipase (LPL) resulting in smaller particles.[8,9] These particles are enriched in cholesterol and are pro-atherogenic.

Very Low-Density Lipoprotein Particles

Very low-density lipoprotein particles are produced by the liver and contain apolipoprotein B-100, C-I, C-II, C-III, and E. The core structural protein is Apo B-100 and each VLDL particle contains one Apo B-100 protein. The size of the VLDL particles varies and when triglyceride production in the liver is increased the secreted VLDL particles are large.

Intermediate-Density Lipoprotein Particles; Very Low-Density Lipoprotein Remnant Particles

Intermediate-density lipoprotein particles are formed by the removal of triglycerides from VLDL by muscle and adipose tissue LPL resulting in the formation of IDL particles which are enriched in cholesterol and are pro-atherogenic.[9] These IDL particles contain apolipoprotein B-100 and E.

Low-Density Lipoprotein Particles

Low-density lipoprotein particles are derived from the metabolism of VLDL and IDL particles and are enriched in cholesterol. Each LDL particle contains one Apo B-100 protein. The majority of the cholesterol and Apo B in the circulation is typically carried on LDL particles. LDL vary in size and density. The levels of small dense LDL particles are increased in association with hypertriglyceridemia, low HDL levels, obesity, type 2 diabetes (ie, in patients with metabolic syndrome). These small dense LDL particles are more pro-atherogenic than large LDL particles for several reasons.[10]

1. Small LDL particles have a decreased affinity for the LDL receptor leading to prolonged retention time in the circulation.
2. Small LDL particles more easily enter the arterial wall than large LDL particles.
3. Small LDL particles bind more avidly than large LDL to intra-arterial proteoglycans, which trap these particles in the arterial wall.
4. Small LDL particles are more easily oxidized, which would allow macrophages to more efficiently take up these particles leading to cholesterol accumulation.

Lipoprotein (a) Particles

Lipoprotein (a) is an LDL particle that has apolipoprotein (a) attached to Apo B-100 via a single disulfide bond.[11–13] Lp (a) contain Apo (a) and Apo B-100 in a 1:1 M ratio. Apo (a) is made in the liver. The size of Lp(a) particles can vary greatly based on the size of apolipoprotein (a). Apo (a) contains multiple kringle motifs that are similar to the kringle repeats in plasminogen. The number of kringle repeats can vary greatly and thus the molecular weight of apo (a) can range from approximately 250,000 to 800,000. The levels of Lp (a) in plasma can vary 1000-fold ranging from undetectable to greater than 100 mg/dl. Lp (a) levels. The levels of Lp (a) largely reflect Lp (a) production rates, which are primarily genetically regulated. Individuals with low molecular weight Apo (a) proteins tend to have higher levels of Lp (a) while individuals with high molecular weight Apo (a) tend to have lower levels. It is thought that the secretion of high molecular weight Apo (a) by the liver is less efficient. LDL receptors do not seem to play a major role in Lp (a) clearance while the kidney seems to play an important role as kidney disease is associated with delayed clearance and elevations in Lp (a) levels. Apo (a) is an inhibitor of fibrinolysis and enhances the uptake of lipoproteins by macrophages, both of which could account for the increased risk of atherosclerosis in individuals with elevated Apo (a) levels. Additionally, Lp (a) is the major lipoprotein carrier of oxidized phospholipids, which could also increase the risk of atherosclerosis. The physiologic function of Apo (a) is unknown. Apo (a) is found in primates but not in other species.

APOLIPOPROTEINS

Apolipoproteins play an essential role in lipoprotein metabolism (**Table 3**). They have 4 key functions.[14,15]

1. Guiding the synthesis of lipoproteins
2. Serving in a structural role
3. Serving as ligands for lipoprotein receptors
4. Activating or inhibiting enzymes involved in the metabolism of lipoproteins

Apolipoprotein A-I

Apo A-I is the major structural protein of HDL accounting for approximately 70% of HDL protein.[16] Apo A-I is an activator of lecithin: cholesterol acyltransferase (LCAT),

Table 3
Apolipoproteins

Apolipoprotein	MW	Primary Source	Lipoprotein Association	Function
Apo A-I	28,000	Liver, Intestine	HDL, chylomicrons	Structural protein for HDL, Activates LCAT
Apo A-II	17,000	Liver	HDL, chylomicrons	Structural protein for HDL, Activates hepatic lipase
Apo A-IV	45,000	Intestine	HDL, chylomicrons	Unknown
Apo A-V	39,000	Liver	VLDL, chylomicrons, HDL	Promotes LPL-mediated TG lipolysis
Apo B-48	241,000	Intestine	Chylomicrons	Structural protein for chylomicrons
Apo B-100	512,000	Liver	VLDL, IDL, LDL, Lp (a)	Structural protein, Ligand for LDL receptor
Apo C-I	6600	Liver	Chylomicrons, VLDL, HDL	Activates LCAT
Apo C-II	8800	Liver	Chylomicrons, VLDL, HDL	Cofactor for LPL
Apo C-III	8800	Liver	Chylomicrons, VLDL, HDL	Inhibits LPL and uptake of lipoproteins
Apo E	34,000	Liver	Chylomicron remnants, IDL, HDL	Ligand for LDL receptor
Apo (a)	250,000–800,00	Liver	Lp (a)	Inhibits plasminogen activation

From Feingold KR. Introduction to Lipids and Lipoproteins. 2021 Jan 19. In: Feingold KR, Anawalt B, Boyce A, Chrousos G, de Herder WW, Dhatariya K, Dungan K, Hershman JM, Hofland J, Kalra S, Kaltsas G, Koch C, Kopp P, Korbonits M, Kovacs CS, Kuohung W, Laferrère B, Levy M, McGee EA, McLachlan R, Morley JE, New M, Purnell J, Sahay R, Singer F, Sperling MA, Stratakis CA, Trence DL, Wilson DP, editors. Endotext [Internet]. South Dartmouth (MA): MDText.com, Inc.; 2000–.

an enzyme that converts free cholesterol into cholesteryl ester, and interacts with receptors and transporters including ATP-binding cassette protein A1 (ABCA1), ABCG1, and class B, type I scavenger receptor (SR-B1). Apo A-1 is synthesized in both the liver and intestine. High levels of Apo A-I are associated with a decreased risk of atherosclerosis.

Apolipoprotein A-II

Apo A-II is the second most abundant protein carried on HDL accounting for approximately 20% of HDL protein.[17] The role of Apo A-II in lipid metabolism is not well understood. Apo A-II is synthesized in the liver and high levels are a strong predictor of an increased risk for atherosclerosis.

Apolipoprotein A-IV

Apo A-IV is associated with chylomicrons and HDL, but is also found in the lipoprotein-free fraction.[18] The role of Apo A-IV in lipoprotein metabolism remains to be determined but it may have a role in regulating food intake. Apo A-IV is synthesized in the intestine during fat absorption.

Apolipoprotein A-V

Apo A-V is carried on triglyceride-rich lipoproteins and is an activator of LPL-mediated lipolysis and thus plays an important role in the clearance of triglyceride-rich lipoproteins.[19,20] Apo A-V is synthesized in the liver.

Apolipoprotein B-48

Apo B-48 is the major structural protein of chylomicrons and chylomicron remnants and there is a single apo B-48 protein per chylomicron or chylomicron remnant particle.[21] Apo B-48 is synthesized in the intestine and a single apolipoprotein B gene is expressed in both the liver and intestine. The intestinal Apo B protein is approximately ½ the size of the liver due to mRNA editing. The apobec-1 editing complex, which edits mRNA, is expressed in the intestine and edits a specific cytidine to uracil in Apo B mRNA resulting in a stop codon that leads to the cessation of protein translation and a shorter Apo B protein (Apo B-48). The portion of Apo-B that is recognized by the LDL receptor is not contained in Apo-B48 and Apo B-48 is not recognized by the LDL receptor.

Apolipoprotein B-100

Apo B-100 is the major structural protein of VLDL, IDL, and LDL and there is a single molecule of Apo B-100 per VLDL, IDL, LDL, and Lp(a) particle. Apo B-100 is synthesized in the liver. Apo B-100 is recognized by the LDL receptor and therefore plays an important role in the clearance of Apo B-100 containing lipoprotein particles. Certain mutations in Apo B-100 result in decreased binding to the LDL receptor and familial hypercholesterolemia. Elevated levels of Apo B-100 are associated with an increased risk of developing atherosclerosis.

Apolipoprotein C

The C apolipoproteins are synthesized primarily in the liver. Apo C apolipoproteins are found in association with chylomicrons, VLDL, and HDL and freely exchange between these particles.[22–24]

Apo C-II is a cofactor for LPL and stimulates triglyceride hydrolysis and the clearance of triglyceride-rich lipoproteins.[22,25] Individuals who are homozygous for loss of function mutations in Apo C-II have markedly elevated triglyceride levels due to a failure to clear triglyceride-rich lipoproteins.

Apo C-III inhibits the activity of LPL[26] and inhibits the interaction of triglyceride-rich lipoproteins with their receptors.[23] Loss of function mutations in Apo C-III result in decreases in serum triglyceride levels and a decreased risk of cardiovascular disease. Furthermore, inhibition of Apo C-III leads to a decrease in serum triglyceride levels even in patients deficient in LPL, indicating that the ability of Apo C-III to decrease serum triglyceride levels is not entirely mediated by regulating LPL activity.[27]

Apolipoprotein E

The liver and intestine are the primary sources of circulating Apo E but Apo E is synthesized in many tissues.[28] Apo E is associated with chylomicrons, chylomicron remnants, VLDL, IDL, and a subgroup of HDL particles and exchanges between lipoprotein particles. There are 3 common genetic variants of Apo E (Apo E2, E3, and E4) and Apo E3 is the most common form. Apo E2 differs from Apo E3, by a single amino acid substitution whereby cysteine substitutes for arginine at residue 158 and Apo E4 differ from Apo E3 at residue 112 whereby arginine substitutes for cysteine. Apo E3 and E4 are recognized by the LDL receptor while Apo E2 is poorly recognized.

Individuals who are homozygous for Apo E2 can develop familial dysbetalipoproteinemia. Individuals with Apo E4 have an increased risk of both Alzheimer's disease and atherosclerosis.

TRANSFER PROTEINS AND ENZYMES: KEY ROLES IN LIPOPROTEIN METABOLISM
Cholesteryl Ester Transfer Protein

In the plasma, cholesteryl ester transfer protein (CETP) mediates the transfer of cholesteryl esters from HDL to VLDL, chylomicrons, and LDL and the linked transfer of triglycerides from these particles to HDL.[29] CETP is synthesized in the liver. Inhibition of CETP activity leads to a decrease in LDL cholesterol and an increase in HDL cholesterol.

Lecithin: Cholesterol Acyltransferase

LCAT catalyzes the synthesis of cholesteryl esters in HDL particles by facilitating the transfer of fatty acid from position 2 of lecithin to cholesterol.[30] The formation of cholesteryl esters allows for the transfer of the free cholesterol from the surface of the HDL particle to the core of the HDL particle. This decrease in the free cholesterol concentration on the surface of HDL particles allows for the uptake of free cholesterol by HDL particles facilitating the efflux of cholesterol from cells. LCAT is synthesized in the liver. Patients with decreased LCAT activity have decreased HDL cholesterol levels.

Lipoprotein Lipase

LPL is synthesized in muscle, heart, and adipose tissue, then secreted and attached to the endothelium of capillaries.[31] LPL hydrolyzes the triglycerides carried in triglyceride-rich lipoproteins, chylomicrons, and VLDL, to fatty acids, which are then taken up by adipocytes or muscle cells. The removal of triglycerides results in the conversion of chylomicrons into chylomicron remnants and VLDL into IDL (VLDL remnants). Apo C-II is an essential cofactor for LPL activity and Apo A-V also plays an important role in the activation of LPL. In contrast, Apo C-III and Apo A-II inhibit LPL activity. LPL expression is stimulated by insulin and in patients with poorly controlled diabetes LPL activity is reduced, which can decrease the clearance of triglyceride-rich lipoproteins leading to hypertriglyceridemia. Patients who are homozygotes for loss of function mutations In LPL have marked elevations in plasma triglyceride levels.

Hepatic Lipase

Hepatic lipase is synthesized in the liver and localized at the sinusoidal surface of hepatocytes.[32] Hepatic lipase catalyzes the hydrolysis of triglycerides and phospholipids in IDL and LDL producing smaller lipoprotein particles (IDL is converted to LDL; large LDL is converted to small LDL). Hepatic lipase also catalyzes the hydrolysis of triglycerides and phospholipids in HDL producing smaller HDL particles.

Endothelial Lipase

Endothelial lipase plays a key role in hydrolyzing the phospholipids in HDL.[33]

Microsomal Triglyceride Transfer Protein

Microsomal triglyceride transfer protein is expressed primarily in the liver and small intestine and plays a crucial role in the synthesis of lipoproteins in these tissues. MTP mediates the transfer of triglycerides to apolipoprotein B-100 in the liver to form VLDL and to apolipoprotein B-48 in the intestine to form chylomicrons.[34] Patients homozygous for loss of function mutations in MTP have very low plasma lipid levels (abetalipoproteinemia).

LIPOPROTEIN RECEPTORS AND LIPID TRANSPORTERS: KEY ROLES IN LIPOPROTEIN METABOLISM

Low-Density Lipoprotein Receptor

The LDL receptor is present in most tissues but the expression of LDL receptors in the liver plays a key role in determining plasma LDL levels.[35] A low number of hepatic LDL receptors is associated with high plasma LDL levels while a high number of hepatic LDL receptors is associated with low plasma LDL levels. The LDL receptor recognizes Apo B-100 and Apo E and thereby mediates not only the uptake of LDL but also chylomicron remnants and VLDL remnants (IDL). Lipoprotein particle uptake occurs via endocytosis of the LDL receptor and the attached lipoprotein particle (**Fig. 3**). After internalization, the lipoprotein particle is degraded in lysosomes and the cholesterol is released. The number of LDL receptors is regulated by cellular cholesterol levels.[36] When cellular cholesterol levels are low the transcription factor SREBP is transported from the endoplasmic reticulum to the Golgi whereby proteases cleave and activate SREBP, which then migrates to the nucleus and stimulates the expression of LDL receptors and many of the enzymes that synthesize cholesterol including HMGCoA reductase. Conversely, when cellular cholesterol levels are increased SREBP remains in the endoplasmic reticulum in an inactive form and the expression of LDL receptors is low. As discussed later PCSK9 regulates the rate of degradation of LDL receptors. Loss of function mutation in the LDL receptor is the most common cause of familial hypercholesterolemia.

Low-Density Lipoprotein Receptor-Related Protein 1

Lipoprotein receptor-related protein (LRP-1) is expressed in multiple tissues including the liver and is a member of the LDL receptor family.[37] Apo E is a ligand for LRP-1. LRP-1 mediates the hepatic uptake of Apo E containing lipoproteins (chylomicron remnants and VLDL remnants (IDL)).

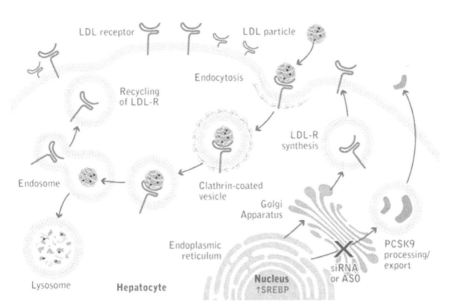

Fig. 3. Ldl receptor pathway. (*Adapted from* Lambert G, Sjouke B, Choque B, Kastelein JJ, Hovingh GK. The PCSK9 decade. J Lipid Res. 2012 Dec;53(12):2515-24.)

Niemann-Pick C1-like 1

Niemann-Pick C1-like 1 (NPC1L1) is expressed in the small intestine and mediates the uptake of dietary cholesterol and plant sterols from the intestinal lumen into the intestinal cell.[38] NPC1L1 is also expressed in the liver whereby it mediates the movement of cholesterol from hepatocytes into the bile.

Class B Scavenger Receptor B1

Scavenger receptor B1 (SR-B1) is expressed in many cells including the liver, adrenal glands, ovaries, testes, and macrophages.[39] In the liver and steroid producing cells (adrenal glands, ovaries, testes), it facilitates the selective uptake of cholesteryl esters from HDL particles. In macrophages and other cells, it mediates the efflux of cholesterol from the cell to HDL particles.

ATP-Binding Cassette Transporter A1

ATP-binding cassette transporter A1 (ABCA1) is expressed in hepatocytes, intestinal cells, macrophages, and many other cells.[40] It mediates the efflux of cholesterol and phospholipids from cells to small lipid-poor HDL particles (pre–beta-HDL).

ATP-Binding Cassette Transporter G1

ATP-binding cassette transporter G1 (ABCG1) is expressed in many different cell types and mediates the efflux of cholesterol from cells to mature HDL particles.[41]

ATP-Binding Cassette Transporter G5 and G8

ATP-binding cassette transporter G5 and G8 (ABCG5 and ABCG8) form a heterodimer and are expressed in the liver and intestine.[42] In the intestine, ABCG5/ABCG8 facilitates the movement of cholesterol and plant sterols from inside the enterocyte into the intestinal lumen thereby decreasing the absorption of cholesterol and limiting the uptake of dietary plant sterols. In the liver, ABCG5/ABCG8 facilitates the movement of cholesterol and plant sterols into the bile resulting in the transport of plant sterols and cholesterol to the intestine.

EXOGENOUS LIPOPROTEIN PATHWAY
Absorption of Dietary Fat

The exogenous lipoprotein pathway is initiated in the small intestine (**Fig. 4**).[43–46] Intestinal lipases hydrolyze dietary triglycerides (approximately 100 g per day) to free fatty acids and monoacylglycerol and these are emulsified with bile acids, plant sterols, cholesterol, and fat-soluble vitamins to form micelles. The fatty acids in the intestinal lumen are mainly from the diet while the cholesterol in the intestinal lumen is mainly derived from bile (approximately 800–1200 mg of cholesterol from bile vs 200–500 mg from diet). Approximately 100 to 150 mg of plant sterols are ingested per day. The cholesterol, plant sterols, fatty acids, monoacylglycerol, and fat-soluble vitamins contained in the micelles are transported into the intestinal cells. NPC1L1 facilitates the uptake of cholesterol and plant sterols from the intestinal lumen into intestinal cells (**Fig. 5**). Ezetimibe binds to NPC1L1 and inhibits the absorption of cholesterol and plant sterols. Cholesterol and plant sterols in the intestinal cell may be converted to sterol esters by acyl-CoA cholesterol acyltransferase (ACAT), which attaches a fatty acid to the sterol or be transported back into the intestinal lumen, a process mediated by ABCG5 and ABCG8. The synthesis of plant sterol esters does not occur as efficiently as the synthesis of cholesteryl esters because plant sterols are poor substrates for ACAT compared with cholesterol. In humans, less than 5%

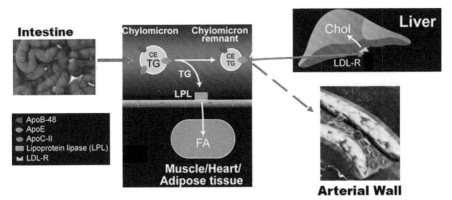

Fig. 4. Exogenous lipoprotein pathway. (*Modified from* Feingold KR. Introduction to Lipids and Lipoproteins. 2021 Jan 19. In: Feingold KR, Anawalt B, Boyce A, Chrousos G, de Herder WW, Dhatariya K, Dungan K, Hershman JM, Hofland J, Kalra S, Kaltsas G, Koch C, Kopp P, Korbonits M, Kovacs CS, Kuohung W, Laferrère B, Levy M, McGee EA, McLachlan R, Morley JE, New M, Purnell J, Sahay R, Singer F, Sperling MA, Stratakis CA, Trence DL, Wilson DP, editors. Endotext [Internet]. South Dartmouth (MA): MDText.com, Inc.; 2000–.)

of dietary plant sterols are absorbed. Mutations in either ABCG5 or ABCG8 result in increased absorption of dietary plant sterols (20%–30% absorbed vs < 5% in normal subjects) resulting in sitosterolemia. Thus, ACAT and ABCG5 and ABCG8 serve as gatekeepers and block the uptake of plant sterols and likely also play an important role in determining cholesterol absorption (humans absorb approximately 50% of dietary cholesterol with a range of 25%–75%).

The absorption of free fatty acids is not well understood but it is likely that both passive diffusion and specific transporters play a role. CD36, a fatty acid transporter, is strongly expressed in the proximal third of the intestine and is localized to the villi. This transporter likely plays a role in fatty acid uptake by intestinal cells but is not essential as humans and mice deficient in this protein do not have fat malabsorption.

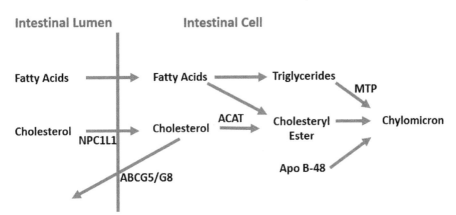

Fig. 5. Formation of chylomicrons by intestinal cells. (*Adapted from* Feingold KR. Introduction to Lipids and Lipoproteins. 2021 Jan 19. In: Feingold KR, Anawalt B, Boyce A, Chrousos G, de Herder WW, Dhatariya K, Dungan K, Hershman JM, Hofland J, Kalra S, Kaltsas G, Koch C, Kopp P, Korbonits M, Kovacs CS, Kuohung W, Laferrère B, Levy M, McGee EA, McLachlan R, Morley JE, New M, Purnell J, Sahay R, Singer F, Sperling MA, Stratakis CA, Trence DL, Wilson DP, editors. Endotext [Internet]. South Dartmouth (MA): MDText.com, Inc.; 2000–.)

In CD36 deficient mice the absorption of fatty acids is enhanced in the distal intestine, suggesting that other pathways compensate for the absence of CD36. Fatty acid transport protein 4 (FATP4), another fatty acid transporter, is also highly expressed in the intestine but mice deficient in FATP4 do not have abnormalities in fat absorption. It is likely that there are multiple pathways for the absorption of fatty acids. The pathways by which monoacylglycerols are absorbed by intestinal cells are unknown.

Formation of Chylomicron Particles

The fatty acids and monoacylglycerols that are absorbed are used in intestinal cells to synthesize triglycerides.[43,46] Monoacylglycerol acyltransferase (MGAT) and diacylglycerol transferase (DGAT) are the key enzymes in triglyceride synthesis. MGAT catalyzes the addition of a fatty acid to monoacylglycerol while DGAT catalyzes the addition of a fatty acid to diacylglycerol resulting in triglyceride formation. The cholesterol in the intestine is esterified to cholesteryl esters by ACAT. In the endoplasmic reticulum of intestinal cells, the triglycerides and cholesteryl esters are packaged into chylomicrons. The formation of chylomicrons in the endoplasmic reticulim requires the synthesis of Apo B-48 (see **Fig. 5**). The movement of lipid in the endoplasmic reticulum to Apo B-48 is mediated by MTP. The absence of MTP activity results in the failure to form chylomicrons and VLDL (abetalipoproteinemia). Lomitapide inhibits MTP activity and is approved to treat patients with homozygous Familial Hypercholesterolemia.

Metabolism of Chylomicron Particles

The chylomicrons synthesized in the intestine are secreted into the lymph and delivered via the thoracic duct to the systemic circulation, rather than to the liver via the portal vein.[22,26,31,47–51] This enhances the delivery of the nutrients to muscle and adipose tissue. LPL is synthesized in myocytes and adipocytes and transported to the luminal surface of capillaries. The stabilization and movement of LPL from muscle cells and adipocytes to the capillary endothelial cell surface is facilitated by Lipase maturation factor 1. Glycosylphosphatidylinositol anchored high-density lipoprotein binding protein 1 (GPIHBP1) binds LPL and transports LPL to the capillary lumen and anchors it to the capillary endothelium. Apo C-II, carried on the chylomicrons, activates LPL, leading to the hydrolysis of the triglycerides in the chylomicrons resulting in the formation of free fatty acids, which are taken up by muscle cells and adipocytes and used for either energy production or storage. The uptake of fatty acids into adipocytes and muscle cells is facilitated by fatty acid transport proteins (FATPs) and CD36. A portion of the free fatty acids released from the hydrolysis of triglycerides in chylomicrons bind to albumin and can be transported to other tissues. Apo A-V also plays a role in activating LPL activity. Mutations in LPL, Apo C-II, GPIHPB1, lipase maturation factor 1, and Apo A-V can result in marked hypertriglyceridemia (familial chylomicronemia syndrome). In addition, Apo C-III inhibits LPL activity and loss of function mutations in this gene are associated with increases in LPL activity and decreases in plasma triglyceride levels. Similarly, angiopoietin-like protein 3 and 4, which target LPL for inactivation, also regulate LPL activity. Loss of function mutations in angiopoietin-like protein 3 and 4 are associated with decreases in plasma triglyceride levels.

The hydrolysis of the triglycerides carried in the chylomicrons results in a marked decrease in the size of the chylomicrons resulting in the formation of chylomicron remnants, which are enriched in cholesteryl esters and acquire Apo E. As chylomicrons decrease in size phospholipids and apolipoproteins (Apo A and C) on the surface of the chylomicrons are transferred to other lipoproteins, primarily HDL. The transfer of Apo C-II from chylomicrons to HDL decreases the ability of LPL to further breakdown triglycerides. The liver is the primary site whereby chylomicrons are removed from circulation. The Apo E carried on the chylomicron remnants bind to the LDL receptor and other hepatic receptors such as LRP-1 and syndecan-4 and the entire particle is taken up by the hepatocytes. Apo E is important for this process and polymorphisms in Apo E (for example the Apo E2 isoform) can result in decreased chylomicron remnant clearance and elevations in plasma cholesterol and triglyceride levels (familial dysbetalipoproteinemia).

The exogenous lipoprotein pathway results in the efficient transfer of dietary triglycerides (fatty acids) to muscle and adipose tissue for energy utilization and storage. In individuals with normal lipid metabolism, this pathway can transfer large amounts of dietary fat from the intestine to muscle and adipose tissue (100 g or more per day) without resulting in marked increases in plasma triglyceride levels. Dietary cholesterol is primarily delivered to the liver whereby it can be used in the synthesis of VLDL or bile acids, or secreted back to the intestine via secretion into the bile.

ENDOGENOUS LIPOPROTEIN PATHWAY
Formation of Very Low-Density Lipoprotein Particles Particles

In the liver, MTP mediates the transfer of cholesterol and triglycerides to newly synthesized Apo B-100 in the endoplasmic reticulum, a process that is similar to the formation of chylomicron particles in the intestine (**Fig. 6**).[34,52,53] The rate of VLDL particle formation is determined by the supply of triglycerides and when the supply of

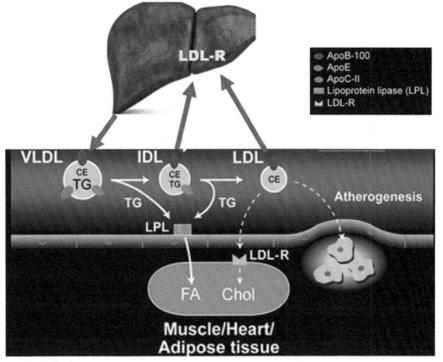

Fig. 6. Endogenous lipoprotein pathway. (*Adapted from* Feingold KR. Introduction to Lipids and Lipoproteins. 2021 Jan 19. In: Feingold KR, Anawalt B, Boyce A, Chrousos G, de Herder WW, Dhatariya K, Dungan K, Hershman JM, Hofland J, Kalra S, Kaltsas G, Koch C, Kopp P, Korbonits M, Kovacs CS, Kuohung W, Laferrère B, Levy M, McGee EA, McLachlan R, Morley JE, New M, Purnell J, Sahay R, Singer F, Sperling MA, Stratakis CA, Trence DL, Wilson DP, editors. Endotext [Internet]. South Dartmouth (MA): MDText.com, Inc.; 2000–.)

triglycerides is not abundant the newly synthesized Apo B-100 is rapidly degraded. When the supply of triglycerides is abundant the Apo B-100 is protected from degradation. Thus, the rate of formation and secretion of VLDL particles is determined by the availability of triglycerides and not the rate of synthesis of Apo B-100. Additionally, the size of the VLDL particles is determined by the availability of triglycerides. When triglycerides are abundant the VLDL particles are large.

The levels of fatty acids available for the synthesis of triglycerides are the main determinant of the number of triglycerides in the liver. The major sources of fatty acids are (a) de novo fatty acid synthesis, (b) the hepatic uptake of triglyceride-rich lipoproteins, and (c) the flux of fatty acids from adipose tissue to the liver. Diabetes, obesity, and metabolic syndrome are common causes of an increase in hepatic triglyceride levels and the increased secretion of VLDL.

The early addition of lipid to Apo B-100 particles is mediated by MTP while other pathways that do not require MTP add additional lipid. The details by which newly synthesized VLDL particles are secreted by the liver remain to be elucidated.

Metabolism of Very Low-Density Lipoprotein Particles Particles

In peripheral tissues, the triglycerides carried on the VLDL particles are hydrolyzed by LPL and fatty acids are released, a process that is very similar to that described above for chylomicrons (see **Fig. 6**).[9,47] VLDL and chylomicron particles compete for clearance by the LPL system. The removal of triglycerides by LPL from VLDL particles results in the formation of VLDL remnants (IDL), which are enriched in cholesteryl esters. VLDL remnant particles are removed from the circulation by the liver via binding of Apo E to LDL and LRP-1 receptors similar to the removal of chylomicron remnants. In contrast to chylomicron remnants where the vast majority are rapidly cleared from the circulation by the liver only a portion of VLDL remnant particles are removed (approximately 50% but varies). The residual triglycerides in the VLDL remnant particles are hydrolyzed by hepatic lipase leading to the formation of LDL particles. LDL particles contain mainly cholesteryl esters and Apo B-100 as the vast majority of triglycerides have been removed and exchangeable apolipoproteins are transferred from the VLDL remnant particles to other lipoproteins. Thus, VLDL metabolism results in the formation of LDL.

Metabolism of Low-Density Lipoprotein Particles

The rate of LDL clearance and the rate of LDL production are primarily regulated by the number of hepatic LDL receptors and thus the number of hepatic LDL receptors is the main determinant of plasma LDL levels.[35,54–56] High LDL receptor activity decreases the conversion of VLDL remnants to LDL while low LDL receptor activity increases the conversion of VLDL remnants to LDL (ie, increased LDL production). Additionally, approximately 70% of circulating LDL is cleared by LDL receptors in the liver with the remainder taken up by extrahepatic tissues. Thus, an increase in LDL receptors in the liver will increase LDL clearance resulting in a decrease in plasma LDL levels, whereas a decrease in liver LDL receptors will decrease LDL clearance resulting in an increase in plasma LDL levels. Thus, the number of LDL receptors in the liver plays a major role in regulating plasma LDL levels. Many of the drugs used to lower plasma LDL levels, such as statins, ezetimibe, PCSK9 inhibitors, and bempedoic acid lower plasma LDL levels by increasing the number of hepatic LDL receptors.

The cholesterol content of the liver is the primary regulator of the number of hepatic LDL receptors. Low cholesterol levels in the liver lead to the transport of inactive sterol regulatory element-binding proteins (SREBPs), which are transcription factors that stimulate the expression of LDL receptors and other key genes involved in cholesterol and fatty acid metabolism, from the endoplasmic reticulum to the Golgi whereby proteases cleave the SREBPs into active transcription factors. These active SREBPs transfer to the nucleus whereby they increase the transcription of LDL receptor mRNA and upregulate other genes, including HMG-CoA reductase and other proteins required for cholesterol synthesis. When hepatic cholesterol is high inactive SREBPs remain in the endoplasmic reticulum and the synthesis of LDL receptors is not increased. Thus, LDL receptor activity is regulated by cellular cholesterol levels with high cellular cholesterol levels leading to decreased LDL receptor activity and decreased clearance of LDL particles from the circulation and low cellular cholesterol levels leading to increased LDL receptor activity and the increased clearance of LDL particles from the circulation. Statins, ezetimibe, and bempedoic acid decrease hepatic cholesterol levels thereby increasing LDL receptor levels and decreasing plasma LDL levels.

Finally, PCSK9 is a secreted protein that binds to the LDL receptor and increases LDL receptor degradation in the lysosomes. Gain of function mutations in PCSK9 lead to decreased LDL receptor activity and elevations in LDL levels while loss of function mutations in PCSK9 result in increased LDL receptor activity and decreased LDL levels. Drugs that inhibit PCSK9 decrease LDL receptor degradation leading to an increase in hepatic LDL receptors resulting in a decrease in plasma LDL levels.

METABOLISM OF HIGH-DENSITY LIPOPROTEIN PARTICLES AND REVERSE CHOLESTEROL TRANSPORT
Formation of High-Density Lipoprotein Particles

The formation of mature HDL particles requires several steps (**Fig. 7**).[30,39–41,57–59] The initial step is the synthesis of Apo A-I, the main structural protein of HDL, in the liver and intestine. The liver and intestine secrete Apo A-1 which then acquires cholesterol and phospholipids that are effluxed from hepatocytes and enterocytes leading to the formation of pre–beta-HDL. ABCA1 facilitates the efflux of cholesterol and phospholipids and patients with loss of function mutations in ABCA1 are unable to add lipid to the newly secreted Apo A-I resulting in the rapid degradation of Apo A-I and very low HDL levels. In mice, targeted knock-outs of ABC1 in the liver result in an 80% decrease in HDL levels while targeted knock-outs in the intestine result in a 30% decrease in HDL levels. ABCA1 is expressed in numerous tissues allowing these tissues to also contribute cholesterol and phospholipids to lipid-poor Apo A-I particles.

During the metabolism of triglyceride-rich lipoproteins cholesterol and phospholipids may be transferred from chylomicrons and VLDL to newly formed HDL, which explains the observation that patients with high plasma triglyceride levels due to decreased metabolism of triglyceride-rich lipoprotein often also have low HDL levels. The metabolism of triglyceride-rich lipoproteins also results in the transfer of apolipoproteins to HDL from these triglyceride-rich lipoproteins. The movement of phospholipids between lipoproteins is facilitated by phospholipid transfer protein (PLTP) and mice lacking PLTP have a large reduction in HDL and Apo A-I levels.

High-Density Lipoprotein Cholesteryl Esterification

As noted earlier free cholesterol is localized on the surface of lipoprotein particles including HDL while the bulk of the cholesterol is in the core of HDL in the form of cholesteryl esters. Free cholesterol is effluxed from cells to HDL and to form mature large spherical HDL particles, this free cholesterol must be esterified. LCAT is an HDL-associated enzyme that catalyzes the transfer of fatty acid from phospholipids to free cholesterol resulting in the synthesis of cholesteryl esters which migrate from

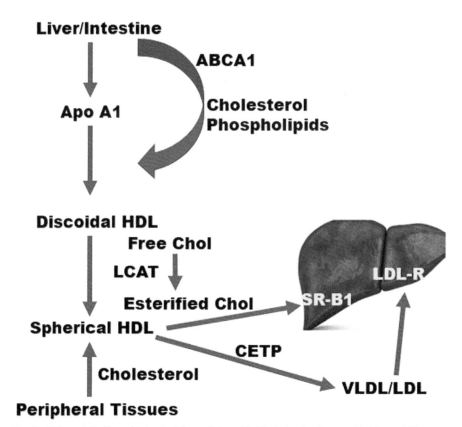

Fig. 7. Hdl metabolism. (*Adapted from* Feingold KR. Introduction to Lipids and Lipoproteins. 2021 Jan 19. In: Feingold KR, Anawalt B, Boyce A, Chrousos G, de Herder WW, Dhatariya K, Dungan K, Hershman JM, Hofland J, Kalra S, Kaltsas G, Koch C, Kopp P, Korbonits M, Kovacs CS, Kuohung W, Laferrère B, Levy M, McGee EA, McLachlan R, Morley JE, New M, Purnell J, Sahay R, Singer F, Sperling MA, Stratakis CA, Trence DL, Wilson DP, editors. Endotext [Internet]. South Dartmouth (MA): MDText.com, Inc.; 2000–.)

the surface of HDL particles into the core. Apo A-I is an activator of LCAT. In humans, LCAT deficiency leads to very low HDL cholesterol and Apo A-I levels and a large number of small HDL particles.

Metabolism of High-Density Lipoprotein Particles

The size and composition of HDL particles are determined by lipases and transfer proteins. CETP mediates the transfer of cholesteryl esters in the core of HDL particles to Apo B containing lipoproteins in exchange for triglycerides. The triglycerides transferred to HDL may be metabolized by hepatic lipase resulting in small HDL particles. Apo A-I more easily disassociates from small HDL resulting in increased Apo A-I degradation. Humans deficient in CETP activity have large HDL particles and very high HDL cholesterol levels. As one would expect the absence of CETP also results in a decrease in LDL cholesterol levels. Genetic deficiency of hepatic lipase results in larger HDL particles and a modest elevation in HDL cholesterol levels. The phospholipids carried on HDL particles are hydrolyzed by endothelial cell lipase. In mice decreased endothelial lipase activity results in increased HDL cholesterol levels while increased endothelial lipase activity results in decreased HDL cholesterol levels.

HDL cholesterol is primarily delivered to the liver. SR-B1, which promotes the selective uptake of HDL cholesterol mediates the uptake of HDL cholesterol by the liver. HDL particles bind to hepatic SR-BI and the cholesterol in HDL is transported into the liver without the internalization of the HDL particle. This results in a cholesterol depleted smaller HDL particle, which is then released back into the circulation. Mice deficient in SR-B1 have a marked increase in HDL cholesterol levels and interestingly, the risk of atherosclerosis is increased despite the increase in HDL cholesterol levels due to a decrease in reverse cholesterol transport. In mice, the importance of the hepatic SR-BI pathway is well defined but the role in humans is less certain. In mice, the transport of cholesterol from peripheral tissues to the liver is dependent solely on SR-BI while in humans CETP transports cholesterol from HDL to Apo B containing lipoproteins, which can serve as an alternative pathway for the transport cholesterol to the liver. In humans' polymorphisms in the SR-BI gene influence HDL cholesterol levels but have only a minimal effect on atherosclerosis.

Apo A-I is metabolized independently of HDL cholesterol with most of the Apo A-I catabolized by the kidneys with the remainder catabolized by the liver. The kidney filters lipid-free or lipid-poor Apo A-I which is then taken up by the renal tubules. The size of the Apo A-I particle determines whether it can be filtered by the kidneys and hence the degree of lipidation of Apo A-I determines the rate of metabolism. Lipid-poor HDL lead to the rapid catabolism of Apo A-1 by the kidney. Conditions or disease states that result in lipid-poor HDL are associated with low HDL and Apo A-I levels. In the renal tubule, Apo A-I binds to cubilin, which in association with megalin, a member of the LDL receptor gene family, results in the uptake and degradation of filtered Apo A-I by renal tubular cells. The mechanisms by which the liver catabolizes Apo A-I are poorly defined. Apo E containing HDL particles may be taken up by the LDL receptor and other Apo E receptors in the liver and degraded.

Reverse Cholesterol Transport

Peripheral cells accumulate cholesterol via de novo cholesterol synthesis and the uptake of cholesterol from circulating lipoproteins.[60–65] Only a few specialized cells have mechanisms to decrease cellular cholesterol levels. Intestinal cells can secrete cholesterol into the intestinal lumen and sebocytes and keratinocytes can secret cholesterol onto the skin surface. Adrenal, testicular, and ovarian cells can convert cholesterol into steroid hormones. Other cells can only decrease cellular cholesterol via reverse cholesterol transport. The ability of macrophages in the arterial wall to efficiently remove cholesterol by reverse cholesterol transport pathway may play an important role in the prevention of atherosclerosis.

The efflux of cellular cholesterol to lipid-poor pre–beta-HDL particles is mediated by ABCA1 while efflux of cellular cholesterol to mature HDL particles is mediated by ABCG1 (**Fig. 8**). SR-B1 and passive diffusion may also contribute to the efflux of cellular cholesterol to mature HDL particles. ABCA1 and ABCG1 are upregulated by the activation of LXR, a nuclear hormone transcription factor that is activated by oxysterols. As cellular cholesterol rises the formation of oxysterols is enhanced resulting in the activation of LXR which stimulates the expression of ABCA1 and ABCG1 resulting in an increase in the efflux of cholesterol from cells to HDL.

miR-33 is a microRNA that is embedded within the SREBP2 gene which targets ABCA1 and ABCG1 mRNA for degradation. As the cellular cholesterol levels increase the expression of SREBP2 decreases resulting in a decrease in LDL receptor and cholesterol synthesis and a decrease in miR-33 levels. The decrease in miR-33 will lead to an increase in the expression of ABCA1 and ABCG1 resulting in increased cholesterol efflux which coupled with the decrease in LDL receptor activity and

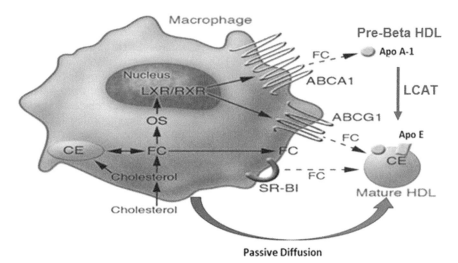

Fig. 8. Cholesterol efflux from macrophages. (*Modified from* Rader DJ. Molecular regulation of HDL metabolism and function: implications for novel therapies. J Clin Invest. 2006 Dec;116(12):3090-100.)

cholesterol synthesis will decrease cellular cholesterol levels. Conversely, a decrease in cellular cholesterol levels will increase SREBP2 expression resulting in an increase in LDL receptor activity and cholesterol synthesis increasing cholesterol accumulation, and an increase in miR-33, resulting in the decreased expression of ABCA1 and ABCG1 and a reduction in cholesterol efflux. Together these changes in cholesterol accumulation mediated by the LDL receptor and cholesterol synthesis and cholesterol efflux mediated by ABCA1 and ABCG1 will maintain cellular cholesterol homeostasis.

There are 2 pathways for cholesterol carried on HDL to be transported to the liver. HDL can interact with hepatic SR-BI receptors resulting in the selective uptake of cholesterol from HDL particles into the liver or CETP can transfer cholesterol from HDL particles to Apo B lipoprotein particles with the subsequent uptake of Apo B containing lipoproteins by the liver. The cholesterol delivered to the liver can be eliminated from the body by 2 pathways. First, cholesterol can be secreted into the bile, a process facilitated by ABCG5 and ABCG8. ABCG5 and ABCG8 expression is increased by the activation of LXR and therefore an increase in hepatic cholesterol levels results in an increase in oxysterol production thereby increasing LXR activation and the secretion of bile acid. Second, cholesterol can be converted to bile acids and secreted in the bile.

Studies have suggested that reverse cholesterol transport plays an important role in protecting from the development of atherosclerosis. HDL cholesterol levels may not be indicative of the rate of reverse cholesterol transport as reverse cholesterol transport involves multiple steps and HDL cholesterol levels may not accurately reflect these steps. For example, the ability of HDL to promote cholesterol efflux from macrophages can vary and the same level of HDL cholesterol may not have equivalent abilities to mediate the first step of reverse cholesterol transport.

CLINICS CARE POINTS

- Low HDL-C levels are often due to decreased metabolism of triglyceride-rich lipoproteins, which explains the association of low HDL-C with hypertriglyceridemia

- Hepatic LDL receptors are the major regulator of LDL-C levels and drugs such as statins, ezetimibe, PCSK9 inhibitors, and bempedoic acid lower LDL-C levels by increasing the number of hepatic LDL receptors
- Reverse cholesterol transport is a complex process and the levels of HDL-C may not accurately indicate the activity of reverse cholesterol transport.

ACKNOWLEDGMENTS

The author has no commercial or financial conflicts of interest.

REFERENCES

1. Feingold KR, Grunfeld C. Lipids: a key player in the battle between the host and microorganisms. J Lipid Res 2012;53:2487–9.
2. Nielsen LB, Nielsen MJ, Moestrup SK. Lipid metabolism: an apolipoprotein-derived weapon combating trypanosoma infection. Curr Opin Lipidol 2006;17: 699–701.
3. Feingold KR. The bidirectional link between HDL and COVID-19 infections. J Lipid Res 2021;62:100067.
4. Smith LC, Pownall HJ, Gotto AM Jr. The plasma lipoproteins: structure and metabolism. Annu Rev Biochem 1978;47:751–7.
5. Asztalos BF, Niisuke K, Horvath KV. High-density lipoprotein: our elusive friend. Curr Opin Lipidol 2019;30:314–9.
6. Thakkar H, Vincent V, Sen A, et al. Changing perspectives on hdl: from simple quantity measurements to functional quality assessment. J Lipids 2021;2021: 5585521.
7. Vaisar T, Pennathur S, Green PS, et al. Shotgun proteomics implicates protease inhibition and complement activation in the antiinflammatory properties of HDL. J Clin Invest 2007;117:746–56.
8. Julve J, Martin-Campos JM, Escola-Gil JC, et al. Advances in biology, pathology, laboratory testing, and therapeutics. Clin Chim Acta 2016;455:134–48.
9. Chait A, Ginsberg HN, Vaisar T, et al. Remnants of the triglyceride-rich lipoproteins, diabetes, and cardiovascular disease. Diabetes 2020;69:508–16.
10. Berneis KK, Krauss RM. Metabolic origins and clinical significance of LDL heterogeneity. J Lipid Res 2002;43:1363–79.
11. Kostner KM, Kostner GM. Lipoprotein (a): a historical appraisal. J Lipid Res 2017; 58:1–14.
12. Schmidt K, Noureen A, Kronenberg F, et al. Structure, function, and genetics of lipoprotein (a). J Lipid Res 2016;57:1339–59.
13. Nordestgaard BG, Langsted A. Lipoprotein (a) as a cause of cardiovascular disease: insights from epidemiology, genetics, and biology. J Lipid Res 2016;57: 1953–75.
14. Mahley RW, Innerarity TL, Rall SC Jr, et al. Plasma lipoproteins: apolipoprotein structure and function. J Lipid Res 1984;25:1277–94.
15. Breslow JL. Human apolipoprotein molecular biology and genetic variation. Annu Rev Biochem 1985;54:699–727.
16. Frank PG, Marcel YL. Apolipoprotein A-I: structure-function relationships. J Lipid Res 2000;41:853–72.
17. Chan DC, Ng TW, Watts GF. Apolipoprotein A-II: evaluating its significance in dyslipidaemia, insulin resistance, and atherosclerosis. Ann Med 2012;44:313–24.

18. Wang F, Kohan AB, Lo CM, et al. Apolipoprotein A-IV: a protein intimately involved in metabolism. J Lipid Res 2015;56:1403–18.

19. Hubacek JA. Apolipoprotein A5 fifteen years anniversary: lessons from genetic epidemiology. Gene 2016;592:193–9.

20. Sharma V, Forte TM, Ryan RO. Influence of apolipoprotein A-V on the metabolic fate of triacylglycerol. Curr Opin Lipidol 2013;24:153–9.

21. Anant S, Davidson NO. Molecular mechanisms of apolipoprotein B mRNA editing. Curr Opin Lipidol 2001;12:159–65.

22. Wolska A, Dunbar RL, Freeman LA, et al. Apolipoprotein C-II: New findings related to genetics, biochemistry, and role in triglyceride metabolism. Atherosclerosis 2017;267:49–60.

23. Ramms B, Gordts P. Apolipoprotein C-III in triglyceride-rich lipoprotein metabolism. Curr Opin Lipidol 2018;29:171–9.

24. D'Erasmo L, Di Costanzo A, Gallo A, et al. A multifaceted protein in cardiometabolic disease. Metabolism 2020;113:154395.

25. Wolska A, Reimund M, Remaley AT. Apolipoprotein C-II: the re-emergence of a forgotten factor. Curr Opin Lipidol 2020;31:147–53.

26. Taskinen MR, Boren J. Why Is Apolipoprotein CIII emerging as a novel therapeutic target to reduce the burden of cardiovascular disease? Curr Atheroscler Rep 2016;18:59.

27. Witztum JL, Gaudet D, Freedman SD, et al. Volanesorsen and Triglyceride Levels in Familial Chylomicronemia Syndrome. N Engl J Med 2019;381:531–42.

28. Mahley RW. Apolipoprotein E: from cardiovascular disease to neurodegenerative disorders. J Mol Med (Berl) 2016;94:739–46.

29. Shrestha S, Wu BJ, Guiney L, et al. Cholesteryl ester transfer protein and its inhibitors. J Lipid Res 2018;59:772–83.

30. Ossoli A, Simonelli S, Vitali C, et al. Role of LCAT in Atherosclerosis. J Atheroscler Thromb 2016;23:119–27.

31. Olivecrona G. Role of lipoprotein lipase in lipid metabolism. Curr Opin Lipidol 2016;27:233–41.

32. Kobayashi J, Miyashita K, Nakajima K, et al. Hepatic lipase: a comprehensive view of its role on plasma lipid and lipoprotein metabolism. J Atheroscler Thromb 2015;22:1001–11.

33. Yasuda T, Ishida T, Rader DJ. Update on the role of endothelial lipase in high-density lipoprotein metabolism, reverse cholesterol transport, and atherosclerosis. Circ J 2010;74:2263–70.

34. Hooper AJ, Burnett JR, Watts GF. Contemporary aspects of the biology and therapeutic regulation of the microsomal triglyceride transfer protein. Circ Res 2015;116:193–205.

35. Goldstein JL, Brown MS. The LDL receptor. Arterioscler Thromb Vasc Biol 2009;29:431–8.

36. Goldstein JL, DeBose-Boyd RA, Brown MS. Protein sensors for membrane sterols. Cell 2006;124:35–46.

37. van de Sluis B, Wijers M, Herz J. News on the molecular regulation and function of hepatic low-density lipoprotein receptor and LDLR-related protein 1. Curr Opin Lipidol 2017;28:241–7.

38. Jia L, Betters JL, Yu L. Niemann-pick C1-like 1 (NPC1L1) protein in intestinal and hepatic cholesterol transport. Annu Rev Physiol 2011;73:239–59.

39. Trigatti BL. SR-B1 and PDZK1: partners in HDL regulation. Curr Opin Lipidol 2017;28:201–8.

40. Wang S, Smith JD. ABCA1 and nascent HDL biogenesis. Biofactors 2014;40: 547–54.
41. Baldan A, Tarr P, Lee R, et al. ATP-binding cassette transporter G1 and lipid homeostasis. Curr Opin Lipidol 2006;17:227–32.
42. Patel SB, Graf GA, Temel RE. ABCG5 and ABCG8: more than a defense against xenosterols. J Lipid Res 2018;59:1103–13.
43. Abumrad NA, Davidson NO. Role of the gut in lipid homeostasis. Physiol Rev 2012;92:1061–85.
44. D'Aquila T, Hung YH, Carreiro A, et al. Recent discoveries on absorption of dietary fat: Presence, synthesis, and metabolism of cytoplasmic lipid droplets within enterocytes. Biochim Biophys Acta 2016;1861:730–47.
45. Hussain MM. Intestinal lipid absorption and lipoprotein formation. Curr Opin Lipidol 2014;25:200–6.
46. Kindel T, Lee DM, Tso P. The mechanism of the formation and secretion of chylomicrons. Atheroscler Suppl 2010;11:11–6.
47. Dallinga-Thie GM, Franssen R, Mooij HL, et al. The metabolism of triglyceride-rich lipoproteins revisited: new players, new insight. Atherosclerosis 2010;211:1–8.
48. Dijk W, Kersten S. Regulation of lipid metabolism by angiopoietin-like proteins. Curr Opin Lipidol 2016;27:249–56.
49. Fong LG, Young SG, Beigneux AP, et al. GPIHBP1 and Plasma Triglyceride Metabolism. Trends Endocrinol Metab 2016;27:455–69.
50. Peterfy M. Lipase maturation factor 1: a lipase chaperone involved in lipid metabolism. Biochim Biophys Acta 2012;1821:790–4.
51. Young SG, Fong LG, Beigneux AP, et al. GPIHBP1 and Lipoprotein Lipase, Partners in Plasma Triglyceride Metabolism. Cell Metab 2019;30:51–65.
52. Tiwari S, Siddiqi SA. Intracellular trafficking and secretion of VLDL. Arterioscler Thromb Vasc Biol 2012;32:1079–86.
53. Choi SH, Ginsberg HN. Increased very low density lipoprotein (VLDL) secretion, hepatic steatosis, and insulin resistance. Trends Endocrinol Metab 2011;22: 353–63.
54. Brown MS, Radhakrishnan A, Goldstein JL. Retrospective on cholesterol homeostasis: the central role of scap. Annu Rev Biochem 2018;87:783–807.
55. Goldstein JL, Brown MS. A century of cholesterol and coronaries: from plaques to genes to statins. Cell 2015;161:161–72.
56. Horton JD, Cohen JC, Hobbs HH. Molecular biology of PCSK9: its role in LDL metabolism. Trends Biochem Sci 2007;32:71–7.
57. Rosenson RS, Brewer HB Jr, Davidson WS, et al. Cholesterol efflux and atheroprotection: advancing the concept of reverse cholesterol transport. Circulation 2012;125:1905–19.
58. Rye KA, Barter PJ. Cardioprotective functions of HDLs. J Lipid Res 2014;55: 168–79.
59. Mabuchi H, Nohara A, Inazu A. Cholesteryl ester transfer protein (CETP) deficiency and CETP inhibitors. Mol Cells 2014;37:777–84.
60. Zhao Y, Van Berkel TJ, Van Eck M. Relative roles of various efflux pathways in net cholesterol efflux from macrophage foam cells in atherosclerotic lesions. Curr Opin Lipidol 2010;21:441–53.
61. Lee-Rueckert M, Escola-Gil JC, Kovanen PT. HDL functionality in reverse cholesterol transport–Challenges in translating data emerging from mouse models to human disease. Biochim Biophys Acta 2016;1861:566–83.

62. Tall AR. Cholesterol efflux pathways and other potential mechanisms involved in the athero-protective effect of high density lipoproteins. J Intern Med 2008;263: 256–73.
63. Siddiqi HK, Kiss D, Rader D. HDL-cholesterol and cardiovascular disease: rethinking our approach. Curr Opin Cardiol 2015;30:536–42.
64. Moore KJ, Rayner KJ, Suarez Y, et al. The role of microRNAs in cholesterol efflux and hepatic lipid metabolism. Annu Rev Nutr 2011;31:49–63.
65. Ouimet M, Barrett TJ, Fisher EA. HDL and reverse cholesterol transport. Circ Res 2019;124:1505–18.

Lipoprotein Assessment in the twenty-first Century

Diego Lucero, PhD[a],*, Anna Wolska, PhD[b], Zahra Aligabi, MS[a], Sarah Turecamo, BA[b], Alan T. Remaley, MD, PhD[a]

KEYWORDS

- Lipoprotein diagnostic assays • Cardiovascular risk assessment
- Advanced lipoprotein testing • Recommendations for lipoprotein assessment
- LDL-C calculation • HDL functionality • Lipoprotein (a) • Non-HDL cholesterol

KEY POINTS

- Most recent guidelines state that a nonfasting sample is suitable for initial screening of patients for cardiovascular risk. Nonetheless, patients with elevated nonfasting triglycerides should be retested in the fasting state.
- Recent advances in the equations to calculate low-density lipoprotein cholesterol (LDL-C) allow for a more accurate calculation of LDL-C at higher triglyceride levels, which deemphasizes the need for a fasting sample for LDL-C evaluation.
- Measuring apolipoprotein B and non-HDL cholesterol is highly recommended to discern cardiovascular risk especially in hypertriglyceridemia; however, harmonization of cutoff values in different guidelines is still needed.
- Limitations still remain for the accurate measurement of lipoprotein(a) due to its structural complexity; methods that evaluate particle number in units of nanomoles per liter are preferred.
- The advancement and development of measures of different aspects of lipoprotein metabolism, such as HDL functionality, genetic testing, nuclear magnetic resonance, HDL proteomics, and other more advanced testing will likely improve future assessments of cardiovascular risk.

INTRODUCTION

Lipoproteins are a heterogeneous and polydisperse group of particles that transport water-insoluble lipids like cholesterol in plasma. Extensive research over more than 6 decades has demonstrated a causal relationship between elevated cholesterol,

[a] Lipoprotein Metabolism Laboratory, Translational Vascular Medicine Branch, National Heart, Lung, and Blood Institute, National Institutes of Health, 9000 Rockville Pike, Building 10, Room 5D09, Bethesda, MD 20892, USA; [b] Heart Disease Phenomics Laboratory, Epidemiology and Community Health Branch, National Heart, Lung, and Blood Institute. National Institutes of Health, 9000 Rockville Pike, Building 10, Room 5N323, Bethesda, MD 20892, USA
* Corresponding author. National Heart, Lung and Blood Institute, Building 10, Room 5D09, 10 Center Drive, Bethesda, MD 20892-1666.
E-mail address: diego.lucero3@nih.gov

Endocrinol Metab Clin N Am 51 (2022) 459–481
https://doi.org/10.1016/j.ecl.2022.02.009
0889-8529/22/Published by Elsevier Inc.

endo.theclinics.com

particularly when on low-density lipoproteins (LDL), and adverse cardiovascular events such as myocardial infarction.[1] Furthermore, reduction in plasma cholesterol by either lifestyle changes or by specific lipid-lowering medications have been shown to lower cardiovascular events in both primary prevention and in secondary prevention, in patients with preexisting cardiovascular disease. Consequently, the accurate measurement of plasma lipids and other metrics of lipoprotein metabolism by the clinical laboratory has become a critical step in our efforts to prevent atherosclerotic cardiovascular disease (ASCVD). In this article, we will begin with a brief review of lipoprotein metabolism and how it relates to the pathogenesis of atherosclerosis. Next, we will describe the measurement of the various plasma lipids and related measures of lipoproteins that are routinely used as cardiovascular risk markers. Finally, we will conclude with emerging new tests for lipids and lipoproteins and how they can potentially enhance cardiovascular risk assessment in the future.

Lipoprotein Metabolism

Lipoprotein particles are able to transport water-insoluble lipids because they form micelle-like particles. The hydrophobic cholesteryl esters and triglycerides (TG) are in the core of the particle and are shielded from water by a surface monolayer of amphipathic lipids and proteins that contain both polar and hydrophobic groups. The main proteins found on lipoproteins are called apolipoproteins. They often contain secondary structural motifs such as alpha-helices and or beta-sheets that have polar amino acids on one side facing outward to the water, whereas the more hydrophobic amino acids on the other face point inward. Similarly, the amphipathic lipids, which are mostly phospholipids and free cholesterol, are arranged on the surface of the lipoprotein particles so that the more polar parts of the molecules face outward toward the water, whereas the more hydrophobic parts interact with the hydrophobic lipids in the core.

As shown in **Fig. 1**, lipoprotein metabolism can be divided into 3 major pathways. The exogenous (intestinal) (**Fig. 1** [steps I–IV]) and the endogenous (hepatic) pathways (see **Fig. 1** [steps 1–15]) are mediated by apolipoprotein B-containing lipoproteins, namely chylomicrons and very-low density lipoproteins (VLDL).[2] As described in the figure legend, these pathways relate to either the dietary absorption of lipids (exogenous) or to the distribution of plasma lipids between peripheral tissues and the liver (endogenous). These 2 pathways are critical for triglyceride energy metabolism but also for delivery of other lipids to cells for membrane structure.

Many of the current therapeutic targets and those in development for lowering plasma lipids are in the exogenous and endogenous pathways. A prototypical example is 3-hydroxy-3-methylglutaryl-CoA reductase (HMGCR), a rate-limiting step in cholesterol biosynthesis.[1] Statins, the first-line drug for the treatment of hypercholesterolemia, inhibit HMGCR, leading to the compensatory upregulation of hepatic LDL receptor (LDLR) and a lowering of plasma LDL.[1] Proprotein convertase subtilisin/kexin type 9 (PCSK9), a relatively, recently discovered protein, inhibits the recycling of LDLR and has become a therapeutic target of interest because its inhibition increases the hepatic bioavailability of functional LDLR,[3] leading to additional reduction of LDL levels on top of statins. A series of monoclonal antibodies have been developed to inhibit PCSK9[3]; however, the treatment is relatively expensive and requires subcutaneous injection. New alternative therapeutic approaches to block PCSK9 are being actively developed, such as oral administration of antisense oligonucleotides (ASO) and small molecules.[4,5]

Besides elevated LDL cholesterol (LDL-C), increased TG, which are carried mainly on chylomicrons and VLDL, can also promote disease. It has been known for a long

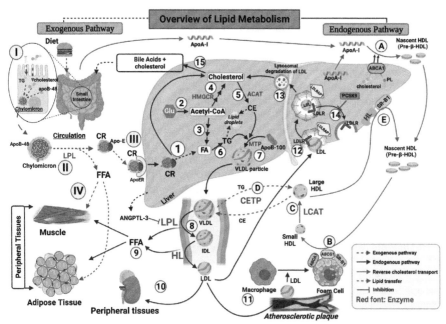

Fig. 1. Overview of lipoprotein metabolism. (I–IV) Exogenous pathway: (*I*) Dietary lipids are absorbed in enterocytes, packed into chylomicrons that are secreted into lymph/blood (II). In circulation, LPL lipolyze chylomicrons into chylomicron remnants (CR) and free fatty acids (FFA). (III) CR, rich in apo-B48 and Apo-E, are internalized by the liver through apo-E receptor (ApoER). (IV) FFA are used or stored in peripheral tissues. (1–10) Endogenous pathway: (1) CR internalized in the liver are degraded into its components. Cholesterol and fatty acids (FA) enlarge their respective hepatic pools. (2) Acetyl-CoA, coming from glucose degradation, is used for: (3) de novo synthesis FA (lipogenesis) or (4) endogenous cholesterol synthesis, regulated by HMGCR. (5) Hepatic free cholesterol is esterified into cholesterol esters (CE) by intracellular Acyl-CoA:cholesterol acyltransferase (ACAT) and (6) FA are esterified into triglycerides (TG). TG and CE are either stored in intracellular lipid droplets or (7) added to nascent apolipoprotein B-100 (apoB-100) by microsomal triglyceride transfer protein (MTP) to form VLDL, which is secreted into circulation. (8) In circulation, TG in VLDL are lipolyzed by lipoprotein lipase (LPL) forming intermediate density lipoprotein (IDL). Liver secretes ANGPTL3 that inhibits LPL in peripheral tissues. IDL is then further lipolyzed by hepatic lipase (HL) into LDL. (9) Released FFA are internalized by muscles or adipose tissue for oxidation or storage, respectively. LDL in circulation has 3 main fates: (10) internalization by peripheral tissues with high cholesterol demands (adrenal glands, testis, ovaries), (11) infiltration into the arterial wall, where it suffers modifications and is internalized by macrophages to form foams cells leading to atherosclerosis, or (12) internalization through hepatic LDLR in a clathrin-mediated endocytic process aided by the LDLRAP1. (13) Internalized LDL is degraded in lysosomes and its cholesterol enlarges the hepatic cholesterol pools. (14) LDLR is recycled back to the plasma membrane. This is inhibited by the PCSK9. (15) Excess of hepatic cholesterol is secreted into the intestine as bile acids. HDL metabolism (reverse cholesterol transport) (*A – E*): (*A*) Lipid poor apoA-I is secreted by liver and small intestine. Free lipid poor apoA-I acquires cholesterol and phospholipids (PL) through hepatic ATP binding cassette (ABC) subfamily A member 1 (ABCA1) and forms nascent discoidal high-density lipoprotein (HDL). (*B*) Nascent HDL captures free cholesterol and phospholipids from the surface of foam cells and other peripheral cells through surface transporters (ABCA1, ABC subfamily G member 1 [ABCG1], and Scavenger Receptor class B type I [SR-BI]), forming small spherical HDL particles. (*C*) Lecithin-cholesterol acyltransferase (LCAT) esterifies free cholesterol in small HDL and forms large mature HDL particles. (*D*) Cholesteryl

time that markedly elevated TG (TG > 1000 mg/dL) from either genetic mutations in key enzymes such as lipoprotein lipase or from other metabolic disturbances such as uncontrolled diabetes can cause acute pancreatitis.[6] Recently, more modest forms of hypertriglyceridemia have also been associated with an increase in the risk of ASCVD and have become a target of drug development. For example, angiopoietin-like 3 (ANGPTL3), which is secreted by the liver and inhibits LPL, is an active target for drug development. It was first identified from loss-of-function mutations in *ANGPTL3* that were associated with reduced TG and lower ASCVD risk.[7] Both monoclonal antibodies and ASO against ANGPTL3 are currently being tested in late-stage clinical trials.[7] Another important factor in regulating plasma TG levels is apolipoprotein C-III (apoC-III), protein mainly produced in liver that inhibits LPL activity and hepatic clearance of apoB-containing lipoproteins. Similar to ANGPTL3, loss-of-function mutations in *APOC3* are associated with lower plasma TG and atheroprotection.[8,9] Volanesorsen, an ASO targeting hepatic apoC-III, was approved for the treatment of patients with familial chylomicron syndrome in Europe.[10] Furthermore, the same ASO demonstrated, in a phase 3 clinical trial, to significantly reduce plasma TG in patients with severe multifactorial hypertriglyceridemia and even in patients with LPL mutations.[11]

Besides being a drug target, many of the genes involved in both the exogenous and endogenous pathways are also a cause of inherited dyslipidemias. The best example of this is familial hypercholesterolemia (FH), one of most common inherited disorder worldwide. FH is characterized by mutations in genes encoding for PCSK9, LDLR, and ApoB, leading to high LDL levels and premature ASCVD.[12] Patients with genetic dyslipidemia are at the highest risk for ASCVD due to lifelong exposure to elevated plasma lipids. The early diagnosis allows the prompt intervention and the proactive identification of other family members at risk.[13] The identification of the LDLR adaptor protein 1 (LDLRAP1),[14] a protein required for the correct internalization of hepatic LDLR, and the above-mentioned PCSK9 are the most recent advancements in genetic discovery associated with LDL metabolism.

The third major lipoprotein pathway (see **Fig 1**, Steps A–D) is mediated by high-density lipoproteins (HDL), which contain apoA-I as their major structural protein.[15] Unlike the apoB-containing lipoproteins in the other 2 pathways, HDL is thought to be antiatherogenic because of its ability to remove excess cholesterol from cells and return it to the liver for excretion by the reverse cholesterol transport pathway. Cholesterol on HDL (HDL-C) has been consistently shown in numerous large-scale epidemiologic studies to be inversely related to cardiovascular events but the reason for this strong association is still not known. Based on recent genetic studies, it is not clear that HDL-C is causally related to the development of atherosclerosis, and instead, it may be just a biomarker for a favorable antiatherogenic state. Drugs that raise HDL-C have so far failed to show any benefit in reducing cardiovascular disease.

Lipoproteins in Atherosclerosis

Atherosclerotic plaques, which are collections of lipid-rich cells and extracellular lipids in the vascular wall, can form throughout the arterial vasculature (**Fig. 2**). When present

←─────────────────────────────────

ester transfer protein (CETP) transfers TG from VLDL to HDL and CE from HDL to VLDL. (*E*) At hepatic level, TG and phospholipids in large HDL are lipolyzed by HL, or CE in large HDL is taken up by hepatic SR-BI. This process generates small HDL particles that can either reenter the HDL's metabolic pathway or be filter and excreted through the kidney. Created with BioRender.com.

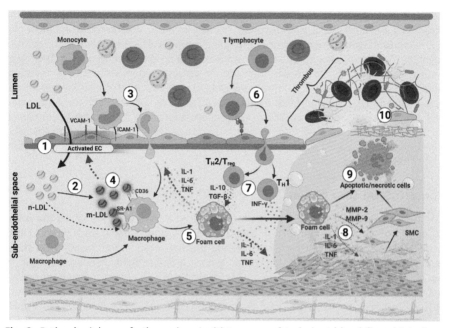

Fig. 2. Pathophysiology of atherosclerosis. (1) In areas of turbulent blood flow, high shear stress induces the activation of endothelial cells (EC) leading to an increase endothelial barrier permeability. In these areas, low-density lipoproteins (LDL) infiltrate into the subendothelial space. (2) In the vessel wall, LDL can undergo modifications, such as oxidation and aggregation (mLDL), becoming more immunogenic and proinflammatory. Oxidation products further stimulate endothelial activation. (3) Activated endothelium express adhesion molecules (vascular cell adhesion molecule 1 [VCAM-1] and intracellular adhesion molecules 1 [ICAM-1]) on the luminal surface. Circulating monocytes interact with adhesion molecules and transmigrate to the subendothelial space where they differentiate into macrophages. (4) Macrophages internalize mLDL by receptor-mediated endocytosis, involving scavenger receptors (SR-A1 and CD36), lectin-like oxidized LDL 1 (LOX-1) receptor, and LDL receptor-related protein 1 (LRP1), and native LDL by fluid-phase endocytosis. (5) Macrophages transform into cholesterol-loaded foam cells that secrete proinflammatory cytokines such as interleukin 1 (IL-1), IL-6, and tumor necrosis factor (TNF), which amplifies the inflammatory response and promote the proliferation of smooth muscle cells (SMC). (6) Adaptative immune cells infiltrate into the lesion area. (7) Although type 1 T helper lymphocytes (T_H1) secrete interferon gamma IFN-γ and exacerbate the inflammation, T_H2 and Treg cells secrete anti-inflammatory cytokines (IL-10 and transforming growth factor beta [TGF-β]) to limit inflammation and SMC proliferation. (8) Inflammation and lipid accumulation continue, and foam cells secrete metalloproteinases (MMP-2 and MMP-9) that degrade the proteoglycan matrix, favoring the migration of SMC. (9) Apoptosis and necrosis of foam cells and SMC lead to the formation of the necrotic core. (10) Plaques with large lipid accumulation and thin fibrous cap are more prone to rupture. Plaque's content is exposed, triggering thrombosis, which can occlude the artery lumen and cause downstream ischemia. Created with BioRender.com.

in coronary vessels, atherosclerotic plaques can impair blood flow to the heart and trigger myocardial infarction, particularly after plaque rupture.[16] When an atherosclerotic plaque is present in the femoral artery or elsewhere, it can cause peripheral vascular disease. When present in the carotid artery, atherosclerotic plaques can cause ischemic stroke. As described in the figure legend, the deposition of LDL into the vessel wall and their subsequent uptake by macrophages is central to the development of atherosclerosis. Subendothelial fatty streaks form first but given the ongoing deposition of LDL and the onset of inflammation, more complex types of plaques can form with a necrotic core containing extracellular cholesterol in the form of crystals. These complex plaques can rupture or become eroded by losing their overlying endothelial cells, which can then trigger platelet thrombosis and the complete occlusion of a small vessel. Subfractions of LDL, such as small dense low-density lipoprotein (sdLDL-C) or modified forms of LDL, such as oxidized LDL or aggregated LDL may be even more prone to causing atherosclerosis.[17] Other apo-B containing lipoproteins have also been implicated in atherogenesis, such as Lipoprotein(a),[18] triglyceride-rich lipoproteins (TRL) such as VLDL and IDL, and their partially lipolyzed forms called remnant lipoproteins.[19]

CONVENTIONAL LIPID TESTING

The determination of the so-called Standard Lipid Panel, which involves the measurement of total cholesterol (TC), TG, and HDL-C and either a calculated LDL-C or a directly measured LDL-C, is currently the first step recommended by most guidelines for the management of patients for cardiovascular disease risk. This is because LDL-C is known to be causally related to ASCVD and the levels of LDL-C are used in almost all guidelines to direct lipid lowering therapy (**Fig. 3**). TC and HDL-C, which can be used to calculate non-HDL-C (cholesterol on all apoB-containing lipoproteins), are also used in most risk equations for estimating a 10-year ASCVD risk score, another key piece of information used for managing patients (see **Fig. 3**). Other tests, which are sometimes referred to as risk enhancer tests, such as apoB and high sensitivity C-reactive protein, a marker of inflammation, can also be used for patients at intermediate risk to decide who to treat with statins or other lipid-lowering medications.

Enzymatic Measurement of Plasma Lipids

Plasma TC and TG represent the cholesterol and triglyceride carried by all circulating lipoproteins. Although the reference method performed by the centers for disease control (CDC) involves the use of mass spectrometry to measure these 2 lipids, they are routinely measured in the clinical laboratory by enzyme-coupled colorimetric reactions. In the first steps, esterified cholesterol or TG are hydrolyzed to free cholesterol or free glycerol by cholesterol esterase or a lipase. Next, in a series of coupled reactions, free cholesterol or glycerol are enzymatically oxidized to generate hydrogen peroxide, which finally reacts to form a chromophore that can be measured spectrophotometrically. Alternatively, glycerol can be quantified by monitoring the formation or disappearance of nicotinamide adenine dinucleotide. The enzymatic/colorimetric methods for total lipids are well standardized, and results are reproducible between different commercial assays. These assays are fully automated, which improves their precision and reproducibility. In general, the coefficient of variance for both, TC and TG, is less than 3%.

Certain components in plasma, such as bilirubin, hemoglobin, and citric acid, if found in high concentrations, can interfere with enzymatic assays. In addition, as all TG assays determine total glycerol, high endogenous free glycerol in plasma, as seen in rare genetic disorders such as glycerol kinase deficiency and sometimes with diabetes, can falsely overestimate plasma TG (pseudohypertriglyceridemia). There are TG assays that account for free glycerol by doing what is called a glycerol blanking step, but are not widely used.[20] Plant sterols that contain a similar structure to cholesterol can also falsely raise TC when measured enzymatically as observed in the rare genetic disorder called sitosterolemia.[21]

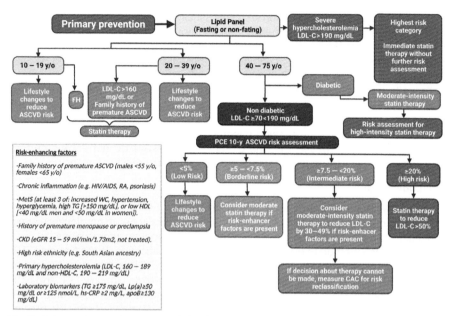

Fig. 3. Primary Prevention approach in the US 2018 Multi-Society Guidelines. LDL-C: low-density lipoprotein cholesterol. ASCVD, atherosclerotic cardiovascular disease; FH, familial hypercholesterolemia; PCE, pooled cohort equations; HIV/AIDS, human immunodeficiency virus/acquired immunodeficiency syndrome; RA, rheumatoid arthritis; MetS, metabolic syndrome; WC, waist circumference; TG, triglycerides; HDL, high-density lipoproteins; CKD, chronic kidney disease; eGFR, estimated glomerular filtration rate; Non-HDL-C, non-HDL cholesterol; Lp(a): lipoprotein (a); hs-CRP, high sensitivity "C" reactive protein. (*Adapted from* Grundy, S.M., et al., 2018 AHA/ACC/AACVPR/AAPA/ABC/ACPM/ADA/AGS/APhA/ASPC/NLA/PCNA Guideline on the Management of Blood Cholesterol: A Report of the American College of Cardiology/American Heart Association Task Force on Clinical Practice Guidelines. Circulation, 2019. 139(25): p. e1082-e1143.)

TG, depending on the fat composition of the meal, can acutely increase in the postprandial state, but the other lipids in the standard lipid panel do not change significantly. As described below, recent advances in equations for estimating LDL-C that are not so affected by TG levels and the development of direct LDL-C tests, as well as the fact that postprandial lipids may be a better predictor of ASCVD risk,[22] has caused most guidelines to state that a nonfasting sample is suitable for initial screening of patients. Patients with elevated nonfasting TG should, however, be retested in the fasting state before making a final decision about therapy.

HDL-Cholesterol

High-density lipoprotein cholesterol represents the cholesterol transported in all the HDL particles in circulation. Because of its inverse association with ASCVD, it is often used for calculating a 10-year ASCVD risk score. It is important to note that an accurate determination of HDL-C is also important when calculating LDL-C and non-HDL-C.[23] The reference method established by the CDC for the measurement of HDL-C consists of a combination of ultracentrifugation and selective precipitation. The first generation of routine HDL-C methods used by clinical laboratories[24] relied on the use of polyanions and divalent cations to selective precipitate of apoB-containing lipoproteins. HDL-C in the supernatant was then measured by enzymatic-colorimetric methods. Because the precipitation step was usually done manually, most clinical laboratories have now switched to fully automated homogenous or direct methods that do not involve the physical separation of HDL from the other lipoproteins. The direct HDL-C methods use a variety of compounds (polyethylene glycol, modified dextran, antibodies, among others) to block or shield apoB-containing lipoproteins from interacting with the enzymes used for measuring cholesterol, so that only cholesterol on HDL is measured.[23] Besides reducing the labor cost, the direct automated assays show better precision than the first-generation HDL-C tests because errors associated with the manual sample processing (pipetting, centrifugation) were eliminated. It is important to note, however, that the direct HDL-C assays do not always perform well when compared with the reference method on dyslipidemic samples.[25]

LDL-Cholesterol

Low-density lipoproteins are causally associated with ASCVD[26]; hence, accuracy and reliability in quantifying plasma levels of LDL-C are central for both cardiovascular risk evaluation and for monitoring the effectiveness of therapeutic interventions.

The reference method to quantify LDL-C is beta-quantification. In the first step, TRL (VLDL, chylomicrons, and their remnants), with a density of less than 1.006 g/mL, are removed by density gradient centrifugation. Other lipoproteins (mainly LDL and HDL, and Lp(a) and IDL if present) remain in the infranatant. In the second step, TC is measured in the infranatant. HDL-C in the infranatant is determined after the precipitation of LDL with heparan/Mn + 2. LDL-C is calculated as the difference between the cholesterol measured in the infranatant minus the HDL-C in the infranatant. It is important to note that cholesterol in IDL and Lp(a) is also quantified as LDL-C. Unlike other methods to evaluate LDL-C, beta-quantification is not affected by triglyceride levels because TRL are removed in the ultracentrifugation step.

Like for HDL-C, methods for measuring LDL-C by selective precipitation with sulfated polyanions have been developed but have never been widely implemented.[27] This is because of analytical interference issues,[28] and as described below, LDL-C can be calculated from the results of a standard lipid panel. More recently, fully automated direct assays for LDL-C have been developed and are in routine use. These direct methods, like the direct HDL-C assays, also rely on a combination of different detergents, polymers, and other agents that either first selectively dissolve or block other plasma lipoproteins, such as VLDL and HDL. Then LDL-C is selectively measured by an enzymatic/colorimetric reaction. Because direct LDL-C assays can sometimes show lack of selectivity on dyslipidemic samples[25,29] and due to cost considerations, many laboratories continue to only report an estimated LDL-C done by a calculation. Some clinical laboratories only use direct LDL-C assays when TG are greater than 400 mg/dL, which as described below can lead to an inaccurate estimate for LDL-C depending on the calculation method.

Equations to Estimate LDL-C

Until recently, the only commonly used method for calculating LDL-C was the Friedewald equation, which was first developed in 1972 to match the results for LDL-C as determined by the beta quantification reference method (**Fig. 4**A).[30,31]

As can be inferred by the equation in **Fig. 4**A, it depends on the fact that in a fasting sample with low chylomicrons or remnant lipoproteins, cholesterol is either on HDL, LDL, or VLDL. The term TG/5 was found to be an estimate of very low-dense lipoprotein cholesterol (VLDL-C), so just by simply subtracting cholesterol from HDL and VLDL, one can obtain a reasonably good estimate on LDL-C from the results of a standard lipid panel.[32]

A

$$LDL\text{-}C = TC - HDL\text{-}C - \frac{TG}{5} \ [mg/dL]$$

B

$$LDL\text{-}C = TC - HDL\text{-}C - \frac{TG}{\text{adjustable factor}} \ [mg/dL]$$

C

$$LDL\text{-}C = \frac{TC}{0.948} - \frac{HDL\text{-}C}{0.971} - \left(\frac{TG}{8.56} + \frac{TG \times non\text{-}HDL\text{-}C}{2140} - \frac{TG^2}{16100} \right) - 9.44 \ [mg/dL]$$

D

$$lbLDL\text{-}C = 1.43 \times LDL\text{-}C - \left(0.14 \times (\ln(TG) \times LDL\text{-}C) \right) - 8.99$$

E

$$sdLDL\text{-}C = LDL\text{-}C - lbLDL\text{-}C$$

Fig. 4. Equations for the calculation of total low-density lipoprotein cholesterol (LDL-C), large buoyant LDL-C (lbLDL-C), and small dense LDL-C (sdLDL-C). (*A*) Friedewald equation. (*B*) Martin-Hopkins equation. (*C*) Sampson-NIH equation. (*D, E*) Equations to estimate lbLDL-C and sdLDL-C. TC, total cholesterol; HDL-C, high-density lipoprotein cholesterol; TG, triglycerides; non-HDL-C, nonhigh-density lipoprotein cholesterol; adjustable factor, median ratio between TG and very low-density lipoprotein cholesterol categorized by TG and non-HDL-C.[35]

Although widely used for many years, a major limitation of the Friedewald equation is that with higher TG levels, the term TG/5 overestimates the amount of VLDL-C, which then leads to an underestimation of LDL-C.[33,34] Considering this issue, it is not recommended to use this equation when TG is greater than 400 mg/dL, but errors related to this problem actually occur at much lower levels of TG. In addition, with the advent of anti-PCSK9 monoclonal antibody therapy[3] and more effective LDL-C lowering, accurate measurement of low LDL-C well below 100 mg/dL has become more clinically relevant. Because the absolute value of LDL-C in these patients is much lower, errors related to this TG issue has been shown to result in the misclassification of patients, which can affect the eligibility of patients for anti-PCSK9 therapy.[35]

Accuracy concerns about the Friedewald equation led to the development of an alternative method called the Martin-Hopkins equation (**Fig. 4B**)[35] that is now recommended by the recent US guidelines as the preferred way to calculate LDL-C, particularly at LDL-C less than 100 mg/dL.[36] As displayed in **Fig. 4B**, it is similar to the Friedewald equation but uses an adjustable factor for dividing TG to estimate VLDL-C.

The adjustable factor can be found in a table of 180 different values that varies depending not just on TG but also on the non-HDL-C value (see **Fig. 4B**). It was empirically found using the vertical auto profile (VAP) method, a density-based procedure for separating lipoproteins, that the optimal adjustment factor is higher when TG is higher but is lower when non-HDL-C is higher. The Martin-Hopkins method for estimating LDL-C has been shown to be superior to the Friedewald equation, particularly for low LDL-C[37] but was not evaluated for TG > 400 mg/dL.

Recently, a newly developed Sampson-NIH equation for LDL-C[38] has been described to be more accurate than both the Friedewald and Martin-Hopkins equations when compared with the beta quantification reference method (**Fig. 4C**).

Unlike the other 2 equations, the Sampson-NIH equation uses higher order mathematical terms that better account for the surface-volume relationships that determine the carrying capacity of TG versus cholesterol on lipoproteins. Its accuracy is also adversely affected by high TG samples but less so than the other equations. It was found to be suitable for TG up to 800 mg/dL. Because this TG level is near the 99th percentile of the population distribution, it reduces the need to obtain a fasting sample and to reflex to a direct LDL-C test when TG > 400 mg/dL. More studies are needed, but several recent studies support that the Sampson-NIH equation is clearly superior to Friedewald equation, particularly at high TG levels.[39,40] Unlike the Martin equation, the Sampson equation should be easier to implement for most Laboratory Information Systems and is in the public domain and does not require any license fees.

Although LDL plays a causal role in atherosclerosis, there is evidence that particular modified forms or subfractions of LDL may be more proatherogenic or at least more strongly associated with ASCVD events. One such potentially more proatherogenic form of LDL is sdLDL-C, and it is widely considered as an emerging risk factor for ASCVD.[26] It is often found in patients with diabetes and/or hypertriglyceridemia and is thought to form as a consequence of TG enrichment of LDL by CETP (see **Fig. 1**), which then leads to more lipolysis and the generation of smaller LDL. sdLDL seems to readily accumulate in the vessel wall potentially because of its smaller size and/or because of its increased propensity for oxidation.[41] It can be measured by several different advanced lipoprotein separation methods, which will be discussed in the next section, but an equation for estimating sdLDL-C from the results of the standard lipid panel was recently described (see **Fig. 4D–E**).[42] Calculating sdLDL-C levels consists of 2 steps. First, large buoyant LDL-C concentrations are estimated based on the interaction term between LDL-C (Sampson-NIH method) and the natural log of TG (see **Fig. 4D**). lbLDL-C is then subtracted from total LDL-C to estimate sdLDL-C (see **Fig. 4E**).

In both univariate and multivariate analysis after adjustment for the conventional risk factors, it was found to be superior to LDL-C and other routine lipid measures for predicting ASCVD,[42] but additional studies will be needed before it can be routinely recommended.

Non-HDL Cholesterol

Non-HDL cholesterol (non-HDL-C) represents the cholesterol transported in all the apoB-containing lipoproteins (LDL, Lp(a), and TRL and their remnants), which are all considered all to be atherogenic.[43] Non-HDL-C is easily calculated from the lipid panel by subtracting HDL-C from the TC and thus does not involve any extra cost. As TG are not used for its calculation, non-HDL-C is more accurate than LDL-C in classifying patients into different risk categories, particularly in hypertriglyceridemia.[44] In fact, non-HDL-C is only limited by the accuracy of the HDL-C measurement at high TG, which is usually acceptable up to ~880 mg/dL (~10 nmol/L) of TG,[45] thereby also making it an attractive alternative to evaluate risk in nonfasting samples. Furthermore, the accumulation of cholesterol-rich remnants in hypertriglyceridemia makes LDL-C a poor predictor of cardiovascular events.[46] Nonetheless, non-HDL-C has some potential limitations. For example, patients with high levels of remnant lipoproteins and low LDL-C and Lp(a) may have low non-HDL-C but still be at an increased risk. In addition, although cholesterol on all the lipoprotein fractions within non-HDL-C are believed to be atherogenic, some such as cholesterol on Lp(a) may be even more proatherogenic.[47] The typical cutoff values for non-HDL-C are defined the same as for LDL-C plus 30 mg/dL, which corresponds to the cutoff value for a desirable VLDL-C. Non-HDL-C levels between 190 and 219 mg/dL is defined as a risk enhancer factor by the 2018 Multi-Society Guidelines.[36] The European Guidelines recommend measuring non-HDL-C and apoB for the primary risk evaluation of patients with high TG and recognized non-HDL-C as a secondary target for ASCVD prevention, defining cutoff values based on the patient's risk category (<85, <100, <130 mg/dL for very high, high, and moderate risk, respectively).[48] Given that it does involve any additional costs and its utility for evaluating risk in hypertriglyceridemic patients and for nonfasting patients, non-HDL-C should be reported as part of the lipid panel by clinical laboratories.

Lipoprotein (a)

Lipoprotein (a) (Lp(a)) is an LDL-like lipoprotein in which apolipoprotein(a), a homolog of plasminogen with multiple repeats of kringles V and IV, is covalently bound to apoB. Kringle IV has 10 different isoforms, but only type 2 (KIV2) is repeated a variable number of times, thus accounting for the size polymorphisms of Lp(a). The number of KIV2 repeats is determined genetically and is inversely correlated with Lp(a) concentrations in plasma.[49] In recent years, epidemiologic and genetic studies demonstrated a causative role of Lp(a) in atherosclerosis and ASCVD[18] and in calcific aortic stenosis[50]; therefore, there is growing interest in its accurate quantification. Cholesterol on Lp(a) is included in the LDL-C computed by conventional methods; however, the direct measurement of Lp(a) has presented several difficulties due to its repeat kringle structure.[49] Methods to determine Lp(a) rely on immunoassays, using antibodies directed to different epitopes on apolipoprotein(a) and apolipoprotein B. Nonetheless, these methods either underestimate or overestimate Lp(a) concentrations, depending on apolipoprotein(a) size. Lp(a) levels are sometimes expressed in mg/dL representing the total circulating mass of both lipid and protein on the particle and are dependent on the size polymorphisms of apolipoprotein(a). Alternatively, Lp(a) can be expressed in nmol/L, which indicates the particle concentration and is not affected by its size. The 2018 Multi-Society Guidelines established a cutoff value for Lp(a) of 50 or 125 nmol/L; therefore, as much as 20% of the total population is at risk because of increased Lp(a). The 2018 Multi-Society Guidelines also recommend measuring Lp(a) in patients with family history of premature ASCVD or personal history of premature heart disease in the absence of other traditional risk factors.[36] If elevated, it is considered as a risk enhancer and suggests the initiation or intensification of lipid-lowering treatment.[36] It is important to note that, unlike LDL-C, Lp(a) levels respond modestly or not at all to treatment with statins or PCSK9 inhibitors.[49] Lp(a) levels also do not respond well to life-style modifications. ASO therapies targeting apolipoprotein(a), in early-stage clinical trials, do markedly lower Lp(a) levels, but their outcome on clinical events is still not known.[51] The successful development of new drugs for lowering Lp(a) will likely create a greater need for its reliable measurement.

Measurement of Apolipoproteins

Apolipoproteins are structural proteins associated with lipoproteins. They can also mediate lipoprotein–receptor interactions, regulate enzymatic activities, or lipoprotein functionality. The apolipoproteins routinely measured in the clinical practice are apolipoprotein B (apoB), a marker for chylomicrons, VLDL, Lp(a), and LDL, and apolipoprotein A-I (apoA-I), a marker for HDL. The methods used to routinely determine apoB and apoA-I are based on nephelometry or turbidimetry. Typically, these tests, which depend on polyclonal antibodies, have better analytical performance than methods to measure or estimate LDL-C and HDL-C. Nonetheless, the clinical utility of apolipoprotein measurement remains debated. In certain circumstances, such as hypertriglyceridemia, ApoB is clearly a better predictor of cardiovascular events than LDL-C[52] In general, when there is discordance between apoB and LDL-C, apoB has been shown to be a better predictor.

The 2018 Multi-Society Guidelines suggest the use of apoB in patients with TG > 200 mg/dL[36]; if elevated, it is considered a risk enhancer and encourages the adoption of a more aggressive lipid-lowering strategy. European Guidelines (ESC/EAS) in 2020 recommended the use of apoB for all patients with diabetes, obesity, metabolic syndrome, or low LDL-C.[48] Furthermore, the European guidelines suggest that apoB, if available, can be used as the primary measurement for screening, diagnosis, and management. Recommendations differ, however, on the appropriate cutoff values for apoB when used to assess ASCVD risk. The US 2018 Multi-Society Guidelines recommend a cutoff value of 130 mg/dL, which equals to 160 mg/dL of LDL-C.[36] The European guidelines, however, defined apoB as a secondary goal of treatment, determining the cutoff values according to the cardiovascular risk categories as less than 65, less than 80, and less than 100 mg/dL for very high, high, and moderate risk, respectively.[48]

From an analytical perspective, one can clearly define apoB unlike LDL-C, which depends on the beta quantification method that includes cholesterol from Lp(a) and remnants in the LDL fraction. Ongoing efforts to develop a reference method for apoB based on mass spectrometry[53] and the growing evidence that apoB is superior to LDL-C[54] will likely lead to its greater use in the initial screening of patients for ASCVD risk.

Remnant Cholesterol

Remnant lipoproteins form as the result of the incomplete catabolism of TRL, such as chylomicrons and VLDL, and are enriched in cholesterol and apoE. Unlike LDL, large chylomicrons and large VLDLs cannot readily penetrate the endothelial wall and become deposited in the subendothelium space. Their accumulation in plasma is associated with high risk of pancreatitis due to lipolysis form pancreatic lipases and the generation of high amounts of free fatty acids with consequent ischemia and damage to the pancreas.[55] However, smaller remnant lipoproteins can easily penetrate the endothelium, be retained in the intima, and get internalized by macrophages through their apoE to form foam cells.[19,56] Epidemiologic and interventional studies have demonstrated a causal relationship between high circulating remnant lipoproteins and ASCVD[56] and may account for the residual ASCVD risk after reaching LDL-C treatment goals. Because LPL starts to lipolyze chylomicrons and VLDL immediately after they enter circulation, all circulating TRL can be considered remnant lipoproteins; therefore, cholesterol in remnant lipoproteins (Rem-C) is sometimes calculated by subtracting LDL-C from non-HDL-C. In the fasting state, this term represents mostly VLDL remnants and IDL, whereas in the postprandial state, it also contains chylomicron remnants. Preferably, LDL-C should be directly measured instead of calculated. If LDL-C is calculated using the Friedewald equation, Rem-C is reduced to TG/5 and becomes entirely dependent on the TG levels without providing additional information over TG for the ASCVD risk assessment.[57]

One of the first methods designed to directly measure Rem-C relied on monoclonal antibodies against apoA-I and apoB100 to separate remnants from other lipoproteins in plasma.[58] A key to this assay was that the anti-apoB antibody specifically bound apoB100 on LDL and large VLDL but did not recognize apoB100 on apoE-rich VLDLs or apoB48 on chylomicrons. Plasma was eluted through an immunoaffinity column where the antibodies retained HDL, LDL, and large VLDL, whereas a fraction of lipoproteins rich in apoE, called "remnant-like lipoproteins," eluted.[58] This method correlated well with TRL remnants, but it required a pretreatment of the sample, limiting the ability to automate this method. More recently, a direct fully automated method to determine Rem-C was developed.[59] In a first step, a specific combination of lipases and surfactants degrade the nonremnant lipoproteins (HDL, LDL, and nonremnant TRL), whereas Rem-C remain unaltered. In a second step, Rem-C is quantified by an enzymatic colorimetric reaction.[59] This method eliminates the pretreatment of the sample and allows its full automatization, improving the method performance, and making it suitable for routine clinical testing. Furthermore, a recent study of the cohort from the Copenhagen General Population Study, found that both, calculated and directly measured Rem-C, efficiently predicted ASCVD events; however, unlike calculated Rem-C, directly measured Rem-C was able to detect approximately 5% of high-risk patients who would not be detected by the standard lipid tests.[60] Interestingly, in the same study, no differences were found when Rem-C was calculated using LDL-C assessed by either Friedewald or Martin equation.[60]

Even though a significant body of evidence supports the role of remnant lipoproteins in atherosclerosis, more work is still needed to advance toward methodology standardization. Moreover, current guidelines focused on plasma cholesterol management have not defined when Rem-C should be evaluated or have established cut-off values.

ADVANCED AND EMERGING LIPID RISK FACTORS

The currently recommended approach by most guidelines, including the latest 2018 Multi-Society Guidelines,[36] still lead to the classification of a large part of the population as at intermediate risk, creating a dilemma about how to best treat these patients. Furthermore, more than half of all patients that present with a myocardial infarction and other forms of ASCVD do not have elevated plasma lipids as defined by the current approaches. This has stimulated much of the research in the development of advanced lipoprotein testing, which are sometimes called new or emerging risk factors, in order to better stratify patients in terms of their risk. Some of these advanced tests are shown in **Table 1**. At this time, these tests are not recommended in the initial assessment of ASCVD risk but could be considered for patients at intermediate risk. Some of these tests are available at specialty reference laboratories for routine diagnostic testing but many are still used exclusively in research studies.

Many of these advanced tests depend on the different physical properties of lipoproteins to resolve lipoproteins into subclasses. For example, nondenaturing gradient gel electrophoresis can resolve LDL into at least 5 different species or subclasses. As already been described, smaller subclasses of LDL, which often occur with hypertriglyceridemia from obesity or diabetes are more strongly associated with ASCVD events. Similarly, HDL can be separated into a variety of different subclasses based on size and density,[61] which may differ in their association with ASCVD. For example, one smaller subspecies of HDL, pre-beta HDL, which is typically identified by electrophoresis is strongly positively associated with ASCVD in contrast to HDL-C.[62] In addition to the different size subclasses, some of these methods also provide the total particle number of each of the major classes. For example, one can determine by nuclear magnetic resonance (NMR) the total particle number of LDL, which is referred to as LDL-P. It has been shown when there is discordance between LDL-P and LDL-C that ASCVD risk is more strongly associated with particle number.[63]

Although HDL-C is useful negative risk predictor, there has been considerable research efforts on how to better measure its antiatherogenic functions. Research in this area has also been stimulated by the failed efforts to develop drugs that raise HDL-C for lowering ASCVD events.[61] Several large epidemiologic studies have demonstrated that cholesterol efflux capacity of HDL is inversely associated with cardiovascular events independently of HDL-C.[64,65] This assay of HDL function, however, involves the use of cells and often radiolabeled cholesterol and is only used for research. Several fluorescent cell-free assays that measure this aspect of HDL

Table 1
Advanced lipoprotein testing methods

Assay Name	Background	Principle	Notes	Availability	Key References
NMR lipoprotein testing for LDL-P†	Originally developed for measuring lipoprotein particle concentrations in the early 1990s	Based on deconvoluting the H-NMR spectra from the resonance signal of methyl groups on lipids	Additional lipoprotein parameters and other metabolites can be measured	Available in United States as the *NMR LipoProfile* through LabCorp (Burlington, NC, USA) Other vendors in Europe and elsewhere	75,76
Ion mobility ES-DMA	Method originally used for measure nanoparticles and macro-ion size in the 1990s and adapted for lipoproteins in 2008	After removing albumin, serum lipoproteins are aerosolized by an electrospray interface and are separated by size in a specialized mass spectrometer.	Complex assay requiring dedicated instrumentation and personnel	Available through Quest Diagnostics (Madison, NJ, USA)	77,78
Tube gel electrophoresis	Early manual method for lipoprotein separation by electrophoresis	Lipoproteins are stained with a cholesterol-specific dye and then separated by charge and size using polyacrylamide gel electrophoresis in tubes	The main limitation is the low reproducibility due to variabilities in gel quality	*LIPOPRINT* available through Quantimetrix (Redondo Beach, CA, USA) https:// quantimetrix.com/ lipoprint/	79,80
Gel permeation-high-performance liquid chromatography	Initial reports of its use for lipoprotein profiling in serum were published in the early 1980s	Lipoproteins are separated according to their size by HPLC using TSK-like columns. Lipids are measured in fractions	Complex assay requiring dedicated instrumentation and personnel	*LipoSEARCH* is offered through a Japanese company called Skylight	81,82

Vertical Auto Profile (VAP) [VAP-II is the upgraded version]	Developed in the 1980s as a semiautomatic method to quantify lipoprotein subclasses	Lipoprotein subclasses are separated based on their flotation properties in a discontinuous density gradient by ultracentrifugation. Lipids are measured in fractions	VAP-II is similar to the VAP-II fingerstick (VAP-II-fs), and while it offers higher resolution and performance, it requires more plasma sample for testing	Originally offered by Atherotech Diagnostics Lab (Birmingham, AL, USA) Now offered through VAP Diagnostics Lab as the VAP® (Vertical Auto Profile) + Lipid Panel	83,84
HDL-proteomic testing	Recently developed test that serves as a surrogate for HDL functionality	This test uses mass spectrometry to detect apolipoproteins associated with HDL (apoA-I, ApoAC-I, ApoC-II, ApoC-III, and ApoC-IV). A score, called HDLfx pCAD, is generated based on the abundance of HDL apolipoproteins and correlates with cholesterol efflux capacity of HDL	May provide additional information beyond HDL-C for predicting risk	HDL Function Panel with HDLfx pCAD Score (HDLfx Test) Cleveland HeartLab	70 85
LDL-TG	Recently developed test for TG content of LDL	Uses polyoxyethylene benzyl phenyl ether (surfactant 1) and polyoxyethylene alkyl ether (surfactant 2) to selectively measure the TG associated with LDL	Fully automated and can run on standard chemistry analyzers	Reagents available from Denka Seiken (Niigata, Japan)	86

function have recently been described and may 1 day be routinely used as a diagnostic test. Other more functional-based assays for LDL, such as LDL aggregation tests are also being developed.[66]

Since the beginning of the search for useful cardiovascular biomarkers more than 50 years ago, a central focus has been on the measurement of cholesterol. New research on measuring the other types of lipids that lipoproteins carry may also lead to new diagnostic tests. For example, a direct fully automated assay for measuring the TG content of LDL has been described and has been shown to be superior to LDL-C.[67] The sphingomyelin content of LDL has also been associated with cardiometabolic risk.[68] Similarly, the measurement of other proteins besides the conventional apolipoproteins that we currently measure may be valuable.[69] For example, a commercial reference assay that measures several proteins on HDL has been reported to closely correlate with its cholesterol efflux capacity and is inversely related to ASCVD events (see **Table 1**).[70]

Although not strictly a lipid or a lipoprotein test, DNA-based tests for the genes that modulate lipid metabolism can be useful in diagnosing patients and their families with genetic disorders, such as for identifying mutations in the LDLR for FH. Polygenetic risk scores based on genes related to lipid metabolism have also been described for assessing ASCVD risk, but a greater predictive ability from these tests may be needed before they are widely used. Many new genes recently have been identified in the vessel wall that do not determine lipoprotein levels per se but are involved in atherogenesis.[71,72] A polygenetic score that includes genes that determine the vascular response to the deposition of LDL could, therefore, be useful in identifying the many patients that develop ASCVD but do not seem to be at risk based on standard plasma lipid tests.

SUMMARY AND PERSPECTIVE

Since the start of this century, the concept of "Precision Medicine" has become a major driving force for much of biomedical research. Precision medicine is particularly applicable to cardiovascular disease, a common disorder, that is affected by not only an individual's lifestyle choices but also their genetic predisposition and a host of environmental factors. In the future, the clinical laboratory testing will likely provide an increasingly important role in deciding who and how to treat patients for cardiovascular disease. Given that many of the new cardiovascular therapies that are being developed are based on large or complex biological molecules that are expensive to produce, some of the new and advanced diagnostic tests being developed may be justified based on economic considerations. Many of the new "omic" technologies with their multiplex format will also likely penetrate routine diagnostic testing. Already one can measure a standard lipid panel, apoB, lipoprotein particle number, lipoprotein subfractions, GlycA (a marker of inflammation), and many other metabolites in a single NMR test.[73,74] The current lipid tests that primarily focus on cholesterol will undoubtedly remain valuable but will likely be augmented in the future by other types of tests as we continue to expand our knowledge of lipoprotein metabolism and cardiometabolic disease.

CLINICS CARE POINTS

- Initial cardiovascular risk assessment can be done in either a fasting or nonfasting state.
- The use of new alternative equations for estimating LDL-C in nonfasting samples or hypertriglyceridemia is preferred over the Friedewald equation.

- In hypertriglyceridemic patients, measurement of apoB or a calculate non-HDL-C is preferred for cardiovascular risk assessment.
- In patients with intermediate cardiovascular risk (7.5%–20% 10-year risk), risk enhancer tests, such as Lp(a), apoB, and high sensitivity "C" reactive protein are useful to determine the need for therapeutic intervention.

DISCLOSURE

The authors have nothing to disclose.

FUNDING SOURCES

This research was supported by the Intramural Research Program of the National Heart, Lung, and Blood Institute (NHLBI) (HL006095) at National Institutes of Health. S.T. was supported by the NIH Medical Research Scholars Program, a public–private partnership supported jointly by the NIH and contributions to the Foundation for the NIH from the Doris Duke Charitable Foundation, the American Association for Dental Research, and the Colgate-Palmolive Company.

REFERENCES

1. Goldstein JL, Brown MS. A century of cholesterol and coronaries: from plaques to genes to statins. Cell 2015;161(1):161–72. https://doi.org/10.1016/j.cell.2015.01.036.
2. Feingold KR. Introduction to Lipids and Lipoproteins. In: Feingold KR, Anawalt B, Boyce A, et al, editors. Endotext [Internet]. South Dartmouth (MA): MDText.com, Inc.; 2000.
3. Barale C, Melchionda E, Morotti A, et al. PCSK9 Biology and Its Role in Athero-thrombosis. Int J Mol Sci 2021;22(11). https://doi.org/10.3390/ijms22115880.
4. Gennemark P, Walter K, Clemmensen N, et al. An oral antisense oligonucleotide for PCSK9 inhibition. Sci Transl Med 2021;13(593). https://doi.org/10.1126/scitranslmed.abe9117.
5. Pettersen D, Fjellstrom O. Small molecule modulators of PCSK9 - A literature and patent overview. Bioorg Med Chem Lett 2018;28(7):1155–60. https://doi.org/10.1016/j.bmcl.2018.02.046.
6. Garg R, Rustagi T. Management of Hypertriglyceridemia Induced Acute Pancreatitis. Biomed Res Int 2018;2018:4721357. https://doi.org/10.1155/2018/4721357.
7. Ling P, Zheng X, Luo S, et al. Targeting angiopoietin-like 3 in atherosclerosis: From bench to bedside. Diabetes Obes Metab 2021;23(9):2020–34. https://doi.org/10.1111/dom.14450.
8. Tg, Hdl Working Group of the Exome Sequencing Project NHL, Blood I, et al. Loss-of-function mutations in APOC3, triglycerides, and coronary disease. N Engl J Med 2014;371(1):22–31. https://doi.org/10.1056/NEJMoa1307095.
9. Jorgensen AB, Frikke-Schmidt R, Nordestgaard BG, et al. Loss-of-function mutations in APOC3 and risk of ischemic vascular disease. N Engl J Med 2014;371(1):32–41. https://doi.org/10.1056/NEJMoa1308027.
10. Paik J. Duggan S. Volanesorsen: First Global Approval. Drugs 2019;79(12):1349–54. https://doi.org/10.1007/s40265-019-01168-z.
11. Gouni-Berthold I, Alexander VJ, Yang Q, et al. Efficacy and safety of volanesorsen in patients with multifactorial chylomicronaemia (COMPASS): a

multicentre, double-blind, randomised, placebo-controlled, phase 3 trial. Lancet Diabetes Endocrinol 2021;9(5):264–75. https://doi.org/10.1016/S2213-8587(21) 00046-2.

12. Benito-Vicente A, Uribe KB, Jebari S, et al. Validation of LDLr Activity as a Tool to Improve Genetic Diagnosis of Familial Hypercholesterolemia: A Retrospective on Functional Characterization of LDLr Variants. Int J Mol Sci 2018;19(6). https://doi.org/10.3390/ijms19061676.

13. Marais AD. Familial hypercholesterolaemia. Clin Biochem Rev 2004;25(1):49–68.

14. Michaely P, Li WP, Anderson RG, et al. The modular adaptor protein ARH is required for low density lipoprotein (LDL) binding and internalization but not for LDL receptor clustering in coated pits. J Biol Chem 2004;279(32):34023–31. https://doi.org/10.1074/jbc.M405242200.

15. Karathanasis SK, Freeman LA, Gordon SM, et al. The Changing Face of HDL and the Best Way to Measure It. Clin Chem 2017;63(1):196–210. https://doi.org/10.1373/clinchem.2016.257725.

16. Virmani R, Kolodgie FD, Burke AP, et al. Lessons from sudden coronary death: a comprehensive morphological classification scheme for atherosclerotic lesions. Arterioscler Thromb Vasc Biol 2000;20(5):1262–75. https://doi.org/10.1161/01.atv.20.5.1262.

17. Libby P. The changing landscape of atherosclerosis. Nature 2021;592(7855): 524–33. https://doi.org/10.1038/s41586-021-03392-8.

18. Wilson DP, Jacobson TA, Jones PH, et al. Use of Lipoprotein(a) in clinical practice: A biomarker whose time has come. A scientific statement from the National Lipid Association. J Clin Lipidol 2019;13(3):374–92. https://doi.org/10.1016/j.jacl.2019.04.010.

19. Salinas CAA, Chapman MJ. Remnant lipoproteins: are they equal to or more atherogenic than LDL? Curr Opin Lipidol 2020;31(3):132–9. https://doi.org/10.1097/MOL.0000000000000682.

20. Jessen RH, Dass CJ, Eckfeldt JH. Do enzymatic analyses of serum triglycerides really need blanking for free glycerol? Clin Chem 1990;36(7):1372–5.

21. Buonuomo PS, Iughetti L, Pisciotta L, et al. Timely diagnosis of sitosterolemia by next generation sequencing in two children with severe hypercholesterolemia. Atherosclerosis 2017;262:71–7. https://doi.org/10.1016/j.atherosclerosis.2017.05.002.

22. Nordestgaard BG, Langsted A, Mora S, et al. Fasting Is Not Routinely Required for Determination of a Lipid Profile: Clinical and Laboratory Implications Including Flagging at Desirable Concentration Cutpoints-A Joint Consensus Statement from the European Atherosclerosis Society and European Federation of Clinical Chemistry and Laboratory Medicine. Clin Chem 2016;62(7):930–46. https://doi.org/10.1373/clinchem.2016.258897.

23. Warnick GR, Nauck M, Rifai N. Evolution of methods for measurement of HDL-cholesterol: from ultracentrifugation to homogeneous assays. Clin Chem 2001; 47(9):1579–96.

24. McNamara JR, Warnick GR, Cooper GR. A brief history of lipid and lipoprotein measurements and their contribution to clinical chemistry. Clin Chim Acta 2006; 369(2):158–67. https://doi.org/10.1016/j.cca.2006.02.041.

25. Miller WG, Myers GL, Sakurabayashi I, et al. Seven direct methods for measuring HDL and LDL cholesterol compared with ultracentrifugation reference measurement procedures. Clin Chem 2010;56(6):977–86. https://doi.org/10.1373/clinchem.2009.142810.

26. Boren J, Chapman MJ, Krauss RM, et al. Low-density lipoproteins cause athero-sclerotic cardiovascular disease: pathophysiological, genetic, and therapeutic in-sights: a consensus statement from the European Atherosclerosis Society Consensus Panel. Eur Heart J 2020;41(24):2313–30. https://doi.org/10.1093/eurheartj/ehz962.

27. Nauck M, Warnick GR, Rifai N. Methods for measurement of LDL-cholesterol: a critical assessment of direct measurement by homogeneous assays versus calculation. Clin Chem 2002;48(2):236–54.

28. Rifai N, Warnick GR, McNamara JR, et al. Measurement of low-density-lipoprotein cholesterol in serum: a status report. Clin Chem 1992;38(1):150–60.

29. Miller WG, Waymack PP, Anderson FP, et al. Performance of four homogeneous direct methods for LDL-cholesterol. Clin Chem 2002;48(3):489–98.

30. Wolska A, Remaley AT. Measuring LDL-cholesterol: what is the best way to do it? Curr Opin Cardiol 2020;35(4):405–11. https://doi.org/10.1097/HCO.0000000000000740.

31. Wilson PWF, Jacobson TA, Martin SS, et al. Lipid measurements in the manage-ment of cardiovascular diseases: Practical recommendations a scientific state-ment from the national lipid association writing group. J Clin Lipidol 2021. https://doi.org/10.1016/j.jacl.2021.09.046.

32. Friedewald WT, Levy RI, Fredrickson DS. Estimation of the concentration of low-density lipoprotein cholesterol in plasma, without use of the preparative ultracen-trifuge. Clin Chem 1972;18(6):499–502.

33. Fukuyama N, Homma K, Wakana N, et al. Validation of the Friedewald Equation for Evaluation of Plasma LDL-Cholesterol. J Clin Biochem Nutr 2008;43(1):1–5. https://doi.org/10.3164/jcbn.2008036.

34. Martin SS, Blaha MJ, Elshazly MB, et al. Friedewald-estimated versus directly measured low-density lipoprotein cholesterol and treatment implications. J Am Coll Cardiol 2013;62(8):732–9. https://doi.org/10.1016/j.jacc.2013.01.079.

35. Martin SS, Blaha MJ, Elshazly MB, et al. Comparison of a novel method vs the Friedewald equation for estimating low-density lipoprotein cholesterol levels from the standard lipid profile. JAMA 2013;310(19):2061–8. https://doi.org/10.1001/jama.2013.280532.

36. Grundy SM, Stone NJ, Bailey AL, et al. 2018 AHA/ACC/AACVPR/AAPA/ABC/ACPM/ADA/AGS/APhA/ASPC/NLA/PCNA Guideline on the Management of Blood Cholesterol: A Report of the American College of Cardiology/American Heart As-sociation Task Force on Clinical Practice Guidelines. Circulation 2019;139(25):e1082–143. https://doi.org/10.1161/CIR.0000000000000625.

37. Martin SS, Giugliano RP, Murphy SA, et al. Comparison of Low-Density Lipopro-tein Cholesterol Assessment by Martin/Hopkins Estimation, Friedewald Estima-tion, and Preparative Ultracentrifugation: Insights From the FOURIER Trial. JAMA Cardiol 2018;3(8):749–53. https://doi.org/10.1001/jamacardio.2018.1533.

38. Sampson M, Ling C, Sun Q, et al. A New Equation for Calculation of Low-Density Lipoprotein Cholesterol in Patients With Normolipidemia and/or Hypertriglyceri-demia. JAMA Cardiol 2020;5(5):540–8. https://doi.org/10.1001/jamacardio.2020.0013.

39. Ginsberg HN, Rosenson RS, Hovingh GK, et al. LDL-C calculated by Friedewald, Martin-Hopkins, or NIH Equation 2 versus beta-quantification: pooled alirocumab trials. J Lipid Res 2021;100148. https://doi.org/10.1016/j.jlr.2021.100148.

40. Higgins V, Leiter LA, Delaney SR, et al. Validating the NIH LDL-C equation in a specialized lipid cohort: Does it add up? Clin Biochem 2022;99:60–8. https://doi.org/10.1016/j.clinbiochem.2021.10.003.

41. Ohmura H, Mokuno H, Sawano M, et al. Lipid compositional differences of small, dense low-density lipoprotein particle influence its oxidative susceptibility: possible implication of increased risk of coronary artery disease in subjects with phenotype B. Metabolism 2002;51(9):1081–7. https://doi.org/10.1053/meta.2002.34695.

42. Sampson M, Wolska A, Warnick R, et al. A New Equation Based on the Standard Lipid Panel for Calculating Small Dense Low-Density Lipoprotein-Cholesterol and Its Use as a Risk-Enhancer Test. Clin Chem 2021;67(7):987–97. https://doi.org/10.1093/clinchem/hvab048.

43. Johannesen CDL, Mortensen MB, Langsted A, et al. Apolipoprotein B and Non-HDL Cholesterol Better Reflect Residual Risk Than LDL Cholesterol in Statin-Treated Patients. J Am Coll Cardiol 2021;77(11):1439–50. https://doi.org/10.1016/j.jacc.2021.01.027.

44. van Deventer HE, Miller WG, Myers GL, et al. Non-HDL cholesterol shows improved accuracy for cardiovascular risk score classification compared to direct or calculated LDL cholesterol in a dyslipidemic population. Clin Chem 2011;57(3):490–501. https://doi.org/10.1373/clinchem.2010.154773.

45. Langlois MR, Nordestgaard BG, Langsted A, et al. Quantifying atherogenic lipoproteins for lipid-lowering strategies: consensus-based recommendations from EAS and EFLM. Clin Chem Lab Med 2020;58(4):496–517. https://doi.org/10.1515/cclm-2019-1253.

46. Fujihara Y, Nakamura T, Horikoshi T, et al. Remnant Lipoproteins Are Residual Risk Factor for Future Cardiovascular Events in Patients With Stable Coronary Artery Disease and On-Statin Low-Density Lipoprotein Cholesterol Levels <70 mg/dL. Circ J 2019;83(6):1302–8. https://doi.org/10.1253/circj.CJ-19-0047.

47. Mortensen MB, Nordestgaard BG. Examine low-density lipoprotein, remnants, and lipoprotein(a) in parallel in high risk patients. Eur Heart J 2021;42(18):1809–10. https://doi.org/10.1093/eurheartj/ehaa969.

48. Mach F, Baigent C, Catapano AL, et al. 2019 ESC/EAS Guidelines for the management of dyslipidaemias: lipid modification to reduce cardiovascular risk. Eur Heart J 2020;41(1):111–88. https://doi.org/10.1093/eurheartj/ehz455.

49. Reyes-Soffer G, Ginsberg HN, Berglund L, et al. Lipoprotein(a): A Genetically Determined, Causal, and Prevalent Risk Factor for Atherosclerotic Cardiovascular Disease: A Scientific Statement From the American Heart Association. Arterioscler Thromb Vasc Biol 2022;42(1):e48–60. https://doi.org/10.1161/ATV.0000000000000147.

50. Santangelo G, Faggiano A, Bernardi N, et al. Lipoprotein(a) and aortic valve stenosis: A casual or causal association? Nutr Metab Cardiovasc Dis 2022;32(2):309–17. https://doi.org/10.1016/j.numecd.2021.10.015.

51. Tsimikas S, Karwatowska-Prokopczuk E, Gouni-Berthold I, et al. Lipoprotein(a) Reduction in Persons with Cardiovascular Disease. N Engl J Med 2020;382(3):244–55. https://doi.org/10.1056/NEJMoa1905239.

52. Behbodikhah J, Ahmed S, Elyasi A, et al. Apolipoprotein B and Cardiovascular Disease: Biomarker and Potential Therapeutic Target. Metabolites 2021;11(10). https://doi.org/10.3390/metabo11100690.

53. Delatour V, Clouet-Foraison N, Gaie-Levrel F, et al. Comparability of Lipoprotein Particle Number Concentrations Across ES-DMA, NMR, LC-MS/MS, Immunonephelometry, and VAP: In Search of a Candidate Reference Measurement Procedure for apoB and non-HDL-P Standardization. Clin Chem 2018;64(10):1485–95. https://doi.org/10.1373/clinchem.2018.288746.

54. Sniderman A, Langlois M, Cobbaert C. Update on apolipoprotein B. Curr Opin Lipidol 2021;32(4):226–30. https://doi.org/10.1097/MOL.0000000000000754.
55. Naqvi SMA, Haider S, Patel A, et al. Hypertriglyceridemia-Induced Pancreatitis Complicated by Diabetic Ketoacidosis. Cureus 2021;13(11):e19985. https://doi.org/10.7759/cureus.19985.
56. Nordestgaard BG. Triglyceride-Rich Lipoproteins and Atherosclerotic Cardiovascular Disease: New Insights From Epidemiology, Genetics, and Biology. Circ Res 2016;118(4):547–63. https://doi.org/10.1161/CIRCRESAHA.115.306249.
57. Duran EK, Pradhan AD. Triglyceride-Rich Lipoprotein Remnants and Cardiovascular Disease. Clin Chem 2021;67(1):183–96. https://doi.org/10.1093/clinchem/hvaa296.
58. Nakajima K, Saito T, Tamura A, et al. Cholesterol in remnant-like lipoproteins in human serum using monoclonal anti apo B-100 and anti apo A-I immunoaffinity mixed gels. Clin Chim Acta 1993;223(1-2):53–71. https://doi.org/10.1016/0009-8981(93)90062-9.
59. Hirao Y, Nakajima K, Machida T, et al. Development of a Novel Homogeneous Assay for Remnant Lipoprotein Particle Cholesterol. J Appl Lab Med 2018;3(1):26–36. https://doi.org/10.1373/jalm.2017.024919.
60. Varbo A, Nordestgaard BG. Directly measured vs. calculated remnant cholesterol identifies additional overlooked individuals in the general population at higher risk of myocardial infarction. Eur Heart J 2021;42(47):4833–43. https://doi.org/10.1093/eurheartj/ehab293.
61. Casula M, Colpani O, Xie S, et al. HDL in Atherosclerotic Cardiovascular Disease: In Search of a Role. Cells 2021;10(8). https://doi.org/10.3390/cells10081869.
62. Pullinger CR, O'Connor PM, Naya-Vigne JM, et al. Levels of Prebeta-1 High-Density Lipoprotein Are a Strong Independent Positive Risk Factor for Coronary Heart Disease and Myocardial Infarction: A Meta-Analysis. J Am Heart Assoc 2021;10(7):e018381. https://doi.org/10.1161/JAHA.120.018381.
63. Cromwell WC, Otvos JD, Keyes MJ, et al. LDL Particle Number and Risk of Future Cardiovascular Disease in the Framingham Offspring Study - Implications for LDL Management. J Clin Lipidol 2007;1(6):583–92. https://doi.org/10.1016/j.jacl.2007.10.001.
64. Rohatgi A, Khera A, Berry JD, et al. HDL cholesterol efflux capacity and incident cardiovascular events. N Engl J Med 2014;371(25):2383–93. https://doi.org/10.1056/NEJMoa1409065.
65. Khera AV, Cuchel M, de la Llera-Moya M, et al. Cholesterol efflux capacity, high-density lipoprotein function, and atherosclerosis. N Engl J Med 2011;364(2):127–35. https://doi.org/10.1056/NEJMoa1001689.
66. Ruuth M, Nguyen SD, Vihervaara T, et al. Susceptibility of low-density lipoprotein particles to aggregate depends on particle lipidome, is modifiable, and associates with future cardiovascular deaths. Eur Heart J 2018;39(27):2562–73. https://doi.org/10.1093/eurheartj/ehy319.
67. Marz W, Scharnagl H, Winkler K, et al. Low-density lipoprotein triglycerides associated with low-grade systemic inflammation, adhesion molecules, and angiographic coronary artery disease: the Ludwigshafen Risk and Cardiovascular Health study. Circulation 2004;110(19):3068–74. https://doi.org/10.1161/01.CIR.0000146898.06923.80.
68. Poss AM, Maschek JA, Cox JE, et al. Machine learning reveals serum sphingolipids as cholesterol-independent biomarkers of coronary artery disease. J Clin Invest 2020;130(3):1363–76. https://doi.org/10.1172/JCI131838.

69. Birner-Gruenberger R, Schittmayer M, Holzer M, et al. Understanding high-density lipoprotein function in disease: recent advances in proteomics unravel the complexity of its composition and biology. Prog Lipid Res 2014;56:36–46. https://doi.org/10.1016/j.plipres.2014.07.003.

70. Natarajan P, Collier TS, Jin Z, et al. Association of an HDL Apolipoproteomic Score With Coronary Atherosclerosis and Cardiovascular Death. J Am Coll Cardiol 2019;73(17):2135–45. https://doi.org/10.1016/j.jacc.2019.01.073.

71. Lucero D, Dikilitas O, Mendelson MM, et al. Transgelin: A New Gene Involved in LDL Endocytosis Identified by a Genome-wide CRISPR-Cas9 Screen. J Lipid Res 2021;100160. https://doi.org/10.1016/j.jlr.2021.100160.

72. Kessler T, Schunkert H. Coronary Artery Disease Genetics Enlightened by Genome-Wide Association Studies. JACC Basic Transl Sci 2021;6(7):610–23. https://doi.org/10.1016/j.jacbts.2021.04.001.

73. Ballout RA, Remaley AT. GlycA: A New Biomarker for Systemic Inflammation and Cardiovascular Disease (CVD) Risk Assessment. J Lab Precis Med 2020;5. https://doi.org/10.21037/jlpm.2020.03.03.

74. Garcia E, Bennett DW, Connelly MA, et al. The extended lipid panel assay: a clinically-deployed high-throughput nuclear magnetic resonance method for the simultaneous measurement of lipids and Apolipoprotein B. Lipids Health Dis 2020;19(1):247. https://doi.org/10.1186/s12944-020-01424-2.

75. Otvos JD. Measurement of lipoprotein subclass profiles by nuclear magnetic resonance spectroscopy. Clin Lab 2002;48(3-4):171–80.

76. Jeyarajah EJ, Cromwell WC, Otvos JD. Lipoprotein particle analysis by nuclear magnetic resonance spectroscopy. Clin Lab Med 2006;26(4):847–70. https://doi.org/10.1016/j.cll.2006.07.006.

77. Caulfield MP, Li S, Lee G, et al. Direct determination of lipoprotein particle sizes and concentrations by ion mobility analysis. Clin Chem 2008;54(8):1307–16. https://doi.org/10.1373/clinchem.2007.100586.

78. Clouet-Foraison N, Gaie-Levrel F, Gillery P, et al. Advanced lipoprotein testing for cardiovascular diseases risk assessment: a review of the novel approaches in lipoprotein profiling. Clin Chem Lab Med 2017;55(10):1453–64. https://doi.org/10.1515/cclm-2017-0091.

79. Noble RP. Electrophoretic separation of plasma lipoproteins in agarose gel. J Lipid Res 1968;9(6):693–700.

80. Warnick GR, McNamara JR, Boggess CN, et al. Polyacrylamide gradient gel electrophoresis of lipoprotein subclasses. Clin Lab Med 2006;26(4):803–46. https://doi.org/10.1016/j.cll.2006.07.005.

81. Okazaki M, Ohno Y, Hara I. High-performance aqueous gel permeation chromatography of human serum lipoproteins. J Chromatogr 1980;221(2):257–64. https://doi.org/10.1016/s0378-4347(00)84310-8.

82. Okazaki M, Yamashita S. Recent Advances in Analytical Methods on Lipoprotein Subclasses: Calculation of Particle Numbers from Lipid Levels by Gel Permeation HPLC Using "Spherical Particle Model. J Oleo Sci 2016;65(4):265–82. https://doi.org/10.5650/jos.ess16020.

83. Chung BH, Segrest JP, Cone JT, et al. High resolution plasma lipoprotein cholesterol profiles by a rapid, high volume semi-automated method. J Lipid Res 1981;22(6):1003–14.

84. Cone JT, Segrest JP, Chung BH, et al. Computerized rapid high resolution quantitative analysis of plasma lipoproteins based upon single vertical spin centrifugation. J Lipid Res 1982;23(6):923–35.

85. Jin Z, Collier TS, Dai DLY, et al. Development and Validation of Apolipoprotein AI-Associated Lipoprotein Proteome Panel for the Prediction of Cholesterol Efflux Capacity and Coronary Artery Disease. Clin Chem 2019;65(2):282–90. https://doi.org/10.1373/clinchem.2018.291922.

86. Ito Y, Ohta M, Ikezaki H, et al. Development and Population Results of a Fully Automated Homogeneous Assay for LDL Triglyceride. J Appl Lab Med 2018; 2(5):746–56. https://doi.org/10.1373/jalm.2017.024554.

Assessment of Cardiovascular Disease Risk
A 2022 Update

Earl Goldsborough III, BS[a], Ngozi Osuji, MD, MPH[a,b],
Michael J. Blaha, MD, MPH[b],*

KEYWORDS

- Risk assessment • Primary prevention • Atherosclerosis • Cardiovascular disease
- Cardiovascular risk • Family history • Coronary artery calcium • Lipoprotein(a)

KEY POINTS

- ASCVD risk assessment is critical for personalizing preventive therapy, targeting the most aggressive interventions to those most likely to benefit, while allowing conservative therapy approaches for those who are low risk.
- The first step in ASCVD risk assessment is the use of a traditional 10-year risk calculator, for example, the Pooled Cohort Equations or the SCORE2 algorithm.
- Next, risk-enhancing factors (otherwise unaccounted for factors that raise risk estimates) should be considered, such as family history.
- Subclinical atherosclerosis testing, notably using coronary artery calcium (CAC), can further personalize risk particularly in borderline to intermediate-risk individuals.
- Lipoprotein(a) is perhaps the most promising serum biomarker and should be considered for one-time measurement in most patients with risk attributable to family history or dyslipidemia.
- 2020 guidelines from the Endocrine Society focus on traditional 10-year risk assessment, risk-enhancing factors, CAC, and lipoprotein(a) testing in clinical practice. Most other tests, including advanced lipid testing and stress testing, are considered much less helpful for routine clinical practice.

INTRODUCTION

Cardiovascular diseases (CVDs) are the leading cause of death worldwide, with atherosclerotic cardiovascular disease (ASCVD) being the dominant cause of total CVD mortality.[1–3] From 1993 to 2019, the global prevalence of CVD nearly doubled[4] and is projected to continue increasing through 2024.[5] In the United States (US), ASCVD is the predominant cause of morbidity and health care expenditure.[6] As

[a] Johns Hopkins University School of Medicine, 600 North Wolfe Street, Baltimore, MD 21287, USA; [b] Division of Cardiology, Department of Medicine, Ciccarone Center for the Prevention of Cardiovascular Disease, Johns Hopkins University School of Medicine, Baltimore, MD, USA
* Corresponding author. Blalock 524D1 JHH, 600 N Wolfe Street, Baltimore, MD 21287.
E-mail address: mblaha1@jhmi.edu

Endocrinol Metab Clin N Am 51 (2022) 483–509
https://doi.org/10.1016/j.ecl.2022.02.005
0889-8529/22/© 2022 Elsevier Inc. All rights reserved.
endo.theclinics.com

such, clinical ASCVD risk assessment is instrumental in constructing a holistic view of patient health. However, this assessment is particularly imperative for patients with a diagnosis of, or under suspicion for, dyslipidemia as these patients portend an increased risk of developing ASCVD.[7–11]

Primary prevention is directed at either the level of the population or the individual,[12] depending on the degree of predisposing risk. Preventive strategies directed at the population emphasize lifestyle modifications (eg, diet improvement, regular exercise, and avoidance of tobacco and secondhand smoke exposure) and are generally indicated for individuals regardless of predisposing risk.[13] Through general recommendations and/or public policy approaches, population-centered approaches focused on mitigating the effect of modifiable risk factors can eschew some risk and derive a net cardiovascular benefit for the general population. However, this generalizability can come at the expense of selectively identifying high-risk groups with prodigious vascular aging who may gain larger benefits and exclusion of very low-risk patients for whom strict adherence to such recommendations would derive little to no net benefit.

Statins are an example of a therapy that may straddle the boundaries between population and individual-level prevention. For example, a meta-analysis on statin efficacy yielded data suggesting that statin use poses minimal risks while significantly reducing ASCVD risk,[14] leading some to propose statin use for almost everyone over the age of 50.[15] While expansion in statin use may be a step forward, it is incomplete. There are individuals in their 40s with predisposing factors for whom statin therapy would be of greater benefit, and there are individuals more than 50 for whom the risk-benefit ratio of initiating statin therapy would not substantiate lifelong preventive therapy. Thus, while general population-level preventive guidelines are an important first step, in routine clinical practice there is a need for guidance at the level of the individual.

Formal ASCVD risk assessments aid in identifying individuals at increased risk of developing ASCVD, stratifying risk into clinically actionable categories, and concomitantly guiding the clinical decision-making process.[16–18] The primary objectives of this review are to:

1. Describe the commonly used ASCVD risk calculators and elucidate ASCVD risk score interpretation.
2. Highlight the role of risk-enhancing factors and family history in interpreting patient risk.
3. Discuss the role of inflammatory markers, coronary artery calcium (CAC) scoring, and lipoprotein A (Lp(a)) in risk assessment.
4. Provide additional context to the most recent Endocrine Society guidelines on Lipid Management in Patients with Endocrine Disorders.

ATHEROSCLEROTIC CARDIOVASCULAR DISEASE RISK ASSESSMENT

Clinical risk assessment can be facilitated via many modalities, with traditional risk calculators, imaging, hybrid risk calculators, serum biomarkers, polygenic risk scores (PRS), and stress testing predominating. However, the gold standard for initial clinical risk assessment remains the traditional risk calculators—notably, the Pooled Cohort Equations (PCE) in the U.S.[13] and the Systemic COronary Risk Evaluation (SCORE) in Europe.[19]

TRADITIONAL ATHEROSCLEROTIC CARDIOVASCULAR DISEASE RISK CALCULATORS

Traditional risk calculators are the recommended first steps for facilitating a clinical risk assessment for individuals with no known ASCVD (ie, no known acute coronary syndrome (ACS), myocardial infarction (MI), stable angina, unstable angina, coronary revascularization, arterial revascularization, stroke, transient ischemic attack (TIA), or peripheral artery disease (PAD) of atherosclerotic etiology).[19,20] Risk calculators are mathematical equations that stratify individuals by prognosticated likelihood of experiencing an atherosclerotic event in future years (eg, 10-year or lifetime estimation). These risk assessments are generally most validated and beneficial in the risk stratification of middle-aged adults.

ASCVD risk calculators are derived from data pooled from multiple cohort studies in the population or populations for which they are indicated. The score derived from the calculator relates to an estimated likelihood of an atherosclerotic event over a defined time period and is concomitant with delegation into an absolute risk category. From this risk stratification, the most appropriate preventive strategy can be identified. These preventive strategies range from risk discussion to lifestyle modifications concurrent with pharmacotherapy.[13]

Pooled Cohort Equations

Since its introduction in 2013, the American College of Cardiology and American Heart Association (ACC/AHA) have endorsed the PCE for primary clinical risk assessment.[13] The PCE is a race- and sex-specific traditional risk calculator, developed and validated by the Working Group of the ACC/AHA, and it is derived from the data of 5 large US cohort studies.[21] It is used in primary risk assessment for non-Hispanic African American and White adults aged 40 to 79 years and in some non-Hispanic African American and White adults as young as 20 years (**Fig. 1**).[20] The PCE should only be used for individuals with no known ASCVD.

It estimates the 10-year risk of developing a first hard ASCVD event (eg, nonfatal MI, stroke death, coronary heart disease (CHD) death) for non-Hispanic African American and White adults aged 40 to 79 years.[21] Additionally, it can estimate the lifetime risk of developing a first hard ASCVD event in non-Hispanic African American and White adults aged 20 to 59 years.[21] For other racial/ethnic groups, it is recommended that the equation for non-Hispanic White adults be used to assess risk and that results be cautiously interpreted.[21]

The risk factors operationalized include chronologic age, sex, total cholesterol (TC), high-density lipoprotein cholesterol (HDL-C), systolic blood pressure (SBP), blood pressure treatment, diabetes mellitus (DM), and current smoking status.[21] Scores are delegated into one of the 4 absolute risk categories: low (<5%), borderline (5%–7.4%), intermediate (7.5%–19.9%), and high (≥20%).[13]

Systemic Coronary Risk Evaluation (Score)

The SCORE has been endorsed by the European Society of Cardiology (ESC) for primary clinical risk assessment in European adults[22] aged 45 to 64 years and is further endorsed by the European Atherosclerosis Society (EAS).[19] SCORE was developed through pooled data from 12 diverse European cohort studies[23] and functions as a country- and sex-specific calculator which estimates the 10-year risk of an incident fatal atherosclerotic event[23] in European adults aged 45 to 64 years.[23] Additionally, it can be used to assess total cardiovascular risk[19] (ie, 10-year risk of both fatal and nonfatal ASCVD events) by multiplying the 10-year cardiovascular mortality SCORE risk by 3.[23]

The risk factors operationalized include age, sex, TC, HDL-C, SBP, smoking status, and nationality. The SCORE differentially uses either a high- or low-risk chart (**Figs. 2 and 3**),[24] dependent on the patient's nationality.[23] SCORE risk is delegated into one of the 4 absolute risk categories: low (<1%), moderate (1 to <5%), high (5 to <10%), and

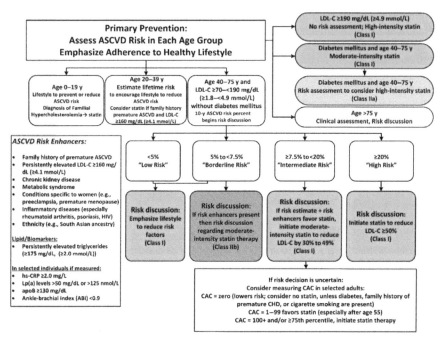

Fig. 1. Primary prevention algorithm in the AHA/ACC Guideline on the Management of Blood Cholesterol. (*From* Grundy SM, Stone NJ, Bailey AL, Beam C, Birtcher KK, Blumenthal RS, Braun LT, de Ferranti S, Faiella-Tommasino J, Forman DE, Goldberg R, Heidenreich PA, Hlatky MA, Jones DW, Lloyd-Jones D, Lopez-Pajares N, Ndumele CE, Orringer CE, Peralta CA, Saseen JJ, Smith SC Jr, Sperling L, Virani SS, Yeboah J. 2018 AHA/ACC/AACVPR/AAPA/ABC/ACPM/ADA/AGS/APhA/ASPC/NLA/PCNA Guideline on the Management of Blood Cholesterol: Executive Summary: A Report of the American College of Cardiology/American Heart Association Task Force on Clinical Practice Guidelines. J Am Coll Cardiol. 2019 Jun 25;73(24):3168-3209.)

very high ($\geq$10%).[23] An additional, unofficial very high-risk group exists for several countries. For these countries, results must be cautiously interpreted, as both low- and high-risk charts are likely to underestimate actual risk.[25]

The 2019 ESC/EAS Guideline on the management of dyslipidemia[19] was published before the development and validation of SCORE2,[26] a revision of the original SCORE.[23] Unlike SCORE, SCORE2 is derived from data of 13 diverse European cohort studies, has more inclusive study endpoints (eg, 10-year incident fatal and nonfatal CVD event), and has an extended age range of 40 to 69 years.[26] Since August 2021, the ESC has recommended the use of SCORE2 for primary risk assessment in the 40 to 69-year groups.[27] **Fig. 1** shows a sample SCORE2 chart.[26]

Other Traditional Atherosclerotic Cardiovascular Disease Risk Calculators

There are numerous traditional risk calculators which have been validated and are used in distinct populations. Notably, the Reynolds CVD Risk Scores for Women[28] and Men[29] can be used in the clinical risk assessment of 10-year incident cardiovascular event (eg, MI, ischemic stroke, coronary revascularization, cardiovascular mortality) for American women and men, more than 45 and 50 years, respectively.[28,29] Both risk scores incorporate lipid profiling and inflammatory markers in their assessment of risk, with the Risk Score for Women having more extensive incorporation of

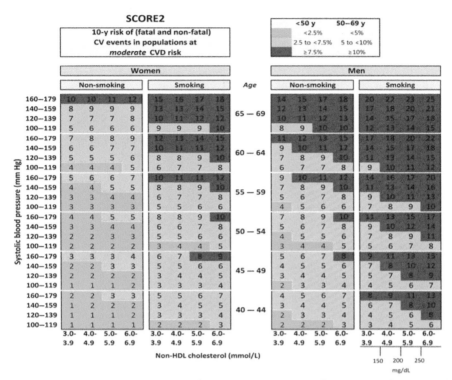

Fig. 2. SCORE2 ASCVD risk calculator for populations with moderate CVD risk. (*Adapted from* SCORE2 working group and ESC Cardiovascular risk collaboration. SCORE2 risk prediction algorithms: new models to estimate 10-year risk of cardiovascular disease in Europe. *Eur Heart J.* 2021;42(25):2439-2454.)

lipid profiling.[28,29] Additionally, multiple QRISK calculators exist for estimating 10-year incident CVD event likelihood (eg, MI, CHD, stroke, TIA) in specific countries such as the United Kingdom.[30–32] The most recent QRISK, the QRISK3, is indicated for British adults as young as 25 years and additionally incorporates atrial fibrillation, chronic kidney disease, and erectile dysfunction in the clinical assessment of ASCVD risk.[32] **Table 1** shows a summary of ASCVD risk calculators.

Specific Populations

A limitation of the PCE and SCORE is their unvalidated utility for clinical risk assessment in adults under the age of 40. To account for this, the ACC recommends measuring traditional risk factors every 4 to 6 years, beginning at age 20 (but without formal global risk assessment)[13]; meanwhile, the ESC/EAS recommends risk factor screening and lipid profiling for men beginning at age 40 and for women beginning at either age 50 or after menopause.[19] This still leaves European adults under the age of 45 without a clinical risk assessment when using SCORE[23] and European adults under the age of 40 bereft of a clinical risk assessment using SCORE2.[26]

Additionally, the ESC/EAS endorse the risk assessment tool, SCORE2-Older Persons (SCORE2-OP) for patients more than 70 years[33] and the ADVANCE and DIAL risk scores and models for patients living with diabetes.[19]

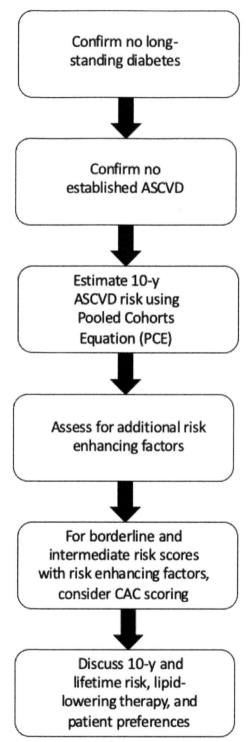

Fig. 3. Steps in initial ASCVD risk assessment. (*Adapted from* Newman CB, Blaha MJ, Boord JB, Cariou B, Chait A, Fein HG, Ginsberg HN, Goldberg IJ, Murad MH, Subramanian S, Tannock LR. Lipid Management in Patients with Endocrine Disorders: An Endocrine Society Clinical Practice Guideline. J Clin Endocrinol Metab. 2020 Dec 1;105(12):dgaa674.)

Table 1
ASCVD traditional risk calculators

Risk Calculator	Indicated Population	Risk-Enhancing Factors Included	Endpoint(s)	Validation	Benefits	Limitations
ASSIGN[116]	Scotland, 30–74 y/o	Age, cigarettes/d, DM, family hx of CHD or stroke, HDL-C, SBP, sex, SIMD score, SS, TC	1—year CVD mortality; incident CHD; incident cerebrovascular disease; coronary artery intervention	No	Incorporates social deprivation to address disproportionate burden; cigarette use is a quantitative variable	Not validated; limited applicable population
China-PAR[117]	Chinese, 35–74 y/o	Women: DM, GR, HDL-C, SBP, SS, WC Men: + family hx ASCVD, urbanization	10-y first nonfatal MI, stroke, stroke death, or CHD death	Yes	Validated in Chinese population; equation for women (C-statistic = 0.811); equation for men (C-statistic = 0.794); predicted rates comparable to observed rates (women [$P = .17$]; men [P-0.16])	Only uses hard ASCVD outcomes as endpoint; does not incorporate CAC scoring; does not incorporate lipid-lowering therapy
Framingham General CVD Risk Score[118]	United States, 30–74 y/o	Age, anti-HTN tx, DM, HDL-C, SBP, SS, TC	Incident CVD (CHD, cerebrovascular disease, peripheral vascular disease, HF)	Yes	Good discrimination (0.763 for men; 0.793 for women)	Data from noncontemporary studies
JBS3[119–122]	Great Britain, >40 y/o	Age, BMI, ethnicity, HDL-C, SBP, sex, Townsend deprivation	10-y and lifetime incident CVD	Yes	Quick; most information is readily available through normal screening	No indication for younger age groups

(continued on next page)

Table 1
(continued)

Risk Calculator	Indicated Population	Risk-Enhancing Factors Included	Endpoint(s)	Validation	Benefits	Limitations
MESA[104]	United States, 45–84 y/o	Age, anti-HTN tx, CAC, DM, family hx of MI, HDL-C, lipid-lowering tx, race/ethnicity, SBP, sex, SS, TC	10-y incident CHD	Yes	Incorporation of CAC increases accuracy (0.80 vs 0.75, $P < .0001$); multi-ethnic, highly powered cohort for the derivation of equation; can identify subclinical CVD	No indication for younger age groups
PCE[13]	United States, non-Hispanic African American, and Whites, 40–79 y/o	Age, anti-HTN tx, DM, HDL-C, race, SBP, sex, SS, TC	10-y (40–79 y/o) or lifetime (20–59 y/o) incident hard ASCVD event	Yes	Quick; reliable; online version is free	Limited age range; limited racial/ethnic representation; data from noncontemporary studies
QRISK[30]	United Kingdom, 35–74 y/o	Age, anti-HTN tx, area measure of deprivation, BMI, family hx of CHD in first-degree relative < 60 y, HDL-C, SBP, sex, SS, TC	10-y first CVD event (MI, CHD, stroke, TIA)	Yes	Incorporates deprivation in risk assessment; incorporates family hx of CHD; better discrimination than Framingham and ASSIGN	Not racial/ethnic specific
QRISK 2[31]	England and Wales, 35–74 y/o	Afib, age, anti-HTN tx, BMI, ethnicity, family hx of CHD in first-degree relative < 60 y, HDL-C, renal disease, RA, SBP, sex, SS, T2DM, Townsend derivation	10-y incident CVD event (CHD, stroke, TIA)	Yes	Ethnic specific; incorporates more risk-enhancing factors than QRISK; better discrimination of high-risk individuals	Does not use MI as an endpoint, unlike in QRISK; validation in a population with similar demographic composition to the population used to derive the equation

Tool	Population	Variables	Outcome	Validated	Discrimination/Performance	Limitations
QRISK 3[32]	England, 25–84 y/o	Afib, age, anti-HTN tx, atypical antipsychotic tx, BMI, CKD, ethnicity, ED ± tx, family hx of CHD in first-degree relative < 60 y, HDL-C, HIV/AIDS, migraine status, RA, renal disease, SBP, SBP sd, severe mental illness, sex, SLE, SS, steroid tablets, T2DM, TC, Townsend deprivation	Incident CVD (CHD, stroke, TIA)	Yes	Good discrimination (Harrell's C statistical of 0.88 for women, 0.86 for men); additional variables better identify high-risk individuals; expanded age range	Validation in a population with similar demographic composition to the population used to derive the equation; limited applicable population; does not incorporate MI as an endpoint
Reynolds CVD Risk Score for Women[28]	United States, women, ≥45 y/o	Age, Apo A1, Apo B-100, hsCRP, parental hx of MI < 60y, SBP, SS, HbA1c if DM, Lp(a) if Apo B-100 ≥ 100 mg/dL	10-y incident CV event (MI, ischemic stroke, coronary revascularization, CV mortality)	Yes	Good discrimination (C-statistic = 0.809); incorporates conditional variables for increased sensitivity	Limited ethnic- and SES-diversity of cohort population used to derive the equation; BP data was self-reported
Reynolds CVD Risk Score for Men[29]	United States, men, ≥50 y/o	Age, HDL-C, hsCRP, parental hx of MI < 60 y, SBP, SS, TC	10-y incident CV event (nonfatal MI, nonfatal stroke, coronary revascularization, CV death)	Yes	Larger C-index compared with traditional model (P < .001); improved accuracy among reclassified individuals	Limited ethnic- and SES-diversity of cohort population used to derive the equation; BP data were self-reported

(continued on next page)

Table 1
(continued)

Risk Calculator	Indicated Population	Risk-Enhancing Factors Included	Endpoint(s)	Validation	Benefits	Limitations
SCORE[23,26,120]	Europeans, 45–64 y/o	Age, HDL-C, SBP, sex, SS, TC	10-y cardiovascular mortality	Yes	Low-risk and high-risk charts for different European countries; data pooled from 12 European cohort studies	Only uses CV mortality as endpoint; minimizes international differences by stratifying country risk categories by geography; data are from cohorts before 1986
SCORE 2[26]	Europeans, 40–69 y/o, no previous CVD or diabetes	Age, HDL-C, SBP, sex, SS, TC	10-y first fatal and nonfatal CVD event	Yes	Data pooled from cohort studies in 13 European countries; includes nonfatal endpoints; uses more recent data than SCORE; moderate-to-good discrimination in external validation (C-indices from 0.67 to 0.81)	High-risk CVD countries had smaller contribution to developing the equation; does not incorporate family hx, medication status, ethnicity, or SES

Abbreviations: Afib, atrial fibrillation; Apo, apolipoprotein; BMI, body mass index; CAC, coronary artery calcium; CHD, coronary heart disease; CKD, chronic kidney disease; ED, erectile dysfunction; GR, geographic region; HbA1c, hemoglobin A1c; HDL-C, high-density lipoprotein-cholesterol; hsCRP, high-sensitivity C-reactive protein; HTN, hypertension; hx, history; Lp(a). lipoprotein a; MI, myocardial infarction; RA, rheumatoid arthritis; SBP, systolic blood pressure; sd, standard deviation; SIMD, Scottish Index of Multiple Deprivation; SLE, systemic lupus erythematosus; SS, smoking status; T2DM, type 2 diabetes mellitus; TC, total cholesterol; TIA, transient ischemic attack; tx, therapy; WC, waist circumference

RISK-ENHANCING FACTORS
Underrepresented Risk-Enhancing Factors

Several risk-enhancing factors (newer risk factors that may elevate risk in particular clinical situations) are not traditionally represented in risk calculators. Some of these include infrequent exercise,[13] unhealthy diet,[13] dyslipidemia,[19] elevated TC in the elderly (ie, >70–75 y),[19,34] family history of premature ASCVD, metabolic syndrome, aspects of the lipid and inflammatory biomarker profiles, and chronic inflammatory conditions (**Table 2**).[20]

Risk Assessment in Specific Populations

Diabetes mellitus

Adults with DM are considered a higher-risk population for developing ASCVD but are no longer considered a "ASCVD risk equivalent."[20] Consequently, for adults aged 40 to 75 years with a diagnosis of DM, while the initiation of statin therapy is indicated before a clinical ASCVD assessment, further risk assessment is required for other decision-making.[20] For example, the intensity of statin and other nonstatin lipid-lowering therapy should match the accumulation of risk factors. Notably, there are DM-specific, independent risk factors that must also be considered in the clinical risk assessment for this population. These include the duration of DM ($\geq$10 y for type 2 DM; $\geq$20 y for type 1 DM), albuminuria ($\geq$30 mcg/mg creatinine); eGFR less than 60 mL/min/1.73 m^2,[2] retinopathy, neuropathy, and ankle-brachial index (ABI) < 0.9.[20]

Endocrine diseases

Various non-DM endocrine diseases, such as persistent Cushing syndrome or untreated thyroid disorders, influence lipid levels, often increasing ASCVD risk. The 10-year ASCVD risk should still be calculated using a traditional risk calculator such as the PCE. However, assessing risk-enhancing factors (ie, insulin-resistance-related risk factors such as metabolic syndrome) is especially salient in adjudicating risk, and when assessing subclinical atherosclerosis, CAC is preferred. Measuring lipoprotein a (Lp(a)) may further enhance short-term and lifetime ASCVD risk prediction

Table 2
Risk-enhancing factors for ASCVD

Family History	Patient Comorbidities	Lipid Testing and Serum Biomarkers
1. Premature ASCVD (eg, males <55 y; females <65 y) 2. High-risk race/ethnicity (eg, S. Asian)	1. Primary hypercholesterolemia 2. Metabolic syndrome 3. Chronic kidney disease 4. Chronic inflammatory conditions (eg, rheumatoid arthritis, HIV/AIDS) 5. Premature menopause 6. Pregnancy-associated conditions which increase the risk of ASCVD (eg, pre-eclampsia)	1. Primary persistent hypertriglyceridemia 2. Elevated hsCRP 3. Elevated Lp(a) 4. Elevated apoB 5. Ankle-brachial index (ABI) < 0.9

Adapted from Grundy SM, Stone NJ, Bailey AL, Beam C, Birtcher KK, Blumenthal RS, Braun LT, de Ferranti S, Faiella-Tommasino J, Forman DE, Goldberg R, Heidenreich PA, Hlatky MA, Jones DW, Lloyd-Jones D, Lopez-Pajares N, Ndumele CE, Orringer CE, Peralta CA, Saseen JJ, Smith SC jr, Sperling L, Virani SS, Yeboah J. 2018 AHA/ACC/AACVPR/AAPA/ABC/ACPM/ADA/AGS/APhA/ASPC/NLA/PCNA Guideline on the Management of Blood Cholesterol: Executive Summary: A Report of the American College of Cardiology/American Heart Association Task Force on Clinical Practice Guidelines. J Am Coll Cardiol. 2019 Jun 25;73(24):3168-3209.

and inform the indication and intensity of low-density lipoprotein C (LDL-C) lowering therapy when in addition to an endocrine disorder there is a personal history of ASCVD or a family history of either ASCVD or high Lp(a).[35]

Women
Clinical risk assessment for women must assess sex-specific disparities in predisposition, exposure, and access to care. Some risk-enhancing factors are sex-specific and include a history of premature menopause (<40 y), preeclampsia,[20] previous preterm delivery,[36] hypertensive pregnancy disorders, depression, and autoimmune diseases such as systemic lupus erythematosus (SLE) and rheumatoid arthritis (RA).[37] Further, traditional risk factors such as DM, obesity, and smoking pose a greater risk of developing ASCVD in women, when compared with men of the same age.[37] Thus, clinical risk assessment in women should not be limited to assessment via traditional risk-enhancing factors but should involve a holistic assessment of individual risk.

Low socioeconomic status
Low socioeconomic status (SES) as well as poor neighborhood socioeconomic factors are associated with poorer cardiovascular health and increased ASCVD adverse events.[20,38,39] The mechanism mediating the increased risk associated with these 2 factors is not well known.[38] Incorporating annual household income to the PCE yielded a modest increase in discrimination (C-Index of 0.739 vs 0.743).[40]

Chronic inflammatory conditions
Chronic inflammatory conditions predispose an individual to increased risk of atherothrombogenesis[41] and ASCVD.[20] It is unclear whether this association is causal or related to shared risk factors, genetic profile, or exposures.[42] Conditions such as inflammatory bowel disease (IBD), periodontitis, RA, psoriasis, and SLE increase the risk of developing ASCVD.[43]

Human immunodeficiency virus
Human immunodeficiency virus (HIV) infection is associated with an increased risk of developing ASCVD in adults $\geq$19 years.[44] For individuals with a low CD4 count (<350 cells/mm^3), it is important to note that a calculated risk may underestimate actual risk.[45]

Race/ethnicity
Race can portend an increased risk of developing ASCVD. A South Asian ancestry is associated with an increased risk of developing ASCVD,[20] incident stroke rates for African Americans are almost twice that of White Americans, and there are many other relationships between race/ethnicity and ASCVD.[46] However, race/ethnicity alone may not account for these differences. Rather, these effects may be further mediated by habitus and lifestyle (eg, exercise). Thus, race/ethnicity-specific guidance should additionally address the habitus and lifestyle of the individual.

Young (<40) and elderly (>75)
Young adults aged less than 40 years are underrepresented in major risk calculators and often considered to be at nonsignificant levels of risk. However, prevalent coronary atherosclerosis as measured using the CAC scoring is considerable in high-risk young adults, with a graded increased odds with increasing risk factor burden.[47] Prevalent CAC is estimated as high as 34.4% in young adults aged 30 to 49 years who are classified as low-risk by a 10-year ASCVD assessment.[48] Imaging seems to be the gold standard for detecting premature coronary atherosclerosis in those younger

than the indicated age for traditional calculators. A recent CAC Percentile Calculator for adults aged 30 to 45 years calculates the estimated probability of a CAC greater than 0 for a given age, sex, and race as well as a CAC percentile ranking with the additional input of an observed CAC score.[49]

For those greater than 75 years, the ACC/AHA only recommends the discussion of preventive therapies appropriate to comorbidities and life expectancy.[13] Moving forward, concise guidelines for initiating or continuing preventive therapy in the elderly are needed.

Family History

Assessment of a family history can improve risk estimation and assist in adjudicating preventive therapy in patients for whom risk stratification is uncertain.[13,50] A family history assessment can be a brief yet invaluable tool. Data suggest only asking about a history of (CHD) in first-degree relatives was as predictive of ASCVD risk as more intensive assessments. Any family history of CHD in a first-degree relative has been associated with an increased relative risk of incident ASCVD[50,51] and CVD mortality.[52] Additionally, it has been shown to be an independent risk factor for ASCVD and to have additive associations with elevated plasma Lp(a).[53] Alone, a family history significant for CHD can indicate benefit from advanced risk assessment. However, it does not substantiate the benefit of high-intensity statin therapy or prophylactic aspirin therapy.[54] Nearly half of the patients in the MESA cohort with a family history significant for CHD had a CAC = 0. However, for those with a significant family history and a non-zero CAC, CAC was a good estimate of ASCVD risk.[54] A family history of CAD was shown to be associated with markers of subclinical atherosclerosis.[55] The ACC/AHA acknowledges a family history of premature ASCVD (eg, male, <55 y; female, <65 y) as a risk-enhancing factor and recommends using such information to revise the 10-year risk estimation.[13] Thus, the assessment of family history can increase the likely benefit from CAC scoring[54] and enhance risk estimation[13] but, alone, should not dictate the intensity of preventive therapy.[13]

Summary of Traditional Risk Atherosclerotic Cardiovascular Disease Assessment

Traditional ASCVD risk calculators are invaluable tools in primary risk assessment. They function to identify and stratify risk, especially in middle-aged adults. Most calculators are readily available online, brief, and of no cost. A universal limitation of these traditional risk calculators is that they are only intended for clinical risk assessment in the population for which they are indicated. As with the PCE, estimated risk from use outside of non-Hispanic African American and White populations should be cautiously interpreted,[21] epitomizing this limitation. Modified versions of the PCE have been developed to address this. In 2020, a Modified PCE were developed and validated for use in American Indian populations.[56] Nonetheless, the original PCE still carry dubious applicability outside strict racial/ethnic categories. Further, the 10-year PCE risk estimation has been shown to be overestimated by approximately 20% across all risk groups.[57] Moreover, the PCE is liable to underestimate risk in select younger populations, on the predication that the accumulation of risk at an early age (eg, <40 y) is not substantial enough to warrant pharmacologic therapy.[58,59] This presumption is often at the expense of those at increased risk for the rapid accumulation of risk factor exposure. Such high-risk groups include those who have a genetic disposition (eg, familial hypercholesterolemia, phytosterolemia, and lipodystrophy), social strain (eg, SES[40,60]), or predisposing medical conditions (eg, HIV,[61] chronic inflammatory disease[62]).

Overall, these calculators are crucial in primary risk assessment, but they should be used as the first step in risk assessment, identifying those who may benefit from advanced risk stratification. **Fig. 2** provides step by step approach to ASCVD risk assessment.[35]

ATHEROSCLEROSIS IMAGING
Coronary Artery Calcium Scoring

Coronary artery calcium (CAC) scoring was first introduced in 1990 as a means of measuring subclinical coronary atherosclerosis burden and, therefore, assessing ASCVD risk[63] through noncontrast computed tomography (CT). As then, multiple studies have substantiated CAC scoring as an effective assessment of ASCVD risk. The Multi-Ethnic Study of Atherosclerosis (MESA) data suggest CAC can effectively stratify CHD risk.[64] In response to the ESC and the American Stroke Association's (ASA) push for the inclusion of stroke in the holistic risk assessment of CVD,[65,66] another study validated CAC as an effective predictor of CVD, rather than solely CHD.[67] Currently, the Endocrine Society strongly endorses CAC in assessing subclinical atherosclerosis.[35]

CAC scoring has been shown to effectively stratify CVD risk in asymptomatic middle-aged-to-elderly men and women with dyslipidemia[68] and to reclassify risk even in patients with LDL-C $\geq$190 mg/dL.[69] It is more predictive of CVD risk than traditional and novel estimators.[70,71] A CAC $\geq$1000 has been shown to be a unique identifier of increased ASCVD risk and benefit from highly aggressive preventive therapy.[72] While the CAC score predicts absolute cardiovascular risk, the CAC score percentile tracks the lifetime risk trajectory.[73] CAC score percentiles are calculated using the MESA CAC Reference Tool and estimate age-, sex-, and race/ethnicity-specific lifetime risk of ASCVD for individuals greater than 45 years.[73]

The ACC/AHA indicate the use of CAC in adjudicating the utility of initiating statin therapy in patients for whom the initial risk assessment, and benefit from statin therapy, derived from the PCE is uncertain (see **Fig. 1**.)[20] In individuals with baseline CAC = 0 whereby an initial conservative approach to prevention is chosen, evidence suggests repeating a CAC scan after 5 to 7 years in low-risk patients, 3 to 5 years in borderline-to-intermediate-risk patients, and in 3 years for high-risk patients or those with diabetes.[74] **Table 3** provides a guide for optimizing absolute CAC scoring versus CAC percentile scoring.[75]

Table 3
Utility of CAC score and CAC percentile in ASCVD risk assessment

CAC Assessment	Population(s) with Unique Perceived Benefit	Unique Benefit
CAC Score	Middle-aged and intermediate-risk patients	Enhanced risk stratification and prognostication of benefit from statin therapy
CAC Percentile	Youth (eg, <40 y)	Prognostication of risk with subclinical risk factor accumulation

Data from Hecht H, Blaha MJ, Berman DS, Nasir K, Budoff M, Leipsic J, Blankstein R, Narula J, Rumberger J, Shaw LJ. Clinical indications for coronary artery calcium scoring in asymptomatic patients: Expert consensus statement from the Society of Cardiovascular Computed Tomography. J Cardiovasc Comput Tomogr. 2017 Mar-Apr;11(2):157-168.

CAC scoring is recommended to aid decision making regarding statin or aspirin initiation in borderline- or intermediate-risk patients for whom the indication to recommend therapy is unclear.[75] The CAC "Agatston" score can either buttress (eg, high CAC score) or weaken (eg, CAC = 0) the indication for initiating statin therapy.[13]

CAC imaging seems to be the most promising means of assessing risk and statin benefit due to its overall increased ability to personalize risk, especially in middle-aged and intermediate-risk populations.[76]

Other Atherosclerosis Imaging Techniques

Carotid ultrasound imaging allows the measurement of the amount of carotid plaque and carotid intima-media thickness (CIMT) to estimate risk.[12] An 8-study meta-analysis demonstrated a 10% to 15% increased risk of MI with every 0.1-mm increase in CIMT[77] and a 2021 study demonstrated the relationship between the amount of carotid plaque and increased risk of chronic CHD and incident CAC.[78] Cardiac computed tomographic angiography (CCTA) can be used to assess risk through identifying and estimating the extent of coronary atherosclerosis, specifically including noncalcified plaque, as well as the degree of coronary stenosis in asymptomatic patients.[12,79] Despite the availability of other atherosclerosis imaging techniques, currently, only CAC scoring is endorsed by the ACC/AHA for clinical risk assessment by imaging due to its excellent performance, low cost, wide availability, and low intrascan variability.[13]

Functional Tests that Imply Atherosclerosis – Stress Testing

Noninvasive cardiac stress testing can be used to enhance risk stratification in intermediate-risk patients. Additionally, when paired with imaging, stress testing can be diagnostic of CAD.[80,81] However, the American Society of Echocardiography indicates its use only for symptomatic patients.[82] Stress testing in asymptomatic individuals reduces its sensitivity and specificity to 45% to 60%.[83]

Plaque burden has been shown to be the main predictor of cardiovascular events and death.[84] This explains the paradigm shift away from the assessment of stenosis severity and ischemia toward the ascertainment of plaque burden by direct subclinical atherosclerosis imaging modalities for risk assessment. Therefore, the role of stress testing in primary prevention is extremely limited.

Summary of Atherosclerosis Imaging for Risk Prediction

Imaging is increasingly favored in clinical risk assessment due to its aptitude in highly personalizing risk assessment. Unlike traditional risk calculators, imaging estimates the accumulated ASCVD risk from both known and unknown risk factors and risk-enhancing factors. By addressing both known and unknown risk factors, imaging offers a more personalized assessment of risk.

However, imaging is much less accessible than traditional risk calculators. Not all health plans cover the cost of CAC scoring,[85] as these are often considered screening examinations.[86] Consequently, the out-of-pocket cost can range from $100 to $400 in the US.[85] Additionally, there is risk from imaging. On average, patients are exposed to 1 to 2 mSv of ionizing radiation during CAC scoring[87] and 5 mSv during CT angiography.[88] This is comparable to the ionizing radiation exposure of a mammogram (<0.3 mSv)[88] and less than the annual background radiation exposure in the US (3.1 mSv).[89] Additionally, there is a risk of a hypersensitivity reaction when using contrast, as in CCTA, presenting CCTA as a less favorable imaging modality for primary prevention.[90] Therefore, imaging has not superseded traditional risk calculators, and remains the preferred "second step" in risk assessment. Stress testing has little to no role for risk assessment in primary prevention.

ADVANCED LIPID TESTING
Overview

Lipid profiling can optimize the adjudication of risk by contributing additional input data as well as assessing atherogenic potential, especially in high-risk asymptomatic individuals. Advanced lipid testing may include the direct measurement of low-density lipoprotein particle number (LDL-P), low-density lipoprotein particle size, apolipoprotein B (apoB), and Lp(a).[91] While such advanced testing is helpful for the diagnosis of genetic dyslipidemias, current guidelines suggest that most tests offer minimal additional benefit for the primary assessment of risk beyond the standard lipid profile.[92] Lp(a) testing is the only advanced lipid test that should be considered for routine use in primary prevention.

Apolipoprotein B

Apolipoprotein B (apoB), a major protein in all atherogenic lipoproteins (eg, chylomicron remnants, VLDL, IDL, LDL, Lp(a))[93] and the major component of LDL and VLDL, is a strong portent of atherogenicity.[20] A meta-analysis using data from 12 studies, demonstrated that apoB was the most potent lipid marker of cardiovascular risk.[94] Measuring apoB levels may be particularly salient in assessing risk in patients with hypertriglyceridemia.[95] It is suggested that apoB be measured if triglycerides $\geq$200 mg/dL, with apoB $\geq$130 mg/dL being a risk-enhancing factor favoring statin therapy.[13,96]

Lipoprotein(a) (Lp(a))

Lp(a) is a largely genetically determined independent risk factor for premature CHD, and an elevated Lp(a) is tantamount to the attributable risk of TC $\geq$240 mg/dL or HDL-C $\leq$35 mg/dL.[24,25,96] Lp(a) $\geq$50 mg/dL is considered a risk-enhancing factor with risk ascending with Lp(a) concentration.[13] Lp(a) has shown risk-enhancing attributes, especially in women with hypercholesterolemia[97] and those of intermediate- or high-CVD/CHD risk.[98] The ACC/AHA recommend measuring Lp(a) when family history is significant for premature ASCVD.[13] Here, it can be used to enhance 10-year risk estimation. Serum Lp(a) is a good predictor of incident ASCVD for middle-aged adults, with a similar associated risk across racial subgroups[99] and is shown to have additive effects with elevated CAC (ie, <100) on the development of incident ASCVD.[100] Elevated Lp(a) in asymptomatic individuals with a family history of premature ASCVD has been associated with increased CAC score[101] and may increase the benefit of CAC scoring in this population. As Lp(a) testing is helpful for the assessment of familial risk, and levels do not change much over one's lifetime, it does not need to be repeated if previously measured in childhood or early adulthood.

Inflammatory Biomarkers – High-Sensitivity C-Reactive Protein

Plasma high-sensitivity C-reactive protein (hsCRP) $\geq$2 mg/dL is a risk-enhancing factor. hsCRP is particularly salient for those at intermediate risk.[13] However, recent data suggest that hsCRP predicts increased ASCVD risk for all PCE risk categories and is independent of atherogenic lipid levels.[102] hsCRP $\geq$2 mg/dL is also a consistent portent of residual inflammatory risk.[103] Following lipid-lowering therapy, hsCRP can further direct pharmacotherapeutic intervention aimed at lowering residual inflammatory risk.[103]

Summary

Lp(a) exhibits the most promise as a routinely used marker and is particularly relevant for middle-aged adults.[99] While promising in adjudicating risk, other forms of advanced lipid testing should be reserved for specific situations and should not be used for routine risk assessment. ApoB may be helpful in enhancing risk estimation in patients with dyslipidemia.[95] hsCRP has declined in popularity and is a relatively weak and nonspecific marker when compared with imaging—especially, CAC scoring.[104] Thus, hsCRP should be used occasionally—particularly, for further risk stratification in patients with metabolic risks, such as in metabolic syndrome.

ENDOCRINE SOCIETY'S 2020 LIPID MANAGEMENT GUIDELINE

The Endocrine Society's 2020 Guideline on Lipid Management in Patients with Endocrine Disorders recommends a 10-year risk estimation via the PCE. CAC is indicated for adjudicating statin therapy for borderline and intermediate-risk individuals with additional risk-enhancing factors and for whom the decision to initiate statin therapy as determined by the PCE score, is uncertain. If baseline CAC = 0, scoring should be repeated every 5 to 7 years (low-risk); 3 to 5 years (borderline-to-intermediate risk); or 3 years (high-risk or with concurrent DM) for patients. CAC scoring is considered the gold standard for assessing subclinical atherosclerosis. Statin therapy is not indicated for all individuals and is determined by a personalized assessment of risk factor burden. For adults with a personal history of ASCVD or family history of either ASCVD or elevated Lp(a), it is recommended that Lp(a) is measured to enhance short- and long-term risk discrimination and clarify the need to increase the pharmacologic intensity of LDL-C lowering. Lp(a) $\geq$50 mg/dL is associated with increased ASCVD risk. Further, the Endocrine Society does not endorse the routine measurement of advanced lipids, including apoB and hsCRP, for risk assessment. Lp(a) testing does not need to be repeated if it was previously measured in childhood or early adulthood.[67]

FUTURE DIRECTIONS
Calculators: Recalibrations and the Future of Hybrid Risk Calculators

Clinical risk assessment must reflect the most contemporaneous data. The PCE and SCORE should be updated, recalibrated, and validated with contemporary data of cohort studies with expanded representation of race/ethnicity, age, and specific (eg, low SES and comorbid chronic inflammatory) conditions. Future versions of already existing ASCVD risk calculators should also be updated with a hybrid risk calculation option incorporating CAC scoring. A recent CAC percentile calculator exhibits an expanded age range.[49] These innovations must continue, and clinical guidelines must be concomitant. More recently, a calculator which estimates the optimal age for incident CAC testing in young adults was derived.[105] Subsequent guidelines should incorporate this calculator into guideline recommendations.

Hybrid risk calculators are calculators which conflate the risk factors operationalized in traditional risk calculators and imaging, such as CAC scoring. The MESA CHD Risk Score is similar to the PCE[21] but includes additional risk factors (eg, CAC score, family history of MI, and whether the patient is currently taking a lipid-lowering medication)[106] in its 10-year assessment of CVD risk. Inclusion of CAC in MESA CHD risk scoring yielded a greater C-statistic (0.80 vs 0.75, $P < .0001$) and discrimination between events and nonevents.[106] As the risk score was derived from data obtained from the MESA Study,[63] the risk score addresses the impact of ethnicity in assessing risk; however, the MESA Study only included ages 45 to 84 years, thus, limiting the generalizability of the MESA CHD Risk Score to individuals within this range.[106] When compared with the Framingham Risk Study (FRS), MESA show a greater ability to predict the severity of CAD in the population and had a better performance in specific subgroups (diabetes, nondiabetes, smoking, male).[107]

Going forward, there needs to be a clarified indication for the routine use of the MESA CHD Risk Score (and the forthcoming MESA CVD Risk Score) in primary risk assessment. Additionally, the development of additional hybrid risk calculators should be encouraged, especially those which operationalize traditionally underrepresented risk factors in their risk estimate.

New and Innovative Uses of Coronary Artery Calcium

Imaging presents as the most efficacious subclinical atherosclerotic assessment and has exciting potential in early risk assessment and monitoring, especially in dyslipidemia. However, it lacks concise indication beyond that of an adjunctive role, despite its enhanced discrimination over traditional risk calculators (eg, Framingham risk score and Reynolds risk score).[108] Potential uses for CAC scoring have been conceptualized but are yet to be incorporated into guidelines (**Fig. 4**).[73]

Risk assessment in conditions like familial hypercholesterolemia could improve from this degree of personalization. It could enhance a benefit-versus-risk analysis of nonstatin pharmacologic interventions (eg, ezetimibe and PCSK9 inhibitors).[20] Additionally, it could be used to indicate benefit for statin initiation and augmentation in younger age groups. Future research will further elucidate the utility of broadened indications for CAC and provide the data necessary to construct risk calculators for specific high- or special-risk populations that could guide advanced preventive therapy choices.

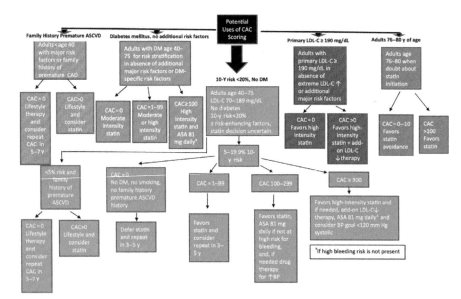

Fig. 4. Potential CAC scoring uses in the NLA Statement on CAC Scoring to Guide ASCVD Prevention. (*Adapted from* Orringer CE, Blaha MJ, Blankstein R, Budoff MJ, Goldberg RB, Gill EA, Maki KC, Mehta L, Jacobson TA. The National Lipid Association scientific statement on coronary artery calcium scoring to guide preventive strategies for ASCVD risk reduction. J Clin Lipidol. 2021 Jan-Feb;15(1):33-60.)

Future of Cardiac Computed Tomographic Angiography

Further, a transition from CAC to CCTA for the assessment of subclinical atherosclerosis may be forthcoming. CCTA visualizes both calcified and noncalcified plaque through the use of intravenous (IV) contrast[79,109,110] and has shown increased prognostic value for major adverse coronary events (MACEs) than CAC in asymptomatic older (>62 y) individuals.[111] However, specific situations where CCTA may be favored over CAC testing are not yet delineated. New technologic advances continue to reduce the radiation dose associated with CCTA, and with emerging technologies such as dual-energy CCTA, IV contrast may one day be optional.

Future of Polygenic Risk Scoring

Additionally, there needs to be a focus on improving risk assessment in young people. Previously, there has been a large emphasis on age in the construction of traditional risk calculators.[112] While age is associated with the accumulation of risk factors,[113] the concept of heart and vascular age may be more appropriate in guiding treatment than chronologic age.[112] Personalized medicine should be emphasized. While CAC scoring can offer this, PRS may be a further progression toward personalized medicine.

PRS have recently emerged as an option for assessing the risk of developing complex traits,[112] including CVDs.[114,115] PRS approximates an individual's susceptibility to developing a complex trait, based on their genotype.[116] Estimates are derived from established associations of genotypic profiles with these traits, as made apparent through the data from genome-wide association studies (GWAS).[116] PRS has a suggested utility in cohorts with predetermined increased risk, especially, early in prognosis to assist in guiding preventive efforts or treatment.[117] However, the National Lipid Association (NLA) does not currently suggest the use of genetic testing in assessing CVD risk, citing a lack of concise clinical indication and formal guidelines, and stating that the use of PRS will only drastically affect the prognosis or treatment of dyslipidemia in select individuals with severe dyslipidemia.[82] The PRS presents itself as a potential CVD risk assessment that offers the unique ability of concise personalization from as early as birth.

CLINICS CARE POINTS

- When initially assessing ASCVD risk, traditional 10-year risk calculators such as the pooled cohort equations (PCE) and Systemic COronary Risk Evaluation 2 (SCORE2) should be used and then augmented with the appraisal of risk-enhancing factors (eg, family history).

- When using the PCE to assess the 10-year ASCVD risk in non-African American (AA) or non-White patients, the equation for non-White individuals should be used and results cautiously interpreted.

- If the indication for initiating statin or aspirin therapy is unclear in patients with borderline- or intermediate-risk, coronary artery calcium (CAC) should be used.

- To reassess the potential benefit of statin or aspirin therapy in primary prevention in patients with initial CAC = 0, CAC scanning should be repeated every 5 to 7 y for low-risk patients; every 3 to 5 y for borderline-to-intermediate-risk patients; and every 3 y for high-risk patients or those with diabetes; risk factors should be assessed at every visit.

- When assessing ASCVD risk in specific populations (eg, women, those with chronic inflammatory conditions or endocrine disorders, racial/ethnic minorities), which portend an increased risk of ASCVD due to factors under-represented in traditional risk calculators, an assessment of risk factors, risk-enhancing factors, and potentially CAC should be used to further arbitrate risk and benefit of preventive therapy.

- When assessing ASCVD risk in the young (<40 y) and elderly (>75 y), consideration of age, sex, and race/ethnicity-specific CAC percentiles are critical for driving nuanced discussion of the net benefit of preventive therapies.
- When considering advanced lipid testing to assess ASCVD risk, measuring lipoprotein(a) (Lp(a)) once has been shown to be the most helpful in further adjudicating risk, especially in women with hypercholesterolemia, those with strong family history, those of intermediate- or high-risk, and middle-aged adults.

ACKNOWLEDGMENTS

M. Blaha reports grants from the NIH, FDA, AHA, Amgen, Novo Nordisk, and Bayer. M. Blaha reports serving on Advisory Boards for Amgen, Novartis, Novo Nordisk, Bayer, Roche, Inozyme, 89Bio, Kaleido, VoxelCloud, Kowa, and emocha health.

DISCLOSURE

E. Goldsborough has no financial disclosures or competing interests to report. N. Osuji has no financial disclosures or competing interests to report.

REFERENCES

1. World Health Organization. Cardiovascular diseases. World Health Organization. Available at: https://www.who.int/health-topics/cardiovascular-diseases/#tab=tab_1. Accessed June 13, 2021.
2. Benjamin EJ, Muntner P, Alonso A, et al. Heart disease and stroke statistics—2019 update: a report from the American Heart Association. Circulation 2019; 139(10). https://doi.org/10.1161/CIR.0000000000000659.
3. European Heart Network. European cardiovascular disease statistics. 2017. Available at: https://ehnheart.org/images/CVD-statistics-report-August-2017.pdf. Accessed December 15, 2021.
4. Roth GA, Mensah GA, Johnson CO, et al. Global burden of cardiovascular diseases and risk factors, 1990–2019. J Am Coll Cardiol 2020;76(25):2982–3021.
5. Roth GA, Nguyen G, Forouzanfar MH, et al. Estimates of global and regional premature cardiovascular mortality in 2025. Circulation 2015;132(13):1270–82.
6. Johnson NB, Hayes LD, Brown K, et al. CDC national health report: leading causes of morbidity and mortality and associated behavioral risk and protective factors—United States, 2005-2013. MMWR Suppl 2014;63:3–27.
7. Yusuf S, Hawken S, Ounpuu S, et al. Effect of potentially modifiable risk factors associated with myocardial infarction in 52 countries (the INTERHEART study): case-control study. Lancet 2004;364(9438):937–52.
8. Wickramasinghe M, Weaver JU. Lipid disorders in obesity. In: Weaver J, editor. Practical guide to obesity medicine. St. Louis, Missouri: Elsevier; 2018. p. 99–108.
9. Pekkanen J, Linn S, Heiss G, et al. Ten-year mortality from cardiovascular disease in relation to cholesterol level among men with and without preexisting cardiovascular disease. N Engl J Med 1990;322(24):1700–7.
10. Urbina EM, Daniels SR. Hyperlipidemia. In: Slap GB, editor. Adolescent medicine. Elsevier; 2008. p. 90–6.
11. Linton MRF, Yancey PG, Davies SS, et al. The role of lipids and lipoproteins in atherosclerosis. [Updated 2019 Jan 3]. In: Feingold KR, Anawalt B, Boyce A, et al, editors. Endotext. South Dartmouth (MA): MDText.com, Inc; 2000.

12. Michos ED, Blaha MJ, Martin SS, et al. Screening for atherosclerotic cardiovascular disease in asymptomatic individuals. In: Delemos J, Omland T, editors. Chronic coronary artery disease: a companion to Braunwald's heart disease. Philadelphia, PA: Elsevier; 2018. p. 459–78.
13. Arnett DK, Blumenthal RS, Albert MA, et al. 2019 ACC/AHA Guideline on the primary prevention of cardiovascular disease. J Am Coll Cardiol 2019;74(10): e177–232.
14. Cholesterol Treatment Trialists' (CTT) Collaborators. The effects of lowering LDL cholesterol with statin therapy in people at low risk of vascular disease: meta-analysis of individual data from 27 randomised trials. Lancet 2012;380(9841): 581–90.
15. Sandesara P, Bogart DB. Almost everyone over 50 should be put on a statin to reduce the risk of cardiovascular disease: a protagonist view. Mo Med 2013; 110(4):332–8.
16. 27th Bethesda Conference. Matching the intensity of risk factor management with the hazard for coronary disease events. September 14-15, 1995. J Am Coll Cardiol 1996;27(5):957–1047.
17. Califf RM, Armstrong PW, Carver JR, et al. 27th Bethesda Conference: matching the intensity of risk factor management with the hazard for coronary disease events. Task Force 5. Stratification of patients into high, medium and low risk subgroups for purposes of risk factor management. J Am Coll Cardiol 1996; 27(5):1007–19.
18. Pearson TA, McBride PE, Miller NH, et al. 27th Bethesda Conference: matching the intensity of risk factor management with the hazard for coronary disease events. Task Force 8. Organization of preventive cardiology service. J Am Coll Cardiol 1996;27(5):1039–47.
19. Mach F, Baigent C, Catapano AL, et al. 2019 ESC/EAS Guidelines for the management of dyslipidaemias: lipid modification to reduce cardiovascular risk. Eur Heart J 2020;41(1):111–88.
20. Grundy SM, Stone NJ, Bailey AL, et al. 2018 AHA/ACC/AACVPR/AAPA/ABC/ ACPM/ADA/AGS/APhA/ASPC/NLA/PCNA Guideline on the management of blood cholesterol: executive summary. J Am Coll Cardiol 2019;73(24):3168–209.
21. Goff DC, Lloyd-Jones DM, Bennett G, et al. 2013 ACC/AHA Guideline on the assessment of cardiovascular risk. J Am Coll Cardiol 2014;63(25):2935–59.
22. European Association of Preventive Cardiology. About HeartScore. HeartScore. Available at: https://www.heartscore.org/el_CY/about-heartscore. Accessed December 15, 2021.
23. Conroy RM, Pyörälä K, Fitzgerald AP, et al. Estimation of ten-year risk of fatal cardiovascular disease in Europe: the SCORE project. Eur Heart J 2003; 24(11):987–1003.
24. Bostom AG, Gagnon DR, Cupples LA, et al. A prospective investigation of elevated lipoprotein (a) detected by electrophoresis and cardiovascular disease in women. The Framingham Heart Study. Circulation 1994;90(4):1688–95.
25. Bostom AG. Elevated plasma lipoprotein(a) and coronary heart disease in men aged 55 years and younger: a prospective study. JAMA 1996;276(7):544.
26. SCORE2 Working Group and ESC Cardiovascular Risk Collaboration, Hageman S, Pennells L, et al. SCORE2 risk prediction algorithms: new models to estimate 10-year risk of cardiovascular disease in Europe. Eur Heart J 2021; 42(25):2439–54.
27. Visseren FLJ, Mach F, Smulders YM, et al. 2021 ESC guidelines on cardiovascular disease prevention in clinical practice. Eur Heart J 2021;42(34):3227–337.

28. Ridker PM, Buring JE, Rifai N, et al. Development and validation of improved algorithms for the assessment of global cardiovascular risk in women: the reynolds risk score. JAMA 2007;297(6):611.

29. Ridker PM, Paynter NP, Rifai N, et al. C-reactive protein and parental history improve global cardiovascular risk prediction: the Reynolds Risk Score for men. Circulation 2008;118(22):2243–51, 4p following 2251.

30. Hippisley-Cox J, Coupland C, Vinogradova Y, et al. Derivation and validation of QRISK, a new cardiovascular disease risk score for the United Kingdom: prospective open cohort study. BMJ 2007;335(7611):136.

31. Hippisley-Cox J, Coupland C, Vinogradova Y, et al. Predicting cardiovascular risk in England and Wales: prospective derivation and validation of QRISK2. BMJ 2008;336(7659):1475–82.

32. Hippisley-Cox J, Coupland C, Brindle P. Development and validation of QRISK3 risk prediction algorithms to estimate future risk of cardiovascular disease: prospective cohort study. BMJ 2017;357:j2099.

33. SCORE2-OP Working Group and ESC Cardiovascular Risk Collaboration, de Vries TI, Cooney MT, et al. SCORE2-OP risk prediction algorithms: estimating incident cardiovascular event risk in older persons in four geographical risk regions. Eur Heart J 2021;42(25):2455–67.

34. Armitage J, Baigent C, Barnes E, et al. Efficacy and safety of statin therapy in older people: a meta-analysis of individual participant data from 28 randomised controlled trials. Lancet 2019;393(10170):407–15.

35. Newman CB, Blaha MJ, Boord JB, et al. Lipid management in patients with endocrine disorders: an Endocrine Society clinical practice guideline. J Clin Endocrinol Metab 2020;105(12):3613–82.

36. Tanz LJ, Stuart JJ, Williams PL, et al. Preterm delivery and maternal cardiovascular disease in young and middle-aged adult women. Circulation 2017;135(6):578–89.

37. Garcia M, Mulvagh SL, Bairey Merz CN, et al. Cardiovascular disease in women: clinical perspectives. Circ Res 2016;118(8):1273–93.

38. Schultz WM, Kelli HM, Lisko JC, et al. Socioeconomic status and cardiovascular outcomes: challenges and interventions. Circulation 2018;137(20):2166–78.

39. Li R, Hou J, Tu R, et al. Associations of mixture of air pollutants with estimated 10-year atherosclerotic cardiovascular disease risk modified by socioeconomic status: the Henan Rural Cohort Study. Sci The Total Environ 2021;793:148542.

40. Colantonio LD, Richman JS, Carson AP, et al. Performance of the atherosclerotic cardiovascular disease pooled cohort risk equations by social deprivation status. JAHA 2017;6(3). https://doi.org/10.1161/JAHA.117.005676.

41. Libby P, Ridker PM. Inflammation and atherothrombosis. J Am Coll Cardiol 2006;48(9):A33–46.

42. Mason JC, Libby P. Cardiovascular disease in patients with chronic inflammation: mechanisms underlying premature cardiovascular events in rheumatologic conditions. Eur Heart J 2015;36(8):482–489c.

43. Hansen PR. Chronic inflammatory diseases and atherosclerotic cardiovascular disease: innocent bystanders or partners in crime? CPD 2018;24(3):281–90.

44. Rosenson RS, Hubbard D, Monda KL, et al. Excess risk for atherosclerotic cardiovascular outcomes among US adults with HIV in the current era. JAHA 2020;9(1). https://doi.org/10.1161/JAHA.119.013744.

45. Feinstein MJ, Hsue PY, Benjamin LA, et al. Characteristics, prevention, and management of cardiovascular disease in people living with HIV: a scientific

statement from the American Heart Association. Circulation 2019;140(2). https://doi.org/10.1161/CIR.0000000000000695.

46. American Heart Association, American Stroke Association. Facts: bridging the gap – CVD health disparities. Heart. Available at: https://www.heart.org/idc/groups/heart-public/@wcm/@hcm/@ml/documents/downloadable/ucm_429240.pdf. Accessed December 15, 2021.

47. Osei AD, Uddin SMI, Dzaye O, et al. Predictors of coronary artery calcium among 20-30-year-olds: The Coronary Artery Calcium Consortium. Atherosclerosis 2020;301:65–8.

48. Miedema MD, Dardari ZA, Nasir K, et al. Association of coronary artery calcium with long-term, cause-specific mortality among young adults. JAMA Netw Open 2019;2(7):e197440.

49. Javaid A, Mitchell JD, Villines TC. Predictors of coronary artery calcium and long-term risks of death, myocardial infarction, and stroke in young adults. JAHA 2021;10(22):e022513.

50. Patel J, Al Rifai M, Scheuner MT, et al. Basic vs more complex definitions of family history in the prediction of coronary heart disease: the Multi-Ethnic Study of Atherosclerosis. Mayo Clin Proc 2018;93(9):1213–23.

51. Lloyd-Jones DM, Nam B-H, D'Agostino RB, et al. Parental cardiovascular disease as a risk factor for cardiovascular disease in middle-aged adults: a prospective study of parents and offspring. JAMA 2004;291(18):2204–11.

52. Bachmann JM, Willis BL, Ayers CR, et al. Association between family history and coronary heart disease death across long-term follow-up in men: the Cooper Center Longitudinal Study. Circulation 2012;125(25):3092–8.

53. Mehta A, Virani SS, Ayers CR, et al. Lipoprotein(a) and family history predict cardiovascular disease risk. J Am Coll Cardiol 2020;76(7):781–93.

54. Patel J, Al Rifai M, Blaha MJ, et al. Coronary artery calcium improves risk assessment in adults with a family history of premature coronary heart disease: results from Multiethnic Study of Atherosclerosis. Circ Cardiovasc Imaging 2015;8(6):e003186.

55. Pandey AK, Pandey S, Blaha MJ, et al. Family history of coronary heart disease and markers of subclinical cardiovascular disease: where do we stand? Atherosclerosis 2013;228(2):285–94.

56. Shara NM, Desale S, Howard BV, et al. Modified pooled cohort atherosclerotic cardiovascular disease risk prediction equations in American Indians. J Nephrol Sci 2020;2(1):5–14.

57. Yadlowsky S, Hayward RA, Sussman JB, et al. Clinical implications of revised pooled cohort equations for estimating atherosclerotic cardiovascular disease risk. Ann Intern Med 2018;169(1):20.

58. Volgman AS, Palaniappan LS, Aggarwal NT, et al. Atherosclerotic cardiovascular disease in South Asians in the United States: epidemiology, risk factors, and treatments: a scientific statement from the American Heart Association. Circulation 2018;138(1). https://doi.org/10.1161/CIR.0000000000000580.

59. Lloyd-Jones DM, Braun LT, Ndumele CE, et al. Use of risk assessment tools to guide decision-making in the primary prevention of atherosclerotic cardiovascular disease: a special report from the American Heart Association and American College of Cardiology. Circulation 2019;139(25). https://doi.org/10.1161/CIR.0000000000000638.

60. Dalton JE, Perzynski AT, Zidar DA, et al. Accuracy of cardiovascular risk prediction varies by neighborhood socioeconomic position: a retrospective cohort study. Ann Intern Med 2017;167(7):456–64.

61. Feinstein MJ, Nance RM, Drozd DR, et al. Assessing and refining myocardial infarction risk estimation among patients with human immunodeficiency virus: a study by the Centers for AIDS Research Network of Integrated Clinical Systems. JAMA Cardiol 2017;2(2):155–62.

62. Ungprasert P, Matteson EL, Crowson CS. Reliability of cardiovascular risk calculators to estimate accurately the risk of cardiovascular disease in patients with sarcoidosis. Am J Cardiol 2017;120(5):868–73.

63. Agatston AS, Janowitz WR, Hildner FJ, et al. Quantification of coronary artery calcium using ultrafast computed tomography. J Am Coll Cardiol 1990;15(4): 827–32.

64. Bild DE, Bluemke DA, Burke GL, et al. Multi-Ethnic Study of Atherosclerosis: objectives and design. Am J Epidemiol 2002;156(9):871–81.

65. Lackland DT, Elkind MSV, D'Agostino R, et al. Inclusion of stroke in cardiovascular risk prediction instruments: a statement for healthcare professionals from the American Heart Association/American Stroke Association. Stroke 2012;43(7): 1998–2027.

66. Piepoli MF, Hoes AW, Agewall S, et al. 2016 European guidelines on cardiovascular disease prevention in clinical practice: the Sixth Joint Task Force of the European Society of Cardiology and other societies on cardiovascular disease prevention in clinical practice (constituted by representatives of 10 societies and by invited experts) developed with the special contribution of the European Association for Cardiovascular Prevention & Rehabilitation (EACPR). Eur Heart J 2016;37(29):2315–81.

67. Budoff MJ, Young R, Burke G, et al. Ten-year association of coronary artery calcium with atherosclerotic cardiovascular disease (ASCVD) events: the multiethnic study of atherosclerosis (MESA). Eur Heart J 2018;39(25):2401–8.

68. Martin SS, Blaha MJ, Blankstein R, et al. Dyslipidemia, coronary artery calcium, and incident atherosclerotic cardiovascular disease: implications for statin therapy from the Multi-Ethnic Study of Atherosclerosis. Circulation 2014;129(1): 77–86.

69. Sandesara PB, Mehta A, O'Neal WT, et al. Clinical significance of zero coronary artery calcium in individuals with LDL cholesterol ≥190 mg/dL: The Multi-Ethnic Study of Atherosclerosis. Atherosclerosis 2020;292:224–9.

70. Greenland P, Blaha MJ, Budoff MJ, et al. Coronary calcium score and cardiovascular risk. J Am Coll Cardiol 2018;72(4):434–47.

71. Yeboah J, McClelland RL, Polonsky TS, et al. Comparison of novel risk markers for improvement in cardiovascular risk assessment in intermediate-risk individuals. JAMA 2012;308(8):788.

72. Peng AW, Mirbolouk M, Orimoloye OA, et al. Long-term all-cause and cause-specific mortality in asymptomatic patients with CAC ≥1,000: results from the CAC Consortium. JACC Cardiovasc Imaging 2020;13(1 Pt 1):83–93.

73. Orringer CE, Blaha MJ, Blankstein R, et al. The National Lipid Association scientific statement on coronary artery calcium scoring to guide preventive strategies for ASCVD risk reduction. J Clin Lipidol 2021;15(1):33–60.

74. Corrigendum to: "Lipid management in patients with endocrine disorders: an Endocrine Society clinical practice guideline. J Clin Endocrinol Metab 2021; 106(6):e2465.

75. Hecht H, Blaha MJ, Berman DS, et al. Clinical indications for coronary artery calcium scoring in asymptomatic patients: expert consensus statement from the Society of Cardiovascular Computed Tomography. J Cardiovasc Comput Tomogr 2017;11(2):157–68.

76. Anderson JL, Le VT, Min DB, et al. Comparison of three atherosclerotic cardio-vascular disease risk scores with and without coronary calcium for predicting revascularization and major adverse coronary events in symptomatic patients undergoing positron emission tomography-stress testing. Am J Cardiol 2020; 125(3):341–8.
77. Lorenz MW, Markus HS, Bots ML, et al. Prediction of clinical cardiovascular events with carotid intima-media thickness: a systematic review and meta-analysis. Circulation 2007;115(4):459–67.
78. Mehta A, Rigdon J, Tattersall MC, et al. Association of carotid artery plaque with cardiovascular events and incident coronary artery calcium in individuals with absent coronary calcification: the MESA. Circ Cardiovasc Imaging 2021;14(4): e011701.
79. Divakaran S, Cheezum MK, Hulten EA, et al. Use of cardiac CT and calcium scoring for detecting coronary plaque: implications on prognosis and patient management. Br J Radiol 2015;88(1046):20140594.
80. Pellikka PA, Arruda-Olson A, Chaudhry FA, et al. Guidelines for performance, interpretation, and application of stress echocardiography in ischemic heart disease: from the American Society of Echocardiography. J Am Soc Echocardiogr 2020;33(1):1–41.e8.
81. Arbab-Zadeh A. Stress testing and non-invasive coronary angiography in patients with suspected coronary artery disease: time for a new paradigm. Heart Int 2012;7(1):e2.
82. Brown EE, Sturm AC, Cuchel M, et al. Genetic testing in dyslipidemia: A scientific statement from the National Lipid Association. J Clin Lipidol 2020. https://doi.org/10.1016/j.jacl.2020.04.011.
83. Burge MR, Eaton RP, Schade DS. The role of a coronary artery calcium scan in type 1 diabetes. Diabetes Technol Ther 2016;18(9):594–603.
84. Mortensen MB, Dzaye O, Steffensen FH, et al. Impact of plaque burden versus stenosis on ischemic events in patients with coronary atherosclerosis. J Am Coll Cardiol 2020;76(24):2803–13.
85. Cigna. Coronary calcium scan: should I have this test? Cigna. Available at: https://www.cigna.com/individuals-families/health-wellness/hw/medical-topics/coronary-calcium-scan-av2072. Accessed December 15, 2021.
86. Cleveland Clinic. Calcium-score screening heart scan. Cleveland Clinic. Available at: https://my.clevelandclinic.org/health/diagnostics/16824-calcium-score-screening-heart-scan. Accessed December 15, 2021.
87. Blaha MJ, Mortensen MB, Kianoush S, et al. Coronary Artery Calcium Scoring. JACC Cardiovascular Imaging 2017;10(8):923–37.
88. American College of Radiology. Radiation dose to adults from common imaging examinations. Available at: https://www.acr.org/-/media/ACR/Files/Radiology-Safety/Radiation-Safety/Dose-Reference-Card.pdf. Accessed December 15, 2021.
89. United States Nuclear Regulatory Commission. Biological effects of radiation. Available at: https://www.nrc.gov/docs/ML0333/ML033390088.pdf. Accessed December 15, 2021.
90. Pradubpongsa P, Dhana N, Jongjarearnprasert K, et al. Adverse reactions to iodinated contrast media: prevalence, risk factors and outcome-the results of a 3-year period. Asian Pac J Allergy Immunol 2013;31(4):299–306.
91. Jacobson TA, Ito MK, Maki KC, et al. National lipid association recommendations for patient-centered management of dyslipidemia: part 1-full report. J Clin Lipidol 2015;9(2):129–69.

92. Davidson MH, Ballantyne CM, Jacobson TA, et al. Clinical utility of inflammatory markers and advanced lipoprotein testing: advice from an expert panel of lipid specialists. J Clin Lipidol 2011;5(5):338–67.

93. Feingold KR. Introduction to lipids and lipoproteins. In: Feingold KR, Anawalt B, Boyce A, et al, editors. Endotext. MDText.com, Inc; 2000. Available at: http://www.ncbi.nlm.nih.gov/books/NBK305896/. Accessed August 1, 2021.

94. Sniderman AD, Williams K, Contois JH, et al. A meta-analysis of low-density lipoprotein cholesterol, non-high-density lipoprotein cholesterol, and apolipoprotein B as markers of cardiovascular risk. Circ Cardiovasc Qual Outcomes 2011; 4(3):337–45.

95. Sniderman AD, Tremblay A, De Graaf J, et al. Phenotypes of hypertriglyceridemia caused by excess very-low-density lipoprotein. J Clin Lipidol 2012;6(5): 427–33.

96. Choi S. The potential role of biomarkers associated with ASCVD risk: risk-enhancing biomarkers. J Lipid Atheroscler 2019;8(2):173–82.

97. Cook NR, Mora S, Ridker PM. Lipoprotein(a) and cardiovascular risk prediction among women. J Am Coll Cardiol 2018;72(3):287–96.

98. Nordestgaard BG, Chapman MJ, Ray K, et al. Lipoprotein(a) as a cardiovascular risk factor: current status. Eur Heart J 2010;31(23):2844–53.

99. Patel AP, Wang M, Pirruccello JP, et al. Lp(a) (lipoprotein[a]) concentrations and incident atherosclerotic cardiovascular disease: new insights from a large national biobank. ATVB 2020. https://doi.org/10.1161/ATVBAHA.120.315291.

100. Mehta A, Vasquez N, Ayers CR, et al. Available at: https://pubmed.ncbi.nlm.nih.gov/35210030/.

101. Verweij SL, de Ronde MWJ, Verbeek R, et al. Elevated lipoprotein(a) levels are associated with coronary artery calcium scores in asymptomatic individuals with a family history of premature atherosclerotic cardiovascular disease. J Clin Lipidol 2018;12(3):597–603.e1.

102. Quispe R, Michos ED, Martin SS, et al. High-sensitivity C-reactive protein discordance with atherogenic lipid measures and incidence of atherosclerotic cardiovascular disease in primary prevention: the ARIC study. JAHA 2020;9(3). https://doi.org/10.1161/JAHA.119.013600.

103. Aday AW, Ridker PM. Targeting residual inflammatory risk: a shifting paradigm for atherosclerotic disease. Front Cardiovasc Med 2019;6:16.

104. Blaha MJ, Budoff MJ, DeFilippis AP, et al. Associations between C-reactive protein, coronary artery calcium, and cardiovascular events: implications for the JUPITER population from MESA, a population-based cohort study. Lancet 2011;378(9792):684–92.

105. Dzaye O, Razavi AC, Dardari ZA, et al. Available at: https://pubmed.ncbi.nlm.nih.gov/34649694/.

106. McClelland RL, Jorgensen NW, Budoff M, et al. 10-Year coronary heart disease risk prediction using coronary artery calcium and traditional risk factors. J Am Coll Cardiol 2015;66(15):1643–53.

107. Wang Y, Lv Q, Wu H, et al. Comparison of MESA of and Framingham risk scores in the prediction of coronary artery disease severity. Herz 2020;45(S1):139–44.

108. Zeb I, Budoff M. Coronary artery calcium screening: does it perform better than other cardiovascular risk stratification tools? Int J Mol Sci 2015;16(3):6606–20.

109. Miller JM, Rochitte CE, Dewey M, et al. Diagnostic performance of coronary angiography by 64-row CT. N Engl J Med 2008;359(22):2324–36.

110. Budoff MJ, Dowe D, Jollis JG, et al. Diagnostic performance of 64-multidetector row coronary computed tomographic angiography for evaluation of coronary

artery stenosis in individuals without known coronary artery disease: results from the prospective multicenter ACCURACY (Assessment by Coronary Computed Tomographic Angiography of Individuals Undergoing Invasive Coronary Angiography) trial. J Am Coll Cardiol 2008;52(21):1724–32.

111. Han D, Hartaigh BÓ, Gransar H, et al. Incremental prognostic value of coronary computed tomography angiography over coronary calcium scoring for major adverse cardiac events in elderly asymptomatic individuals. Eur Heart J Cardiovasc Imaging 2018;19(6):675–83.

112. Martin SS, Abd TT, Jones SR, et al. 2013 ACC/AHA cholesterol treatment guideline. J Am Coll Cardiol 2014;63(24):2674–8.

113. Sniderman AD, Furberg CD. Age as a modifiable risk factor for cardiovascular disease. Lancet 2008;371(9623):1547–9.

114. Singh A. Complex Traits. In: Gellman MD, Turner JR, editors. Encyclopedia of behavioral medicine. New York: Springer; 2013. p. 478–9.

115. Abbate R, Sticchi E, Fatini C. Genetics of cardiovascular disease. Clin Cases Miner Bone Metab 2008;5(1):63–6.

116. Choi SW, Mak TS-H, O'Reilly PF. Tutorial: a guide to performing polygenic risk score analyses. Nat Protoc 2020;15(9):2759–72.

117. Lewis CM, Vassos E. Polygenic risk scores: from research tools to clinical instruments. Genome Med 2020;12(1):44.

118. Woodward M, Brindle P, Tunstall-Pedoe H, SIGN group on risk estimation. Adding social deprivation and family history to cardiovascular risk assessment: the ASSIGN score from the Scottish Heart Health Extended Cohort (SHHEC). Heart 2005;93(2):172–6.

119. Yang X, Li J, Hu D, et al. Predicting the 10-year risks of atherosclerotic cardiovascular disease in Chinese population: the China-PAR project (prediction for ASCVD risk in China). Circulation 2016;134(19):1430–40.

120. D'Agostino RB, Vasan RS, Pencina MJ, et al. General cardiovascular risk profile for use in primary care: The Framingham Heart Study. Circulation 2008;117(6):743–53.

121. Joint British Societies' consensus recommendations for the prevention of cardiovascular disease (JBS3). Heart 2014;100(Suppl 2):ii67, ii1.

122. Joint British Societies for the Prevention of Cardiovascular Disease. JBS3 report. JBS3Risk. Available at: http://www.jbs3risk.com/pages/report.htm. Accessed December 15, 2021.

The Inherited Hypercholesterolemias

Wann Jia Loh, MBBS, BSc[a],*, Gerald F. Watts, DSc, PhD, DM, FRACP, FRCP[b,c]

KEYWORDS

- Inherited hypercholesterolemia • Familial hypercholesterolemia
- Polygenic hypercholesterolemia • Lipoprotein(a) • Familial combined hyperlipidemia

KEY POINTS

- Hypercholesterolemia is greatly influenced by genetic factors.
- Hypercholesterolemic conditions are also dependent on gene–environment interactions.
- Familial hypercholesterolemia (FH) has a high prevalence, is easily diagnosed, and is a treatable and preventable cause of premature atherosclerotic cardiovascular disease (ASCVD). Heterozygous FH is present in 1 in 250 people in the general population.
- FH-mimics include conditions causing high LDL-C (polygenic hypercholesterolemia [PH], familial combined hyperlipidemia [FCH], extreme hyper-lipoprotein(a) levels [hyper-Lp(a)], medications, hypothyroidism) and conditions causing xanthomas (sitosterolemia, cerebrotendinous xanthomatosis (CTX)).
- Hyper-Lp(a) is common, affecting 20% of the population, and under potent genetic control. At markedly elevated plasma levels (5%–10% of the population), it is likely *the* major monogenic risk factor for ASCVD.

INTRODUCTION

Hypercholesterolemias have both genetic and environmental origins.[1] Major monogenic defects include familial hypercholesterolemia (FH) and elevated lipoprotein(a) [Lp(a)]. Polygenic conditions, such as familial combined hyperlipidemia (FCH) and common or polygenic hypercholesterolemia (PH), have by far stronger environmental influences. We review recent advances in understanding these 4 hypercholesterolemic conditions and their clinical care. We also briefly review sitosterolemia and cerebrotendinous xanthomatosis (CTX), as they are important differential diagnoses in FH.

[a] Department of Endocrinology, Changi General Hospital, 2 Simei Street 3, Singapore 529889; [b] School of Medicine, University of Western Australia, 35 Stirling Hwy, Crawley, Western Australia 6009, Australia; [c] Department of Cardiology and Internal Medicine, Royal Perth Hospital, Victoria Square, Perth, Western Australia 6000, Australia
* Corresponding author.
E-mail address: loh.wann.jia@singhealth.com.sg

Endocrinol Metab Clin N Am 51 (2022) 511–537
https://doi.org/10.1016/j.ecl.2022.02.006
0889-8529/22/© 2022 Elsevier Inc. All rights reserved.

FAMILIAL HYPERCHOLESTEROLEMIA
Prevalence

Among inherited hypercholesterolemias, FH is the most clinically important because of its high prevalence, ease of diagnosis, and high phenotypic penetrance leading to premature ASCVD. FH is classified as a Tier 1 condition by the Center for Disease Control and Prevention, meaning that there is very strong evidence that ASCVD is preventable, with a significant impact on public health. Yet only around 10% of patients with FH are diagnosed.[2] FH is 2-fold more common in the general population than previously considered; 1 in 250 have heterozygous FH (HeFH) and 1 in 300,000 homozygous FH (HoFH).[2–5] The prevalence is up to 1% in certain founder populations (Afrikaners, French Canadians, Lebanese), up to 10% of patients with hyperlipidemia and ASCVD, and up to 20% of patients with premature ASCVD.[5,6]

Genetic Defects

FH is a monogenic cause of elevated plasma LDL cholesterol concentration (LDL-C) due to impaired LDL catabolism, with LDL-C ranging from 8 to 26 mmol/L ($\approx$300–1000 mg/dL) in HoFH and 5 to 12 mmol/L (191–460 mg/dL) in HeFH (**Fig. 1**).[7] FH is codominantly inherited with high penetrance.[5,8] About 80% to 85% of FH is caused by *LDLR* gene mutations, with greater than 1200 *LDLR* mutations identified to date. The absence of functional LDL receptors or synthesis of ineffective receptors leads to impaired LDL clearance from plasma.[9] *APOB* gene missense mutations in the LDL receptor-binding domain of apolipoprotein B-100 (otherwise known as familial defective apolipoprotein B-100) account for another 5% to 10%.[2] Gain-of-function mutations in *PCSK9* account for about 1%.[2,5] *PCSK9* encodes proprotein convertase subtilisin/kexin type 9 enzyme, a key player in the hepatic internalization and degradation of LDL receptors. Rarely, mutations in *LDLRAP1,* which encodes LDL receptor adaptor protein 1, cause an autosomal recessive form of FH.[10]

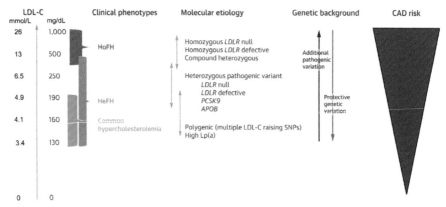

Fig. 1. Phenotypic spectrum of familial hypercholesterolemia. (*From* Sturm AC, Knowles JW, Gidding SS, Ahmad ZS, Ahmed CD, Ballantyne CM, Baum SJ, Bourbon M, Carrié A, Cuchel M, de Ferranti SD, Defesche JC, Freiberger T, Hershberger RE, Hovingh GK, Karayan L, Kastelein JJP, Kindt I, Lane SR, Leigh SE, Linton MF, Mata P, Neal WA, Nordestgaard BG, Santos RD, Harada-Shiba M, Sijbrands EJ, Stitziel NO, Yamashita S, Wilemon KA, Ledbetter DH, Rader DJ; Convened by the Familial Hypercholesterolemia Foundation. Clinical Genetic Testing for Familial Hypercholesterolemia: JACC Scientific Expert Panel. J Am Coll Cardiol. 2018 Aug 7;72(6):662-680; with permission.)

Clinical Diagnostic Criteria and Genetic Testing

The 2 most widely used clinical approaches for diagnosing FH are the Simon Broome Register (SBR) criteria[11] and the Dutch Lipid Clinic Network (DLCN) criteria, with varying weighting given to different criteria (**Table 1**). However, both these criteria and MED-PED criteria were derived for use in Western populations. The LDL-C to diagnose FH should be lower in Asians.[12,13] The Japan Atherosclerosis Society recommends a minimum LDL-C cut-off $\geq$4.7 mmol/L (180 mg/dL) rather than 5 mmol/L (191 mg/dL) and the use of X-ray imaging to determine Achilles tendon hypertrophy to diagnose HeFH[14] (see **Table 1**). The DLCN criteria should not be used in children and adolescents.[15] Secondary causes of raised LDL-C, such as hypothyroidism, use of corticosteroids, extreme cholesterol-raising diets (eg, coconut oil), nephrotic syndrome, and obstructive liver disease, should always be excluded before making a diagnosis of FH.

International guidelines strongly recommend genetic testing for FH in all adult index cases to facilitate diagnosis, prognosis, management, and cascade screening.[12,15–17] Genetic testing for FH should be carried out in an accredited laboratory, ideally using massively parallel sequencing.[15] Tendon xanthomata are present in approximately 13% and corneal arcus in approximately 30% of patients with HeFH.[18] A positive family history of FH is crucial as it increases the yield of diagnosis of the condition.[19] Genetic testing in patients with LDL-C >5 mmol/L alone without other diagnostic criteria for FH or presence of ASCVD, has a very low detection rate of 2% to 3% for pathogenic gene variants.[17] Approximately 30% of patients with probable/definite DLCN criteria test negative for the 3 most common pathogenic variants (*LDLR, APOB, PCSK9*); the reasons include variants of unclear significance, unidentified causative variants, or rare variants not in the genetic test panel (eg, *LDLRAP1*), and PH.[2,15,16] Hence, absence of a positive genetic test does not exclude FH if the phenotypic features are strongly suggestive of the condition.[15,16] Phenotypic FH-mimics include conditions causing xanthomata or xanthelasma such as sitosterolemia, CTX, familial dysbetalipoproteinaemia, and FCH. In patients without phenotypic FH, alternative diagnoses to consider include PH, hyper-Lp(a), and secondary causes of elevated LDL-C. Earlier diagnosis of FH allows for earlier cholesterol-lowering treatment, which can lead to a 10-fold lower risk of ASCVD in adults.[20]

Severity of Coronary Artery Disease

The higher cumulative lifetime exposure of LDL-C increases the risk of ASCVD (mainly coronary artery disease (CAD)) in adults with FH mutations compared with those without. Owing to the accelerated accumulation of LDL starting from birth, in untreated patients with HoFH, CAD starts in early childhood and can lead to premature death due to atherosclerotic CAD before 25 years of age. CAD in untreated HeFH manifests between 30 and 60 years[7]; 30 to 50% untreated individuals with FH have a fatal or nonfatal cardiac event by 50 years of age in men and 60 years of age in women.[2] The relative risk of CAD in patients with FH compared with non-FH in men less than 40 years old is > 20-fold.[21]Among patients with LDL>5 mmol/L (191 mg/dL), CAD risk is increased by more than 3-fold in those with an FH mutation.[17] Thus, diagnosis of FH in patients of young onset CAD and raised LDL-C is essential.[22] The CAD risk in women is lower than in men and increases exponentially after menopause.[21]

Atherosclerotic Cardiovascular Disease Risk

Although LDL is important in the pathogenesis of all ASCVD, the increased risk in FH seems to differ according to the type of ASCVD. The association with CAD is the

Table 1
Clinical criteria for the diagnosis of familial hypercholesterolemia

Clinical criteria for the diagnosis of Familial Hypercholesterolemia

	Simon Broome Register 1991[11]	Dutch Lipid Clinic Network 1990s	MED-PED 1993	CCS 2018[16]	JAS 2018[14]
Likelihood	Definite: a + (b or c) Possible: (a + d) or (a +e)	Definite >8 Probable 6-8 Possible 3-5 Unlikely <3	HeFH is diagnosed if total cholesterol > cut-off	Definite FH: DNA mutation or xanthomas + LDL levels below or LDL≥8.5	HeFH (≥15yr old): LDL ≥6.5mmol/l strongly suggest FH

Criteria

Simon Broome		Score
Total cholesterol (mmol/L)	>7.5 (adult) >6.7 (child)	a a
LDL cholesterol (mmol/L)	>4.9 (adult) >4.0 (child)	a a
Physical	Tendon xanthoma	b
Personal History		
Family history	1° relative or 2° relative: Tendon xanthoma	b
	2° relative<50yr with MI or 1° relative <60yr	d
	1° relative or 2° relative: LDL>7.5 (LDL>6.7 in sibling<16yo)	e
Genetics	LDLR, APOB, or PCSK9 mutation	c

Dutch Lipid	Score
-	
≥8.5 6.5-8.4 5.0-6.4 4.0-4.9	8 5 3 1
Tendon xanthoma Arcus cornealis<45yr	6 4
Premature CAD Premature cerebral or PVD	2 1
1° relative with tendon xanthoma or arcus cornealis OR children<18yr with LDL>95th percentile 1° relative with Premature CAD or vascular disease, or LDL>95th percentile	2 1
LDLR, APOB, or PCSK9 mutation	8

Age	1° FH	2° FH	3° FH	NFH*
<20	5.7	5.9	6.2	7.0
20-29	6.2	6.5	6.7	7.5
30-39	7.0	7.2	7.5	8.8
≥40	7.5	7.8	8.0	9.3

Total cholesterol in mmol/l
1° FH: 1st degree relative with FH
2° FH: 2nd degree relative with FH
3° FH: 3rd degree relative with FH
NFH*: absent family history of FH

Probable FH:
1st degree relative
with LDL>5 or
premature ASCVD
in proband or 1st
degree relative
(men<55yr,
women<65yr)

and

LDL>5   if ≥ 40yr
LDL≥4.5 if 18-40yr
LDL≥4   if <18yr

Diagnostic criteria
for HeFH adults:

1. LDL≥4.7mmol/l

2. Tendon
xanthomas

3. Family history of
FH or premature
CAD (within 2nd
degree relative)

Note:
Xanthelasma is not
included as criteria

Archilles tendon
hypertrophy:
≥9mm on Xray

1° relative: 1st degree relative, 2° relative: 2nd degree relative
MI: myocardial infarction, Premature disease: men aged<55yr, women aged<60yr
PVD: peripheral vascular disease

All units of LDL and non-HDL in mmol/L. To convert LDL cholesterol from mmol/L to mg/dL, multiply by 38.67

All units of LDL and non-HDL are in mmol/L. To convert LDL cholesterol from mmol/L to mg/dL, multiply by 38.67. a and b inside the Table 1 reflects the Score of the clinical criteria for simon broome.

highest. In a large prospective registry study of a Norwegian population with FH, the risk of aortic stenosis was increased in patients with FH compared with the general population, with a standardized incidence ratio of 7.9.[23] However, the risk of ischemic stroke and cerebrovascular disease were not increased in patients with FH in the same population.[24] The Copenhagen General Population study showed that patients with clinical FH by DLCN have increased but different risks of peripheral artery disease and chronic kidney disease.[25]

Not all patients with FH have the same ASCVD risk. Risk factors for severity in FH include (i) clinical risk factors such as degree of untreated LDL-C, age, gender(male), Lp(a) level, diabetes, obesity, hypertension, and smoking and (ii) presence of subclinical atherosclerosis (eg, thickened carotid intima-media thickness, positive coronary calcium score[CAC]).[26] ASCVD risk scores derived from the general population (eg, Framingham, Pooled Cohort Equation, European SCORE) should not be used in patients with FH because the risk is underestimated.[16] Instead, risk scores specific for FH should be used; the SAFEHEART risk equation developed in Spanish patients with FH accurately predicts 5 and 10 yr ASCVD risk[27]; The FH-Risk-Score developed from a prospective cohort study of 5 registries of patients without the history of cardiovascular events also accurately predicts 10 year ASCVD risk in patients with FH without prior ASCVD events.[28] The addition of CAC to the SAFEHEART risk equation further improves the risk prediction of ASCVD.[29]

Models of Care

The models of care for FH should be informed by the best contemporary evidence and specify roles for cardiac and lipid specialists, GPs, and allied health workers.

Implementation practice remains a challenge. Guidelines have evolved to simplify diagnostic pathways, emphasize early detection, and improve ASCVD risk prediction (**Table 2**). Universal screening of children (with child–parent testing) and population genomic screening have been recently promulgated, but the feasibility of implementation and effectiveness of ASCVD risk reduction need to be established.

Therapies

Firstly, lifestyle modification with a heart-healthy diet, regular exercise, antismoking advice, weight regulation, and stress management should be advised for all patients with hyperlipidemia. Secondary causes of elevated LDL-C and other ASCVD risk factors should be treated. There is a progressive shift for lower LDL-C targets in adults with FH (see **Table 2**). The EAS/ESC 2019 guideline recommends LDL less than 1.8 mmol/L (70 mg/dL) for primary prevention and LDL less than 1.4 mmol/L (54 mg/dL) for secondary prevention in patients with FH. In patients with FH and recurrent ASCVD events within 2 years, LDL-C <1 mmol/L (40 mg/dL) is recommended by European and Australian guidelines,[15,30] **Table 2**. The guidelines do not specify different targets for HeFH and HoFH.

High-intensity statin followed by or simultaneously[31] with ezetimibe should be prescribed if LDL-C remains above target. However, most patients with FH cannot attain low LDL-C target levels with maximal tolerated doses of statin, ezetimibe, and diet.[8] Bile acid sequestrants (BAS), niacin, probucol,[14] and fibrates can also lower LDL-C, but their use is hampered by side effects, lower effectiveness compared with statins and insufficient evidence for ASCVD prevention in patients with FH. Bempedoic acid (oral ATP-citrate lyase inhibitor) which can lower LDL-C by 20% was approved by the FDA in 2020 for use in people with HeFH with or without ASCVD even when intolerant to statin. A PCSK9 monoclonal antibody at 2 or 4 weekly injections (eg, evolocumab, alirocumab) recommended for those not achieving LDL-C targets, cause additional lowering of LDL-C around 50% to 60% in HeFH and 25% to 40% in HoFH. PCSK9 inhibition has an additional benefit of approximately 25% lowering of Lp(a)[32] which is often raised in FH. Inclisiran, a small interfering RNA given twice-yearly subcutaneously, lowers LDL-C by around 40% in patients with HeFH.[33] In patients with HoFH and severe HeFH, lipoprotein apheresis remains an important and effective method of lowering LDL-C, Lp(a) and arterial inflammation[34] and enhances the potential benefits of novel treatments. Lomitapide, an inhibitor of MTP, is approved for use in patients with HoFH and reduces LDL-C by approximately 40%.[35] Evinacumab, a monoclonal antibody that inhibits angiopoietin-related protein 3 (ANGPTL3), given via intravenous infusion every 4 weeks, can lower LDL-C by 50% even in HoFH with no LDL receptor activity.[36] Evinacumab was approved for HoFH by the FDA (2021). Ongoing studies including gene editing or vaccines targeting PCSK9[37,38] and ANGPLT3,[39] will likely change the landscape of LDL-lowering in patients with FH and severe hyperlipidemia.

Special Groups

Women with HoFH and HeFH with ASCVD have high-risk pregnancies and should be managed by a multidisciplinary specialist team.[40] BAS and lipoprotein apheresis are approved for use in pregnancy. Statins, fibrates, ezetimibe, and PCSK9 inhibitors are not approved for use in pregnancy although the use of statins in a small group of pregnant women with HoFH was reported to be safe for the fetus.[41] Use of a statin, particularly a hydrophilic statin, pravastatin, in the later trimesters of pregnancy in women with HoFH may be considered as pravastatin does not cross the placenta significantly.[40]

Table 2
Summary of recent guideline and consensus statement concerning treatment targets for primary and secondary prevention in familial hypercholesterolemia (FH)

	Guidelines and Consensus Statements					
	AHA 2015,[12] AHA/ACC/NLA 2018[64]	JAS (Japan) 2018[14]	AACE 2020[135]	Australia 2020[15]	ESC/EAS 2019[30]	CCS 2021[108]
All advocate lowering of LDL by 50% as the initial step (except for AACE 2020 which did not explicitly mention)						
Primary Prevention	LDL-C <2.5 mmol/L Non–HDL-C <2.6 mmol/L	LDL<2.6 mmol/L	LDL-C <1.8 mmol/L Non–HDL-C<2.6 mmol/L ApoB<0.80 g/L	LDL-C <2.5 mmol/L if absent ASCVD LDL-C <1.8 mmol/L if imaging of ASCVD or other major ASCVD risk factors present	LDL-C <1.8 mmol/L Non–HDL-C <2.6 mmol/L ApoB <0.80 g/L	LDL-C <2.5 mmol/L Non–HDL-C <3.2 mmol/L ApoB <0.85 g/L
Secondary Prevention	LDL-C <1.8 mmol/L Non–HDL-C <2.6 mmol/L	LDL<1.8 mmol/L	LDL-C <1.4 mmol/L Non–HDL-C <2.1 mmol/L ApoB<0.7 g/L	LDL-C <1.4 mmol/L Non–HDL-C <2.2 mmol/L ApoB <0.65 g/L Recurrent ASCVD within 2 yr: LDL-C <1.0 mmol/L Non–HDL-C <1.8 mmol/L ApoB <0.5 g/L	LDL-C <1.4 mmol/L Non–HDL-C <2.2 mmol/L ApoB <0.65 g/L Recurrent ASCVD within 2 yr: LDL-C <1.0 Non–HDL-C<1.8 mmol/L ApoB <0.55 g/L	LDL-C <1.8 mmol/L Non–HDL-C <2.4 mmol/L ApoB <0.7 g/L

b. All units of LDL and non-HDL in mmol/L. To convert LDL cholesterol from mmol/L to mg/dL, multiply by 38.67.
Abbreviations: ApoB, apolipoprotein B; LDL-C, low-density lipoprotein cholesterol.

Statins should be initiated early, as young as 8 to 10 years old in children with FH, because this reduces ASCVD risk.[42] The target should be 50% reduction of LDL-C or less than 3.5 mmol/L (130 mg/dL).[43] Ezetimibe, and the PCSK9 inhibitor evolocumab are approved by the FDA for children ≥10 years old with HeFH and HoFH. In 2021, Evinacumab was approved by the FDA in 2021 for children ≥12 years old with HoFH.

Gaps in Care

The major gaps in clinical care include (i) low detection of FH (especially in the young), (ii) access to new therapies (especially HoFH and severe FH), and (iii) the need for improved health policy and financing integrated models of care for FH.

POLYGENIC HYPERCHOLESTEROLEMIA

PH, with a very high polygenic risk score, can masquerade as phenotypic FH. These patients bear multiple common genetic variants that each increases LDL-C by a small amount and collectively have a significant cumulative LDL-C raising effect. Although these traits are highly heritable (50%–80%), they are also readily modifiable by environmental factors and expression of hypercholesterolemia occurs later in life than with monogenic hypercholesterolemias.[1,7] At any given LDL level, patients without FH mutation have lower risk of CAD than those with an FH mutation.[17] However, with novel polygenic risk scores based on millions of SNVs (so-called multigenic risk scores), patients above the 95th percentile have an increased risk of premature myocardial infarction comparable with patients with FH mutations.[44] This is potentially clinically relevant, since the prevalence of PH is 10-fold greater than definite FH.[44,45] Patients with FH mutations *and* a high polygenic risk score have an even higher mean LDL-C than those with monogenic mutations alone,[44] explaining the variability of LDL-C observed in patients despite carrying the same monogenic mutation. As there is overlap between phenotypic FH (by DLCN) and genetic FH, genetic testing for FH and multigenic risk scores for PH could be useful,[45] but this is not usual practice at present.

Gaps in Care

Although utilization of polygenic scores has potential for further risk classification of patients with and without FH, gold standard scoring criteria, and studies evaluating patient outcomes, behavior, and risk stratification are lacking.[46] Unlike monogenic FH, there is a potentially lower detection rate of PH by cascade testing. Further studies may be useful in families with probands with polygenic cholesterol scores above the 95th percentile.[7]

FAMILIAL COMBINED HYPERLIPIDEMIA
Prevalence and Genetics

FCH is more common than FH [0.5%–2%[47] versus 0.3%–0.4%[2]] and is also a frequently missed diagnosis.[30] Unlike FH, FCH is polygenic in origin, mixed hyperlipidemia being due to the interaction of multiple susceptibility genes with environmental factors.[47,48] It typically manifests as the elevation of LDL-C, triglycerides (TG) and apoB, with reciprocal reduction in HDL-C. There is significant phenotypic heterogeneity between and within families.[48] More than 35 genes have now been implicated as FCH susceptibility genes, including *USF1* (regulates hepatic VLDL synthesis), *APOA1* and *CETP* (regulates TG), *LDLR* (effect on LDL clearance) and *HSL* and *PNPLA2* (control of adipose tissue lipolysis and hepatic steatosis).[47] From kindred studies, various dyslipidemic patterns of FCH have been observed, including predominant accumulation of small dense LDLs,[49] increased VLDL production,[49,50] and hypertriglyceridemia due to additional impairment of lipoprotein lipase activity.[51] Metabolic dysregulation in FCH can be related to increased supply of fatty acids to the liver, and overproduction and impaired clearance of apoB-containing particles, which are associated with dysfunctional adipose tissue and hepatic insulin resistance.[47]

Clinical Diagnosis

The Atherosclerosis and Metabolic Diseases Study Group has defined the clinical diagnosis of FCH as hypercholesterolemia [LDL-C greater than 4.1 mmol/L (160 mg/dL), or raised plasma apoB and/or hypertriglyceridemia [TG greater than 2.3 mmol/L (200 mg/dL)] in at least 2 members of the same family.[52] A diagnostic nomogram using total cholesterol, TG and apoB levels for FCH has also been proposed,[53] but this relies on untreated plasma lipid levels and requires validation and simplification for clinical use. Raised apoB level is a useful diagnostic and prognostic factor in patients with FCH.[52–54] The Spanish Foundation for Hypercholesterolemia (2014) proposed phenotypic criteria based on LDL-C greater than 4.14 mmol/L (160 mg/dL) and/or TG greater than 2.25 mmol/L (200 mg/dL)] and at least 2 first-degree relatives with mixed hyperlipidemia.[55] The ESC/EAS guideline suggested the combination of apoB greater than 120 mg/dL and TG greater than 1.5 mmol/L (>133 mg/dL) with a family history of premature CVD to identify patients most likely to have FCH.[30]

The diagnosis of FCH is challenging and requires a clearer definition. FCH overlaps with other common metabolic conditions; such as central obesity,[56] metabolic syndrome,[57] and T2DM,[58] all of which have heritable components. The pattern of dyslipidemia in FCH is similar to that in diabetic dyslipidemia and metabolic syndrome.[52] An important differential diagnosis is familial dysbetalipoproteinemia (ie, type III hyperlipoproteinemia) due to homozygosity for 2 defective apolipoprotein E2 alleles, so-called E2E2 homozygosity. This condition is typically exacerbated by secondary factors, such as insulin resistance, obesity, and metabolic syndrome. This leads to accumulation in the circulation of remnants of TG-rich lipoproteins due to decreased hepatic clearance and manifests as mixed dyslipidemia (typically with equimolar lipid concentrations on a standard lipid profile) and xanthomata.[59] Plasma lipid and lipoprotein concentrations in FCH can fluctuate within an individual over time affecting the precision of diagnosis.[54] The penetrance of FCH increases with age and obesity.[52] Genetic testing does not have a role in the diagnosis of FCH.

Clinical Significance

Patients with FCH are at significantly high ASCVD risk, specifically premature CAD.[57] Risk is dependent on the severity of dyslipidemia and presence of comorbidities, such as metabolic syndrome.[57] Approximately 65% of FCH have metabolic syndrome.[57] Patients with FCH are 6-times more likely to develop T2DM compared with their spouses.[58] Longitudinal studies show that first-degree relatives of patients with FCH have an increased risk of dying from cardiovascular disease.[60,61] Patients with FCH and family members also have an increased risk of hepatic steatosis. USF1 is a key genetic regulator of lipid and glucose metabolism, including processes that induce nonalcoholic fatty liver disease[62] and hypertriglyceridemia,[47] such as the regulation of hepatic synthesis and secretion of VLDL.

Management

The strong association of FCH with CAD makes FCH an important risk-enhancer of ASCVD.[60] In patients at low-to-intermediate absolute risk of ASCVD, the phenotypic diagnosis of FCH (or some of its component criteria) could be used as a risk-enhancing factor. While FCH per se is not highlighted as a risk-enhancer in the recent guidelines,[30,63,64] the factors characterizing FCH that is, presence of family history of premature ASCVD,[64] persistent hypertriglyceridemia,[63,64] metabolic syndrome,[64] and elevated apoB,[64] are *all* risk-enhancing factors supporting statin initiation/intensification in patients with FCH in primary prevention. In the presence of ASCVD, aggressive LDL-C and apoB lowering should be undertaken.[30]

Lifestyle modification should be advised, and secondary causes of elevated LDL-C and other ASCVD risk factors treated aggressively. Statins are the first-line treatment to lower LDL-C in FCH; statins can also lower TG by approximately 10% to 30%.[65] In patients with ASCVD or T2DM with persistent fasting TG $\geq$ 1.7 mmol/L (150 mg/dL), high dose icosapent ethyl, an EPA only omega-3-fatty acid)should be considered to reduce ASCVD risk.[63] Addition of fibrates or icosapent ethyl to a statin may be considered when plasma TG exceed 2.3 mmol/L (200 mg/dL).[31] The European guidelines recommend the use of combination of statin ($\pm$ezetimibe) and fenofibrate for patients with T2DM with TG greater than 2.3 mmol/L (200 mg/dL).[31] RNA therapeutics targeted at apo C-III and ANGPTL3 are currently being tested and developed to profoundly and durably lower hypertriglyceridemia[63] and could in future provide tailored treatment of higher risk patients with FCH receiving a statin.

Gaps in Care

The gaps in the core of FCH include under-detection, absence of definite diagnostic criteria, and lack of accurate methods for ASCVD risk stratification in primary prevention. The role of imaging for subclinical atherosclerosis (eg, CAC) and other biomarkers (eg, Lp(a)) in FCH is unclear. Because FCH is polygenic in nature, with variable penetrance, cascade genetic testing is unlikely to be cost-effective. However, adult relatives of patients with FCH and CAD should be tested with a full plasma lipid profile and assessed for other modifiable risk factors associated with FCH for example, T2DM, HTN, central obesity.

HYPER-LP(A)
Epidemiology

Lp(a) is an LDL-like lipoprotein with a single molecule of apolipoprotein B-100 (apoB) covalently bound to apolipoprotein(a). Partly owing to apoB, the plasminogen-like properties of apo(a), and a high particle content of oxidized phospholipids, Lp(a) has unique proatherogenic, prothrombotic and proinflammatory properties.[66] Epidemiologic, Mendelian randomization and prospective studies across multiple populations conclusively show that Lp(a) increases the risk of CVD events, stroke and calcific aortic valvular stenosis (CAVD).[67-74] Oxidized phospholipids within Lp(a) may be particularly important in the pathogenesis of ASCVD and CAVD.[75]

The distribution of Lp(a) is positively skewed to the right. Lp(a) < 30 mg/dL is considered normal. A large meta-analysis by the Emerging Risk Factors Collaboration of 126,634 participants in 36 prospective studies showed that Lp(a) greater than 30 mg/dL is associated with increased risk of ASCVD.[69] People in the top 20th percentile of the general population are considered to have hyper-Lp(a) (50 mg/dL $\approx$ 100–125 nmol/L), a level above which the risk of ASCVD increases significantly.[76] Extreme plasma concentrations of Lp(a) are associated with high ASCVD[70,74] and CAVD[68] risk. Lp(a) > 95th percentile in the Danish general population ($\geq$120 mg/dL) was associated with a 3- to 4-fold increase in the risk of acute myocardial infarction, with an absolute 10-year risk of 20% and 35% in higher-risk women and men, respectively.[70] Similarly, for CAVD, extreme Lp(a) levels greater than 90 mg/dl were associated with the highest risk of aortic valve stenosis (hazard ratio 2.9).[68] Patients with FH have an increased likelihood of having hyper-Lp(a).[77]

Nongenetic Causes

Because Lp(a) is predominantly under genetic control (70%–90%), the plasma concentration is largely heritable with lesser contributions from dietary saturated fat and carbohydrate, exercise, endocrine changes (eg, pregnancy, menopause, thyroid) and renal function.[66] Lp(a) is synthesized in and secreted exclusively by the liver and the clearance of Lp(a) is by liver and kidney. The plasma concentration of Lp(a) is predominantly determined by the rate of hepatic secretion of the Lp(a) particle.[78] Renal clearance is important as chronic kidney disease, including proteinuria, is associated with elevated Lp(a) levels, with renal transplantation lowering the elevated levels of Lp(a).[79] Other secondary causes of hyper-Lp(a) including overt hypothyroidism,[80] menopause,[81] and nephrotic syndrome.[79] Lp(a) levels are suppressed in obstructive liver disease due to cholestasis.[82] Conditions related to female and male hormones may affect Lp(a); Lp(a) increases in pregnancy and menopause, and is reduced with estrogen and testosterone replacement therapies, but the exact mechanisms are unclear.[81] The LDL receptor may also play a modest role in the clearance of Lp(a) because PCSK9 inhibitors lower plasma Lp(a) by about 25%.[32,83] By contrast, statins tend to have no effect and may even increase Lp(a) concentrations.[84,85] The relationship between ethnicity and Lp(a) is discussed later in discussion.

Genetics

The heritability of Lp(a) is autosomal codominant, with individuals inheriting alleles that determined apo(a) isoform sizes.[86,87] The KIV-2 copy number variation determines apo(a) isoform size, accounting for 25% to 50% variability in Lp(a) concentrations,[72] while single-nucleotide polymorphisms (SNP), in particular rs10455872 in the *LPA* gene, explain 24% to 29% of the variability.[67,88,89] Recent studies show that polygenic risk scores including multiple SNPs derived from GWAS can explain 44% to 63% of the Lp(a) variance.[88–91] Lp(a) is likely the most potent genetic risk factor for CAD, more so than LDL and PCSK9-related variants,[84,92] and arguably the most common monogenic cause of premature ASCVD and the only monogenic risk factor to date for CAVD.[93]

Apart from apo(a) isoforms, the prevalence of *LPA* SNPs is also ethnic-specific.[94] SNP rs10455872 and rs3798220 together may explain 36% of the Lp(a) variance and increased CAD risk in European cohort (OR: 2.57).[67] However, the prevalence of these 2 SNPs differs greatly among other ethnicities[94–97]: Prevalence of SNP rs3798220 varies from 4% (Whites) to 42% (Hispanics), while SNP rs10455872 varies from to less than 2% (Blacks) to 14% (Whites) in population-based Dallas Heart Study,[95] Both SNPs are rare and not associated with Lp(a) in a Chinese population.[96] The population attributable risk of specific threshold of Lp(a) for AMI varies among different ethnicities,[73,94] suggesting the need for further studies to clarify ethnic-specific values and risk thresholds. Currently, the use of apo(a) isoforms and SNPs do not have a clearly defined role in clinical practice.

Issue with Laboratory Measurements

Lp(a) is currently difficult to measure accurately and precisely. This is due to multiple copies of Kringle IV type 2 domain of the apo(a) isoform.[72,78,98] It is technically challenging to create a truly isoform-insensitive or "total particle variation insensitive" assay,[99] so that hitherto none is commercially available. Assays based on Denka reagents calibrated in molar concentration (nmol/L) and traceable to WHO/IFCC reference material are closest to an isoform-insensitive method.[100,101] Conversion factors for mass to molar units is erroneous.[102] Assays that measure Lp(a) by mass (mg/dL) alone have been discouraged.[93,99,103,104]

The estimation of LDL-C would also encompass the contribution from the cholesterol concentration of Lp(a).[84] This is especially problematic with hyper-Lp(a) levels (>80th percentile) as Lp(a) can contribute to 25% to 50% of LDL-C.[105] This could explain why some poor responders to high dose statin have high calculated LDL-C. A novel method has recently been developed to differentiate the cholesterol content of Lp(a) from LDL, VLDL and HDL.[106] This new assay showed that using a correction factor of 30% (derived from Lp(a) mass) for correcting LDL-C is not valid.[106] The formula ([Lp(a) in nmol/L]/[plasma apoB in nmol/L] x 100) can be used to estimate the percentage of apo-B containing lipoproteins that is actually Lp(a) in the plasma.[93] Utility of this approach remains uncertain.

Management

Risk threshold
Regardless of the type of apo(a) isoforms and SNPs, it is the plasma mass or molar concentration of Lp(a) that is most important in predicting ASCVD risk,[91,94] although recent evidence has pointed to a role for Lp(a) polygenic risk scores.[46] Clinical guidelines now tend to define risk threshold using Lp(a) in molar concentration (**Tables 3 and 4**). While the AHA/ACC 2018 guideline recommends a risk threshold of ≥125 nmol/L[107], the NLA 2019 guideline recommends a universal value of 100 nmol/L,[104] **Table 3**. The ESC/EAS 2019 guideline recommends that Lp(a) should be measured at least once in a person's lifetime to identify those with extreme Lp(a) results greater than 430 nmol/L (>180 mg/dL), which has the same ASCVD risk as HeFH, but is 2-fold more prevalent.[30,90] The CCS (2021) recommended measuring Lp(a) once in a lifetime as part of initial lipid screening, without specifying screening of selected groups of people.[108] There is an ongoing discussion on the role of measuring Lp(a) in youth to reduce lifetime ASCVD risk.[109,110] By about 5 years of age, plasma Lp(a) reaches adult levels and may contribute to residual risk despite the optimal reduction of other risk factors.[104,109]

Risk enhancer
As recommended by major international guidelines, Lp(a) is a risk-enhancer that may be useful in improving ASCVD risk prediction in both primary and secondary prevention,[30,64,103,104,108] and specifically FH.[26–28] Elevated Lp(a) may be useful in risk stratification in people with intermediate risk of ASCVD and those with low risk who have a family history of ASCVD.[103,109,111] Treatment decisions may be enabled regarding initiating risk reduction therapy (such as statins) in primary prevention and intensifying therapy (such as adding ezetimibe to a statin, or adding a PCSK inhibitor to a statin plus ezetimibe). In patients with hyper-Lp(a), a thorough history of personal and family history of ASCVD and CAVD should be obtained. Secondary causes of hyper-Lp(a) should be excluded, for example, hypothyroidism and chronic kidney disease. Physical examination may identify arcus cornealis, aortic systolic murmur, and/or signs of PAD. In asymptomatic patients with raised Lp(a) and strong family history of premature ASCVD, a CT calcium score, CT coronary angiography, and/or carotid ultrasound may be considered to assess the presence and burden of ASCVD. If subclinical atherosclerosis is present, this could further enable a decision to initiate/intensify statin therapy to lower LDL-C, initiate aspirin, and optimizing control of other risk factors including diabetes mellitus, hypertension, and smoking. Although diet and exercise do

Table 3
Summary of major cholesterol management guidelines and position statements on Lp(a)

	Mighty Medic Group 2017[136]	AHA/ACC and Group 2018[64]	NLA 2019[104]	EAS/ESC 2019[30]	HEART-UK 2019[103]	AACE 2020[135]	Lipid Association of India 2020[137]	CCS 2021[108] (Canada)
Detection	Targeted screening: • Intermediate/high-risk patients with CVD with premature CVD • FH • Family history of premature CVD without elevated LDL • Recurrent CVD with statin therapy	Targeted screening: • Family history of premature ASCVD • Personal history of ASCVD not explained by major risk factors	Targeted screening: • 1st-degree relatives with premature ASCVD (male<55 yr, female<65 yr) • Personal history of premature ASCVD • Primary severe hypercholesterolemia (LDL ≥190 mg/dL) or suspected FH • Very high-risk ASCVD to better define benefit from PCSK9inhibitor Measurement may be reasonable: • Borderline or intermediate 10 yr ASCVD risk in primary prevention • Less than anticipated LDL lowering to LDL lowering treatment • Family history of high Lp(a) • Calcific valvular aortic stenosis • Recurrent or progressive ASCVD, despite optimal	Universal screening: • At least once in adult person's lifetime to identify Lp(a) > 180 mg/dL (>430 nmol/L) Targeted screening: • Family history of premature CVD • For reclassification in people who are borderline between moderate and high-risk category	Targeted screening: • Personal history of premature ASCVD (<60 yr) • Family history of premature ASCVD (<60 yr) • 1st-degree relative with Lp(a) > 200 nmol/L • FH or other genetic dyslipidemia • Calcific valvular aortic stenosis • Borderline increased but <15% 10 yr risk of CVD	Targeted: • ASCVD especially premature or recurrent despite LDL-lowering • Family history of premature ASCVD and/or high Lp(a) • South Asian or African ancestry, especially family history of ASCVD or increased Lp(a) • 10 yr ASCVD≥10% (primary prevention) to stratify risk • Personal or family history of aortic valve stenosis • refractory elevations of LDL-C despite aggressive LDL-C lowering	Universal screening: • At the time of initial screening at 18 years old Targeted: • premature ASCVD • FH • family history of premature ASCVD and/or high Lp(a) • Recurrent ASCVD • Patients after acute coronary syndrome	Universal screening: • At least once in a lifetime as part of the initial lipid screening

Threshold above which risk increased	>30 mg/dL or >45 nmol/L	≥50 mg/dL or ≥125 nmol/L	≥50 mg/dL or ≥100 nmol/L in Caucasian patients Acknowledges it is unclear what ethnic-specific risk threshold should be	>180 mg/dL or >430 nmol/L equivalent to lifetime ASCVD risk of HeFH	Minor: 32–90 nmol/L Moderate: 90–200 nmol/L High: 200–400 nmol/L Very high: >400 nmol/L	>50 mg/dL	Moderate: 20–49 mg/dL High risk: ≥50 mg/dL	≥50 mg/dL or ≥100 nmol/L
Management	• Niacin or, if refractory, selective apheresis	• Use Lp(a) as a risk-enhancing factor to favor statin initiation	• Use Lp(a) as a risk-enhancing factor to favor more intensive LDL lowering therapy • Niacin is not recommended to reduce ASCVD risk in patients receiving moderate to high intensity and/or ezetimibe and LDL<80 mg/dL • HRT is not recommended to use to lower Lp(a) to reduce ASCVD risk in women	Extreme Lp(a) levels can help reclassify borderline cases between moderate and high-risk	If Lp(a) > 90 nmol/L, • Reduce overall ASCVD risk • Control hyperlipidemia • Consider apheresis if Lp(a) > 150 nmol/L (if LDL-C >3.3 mmol/L despite maximal LDL-lowering therapy) • Aim for non-HDL-C <2.5 mmol/L (100 mg/dL)	• Lipoprotein apheresis in extreme cases • Aggressive lowering LDL-C	• Secondary prevention: consider PCSK9 inhibitor	• Primary prevention: earlier, more intensive health behavior modification and ASCVD risk factors management • Secondary prevention: consider PCSK9inhibitor
Childhood and Adolescent	None specified	None specified	Measurement may be reasonable<20 yr: • Suspected FH • 1st-degree relatives with premature ASCVD • Unknown cause of ischaemic stroke • A parent or sibling with high Lp(a)	None specified	None specified	None specified	Universal screening: • >2 yr old with family history of FH and premature ASCVD	None specified

Table 4
Similarities and differences between FH, FCH, polygenic hypercholesterolemia (PH) and hyper-Lp(a)

Variables	Heterozygous FH (HeFH)	Hyper-Lp(a)	Familial Combined Hyperlipidemia (FCH)	Polygenic Hypercholesterolemia (PH)
Clinical Characteristics				
Main lipoproteins affected	LDL-C	Lp(a)	Apo-B containing particles (LDL-C, VLDL-C) TG-rich lipoproteins	LDL-C
High TG and Low HDL-C	No	No	Yes	No
High LDL-C in early childhood	Yes	No	No	No
Prominent cause of high LDL-C in adults	Yes	No (unless extreme level)	Yes	Yes (most common)
Tendon xanthomata	Yes	No	No	No
Arcus cornealis	Yes	Yes	Yes	Yes
Prevalence and Association				
Prevalence in general population	1 in 250	1 in 5	1 in 100	1 in 20
Prevalence in premature CAD	1 in 10	1 in 6	1 in 5–10	> common than FH[17]
Increased risk of premature CAD	Yes	Yes	Yes, but lower than FH	Yes, but lower than FH
Often associated with HTN and T2DM	No	No	Yes	No
Genetics				
Mode of inheritance	Autosomal codominant	Autosomal codominant	Polygenic	Polygenic
Founder effects described	Yes	No	No	No
Well-defined dominant trait mapped to a major gene locus	Yes	Yes	No	No

	1	2	3	4
Suitable for cascade screening	Yes	Yes	No	No
Current gene testing useful for diagnosis	Yes	No	No	No
Multiplicative interactions with other CAD risk factors	Yes	Yes	Yes	Yes
Management				
Well-defined model of care	Yes	No	No	No
Require lifestyle modification	Yes	Yes	Yes	Yes
Require statins	Yes	No	Yes	Yes
May require ezetimibe	Yes	No	Yes	Yes
May require PCSK9 inhibition	Yes	Yes	Yes	Yes
Often require 3 medications to achieve LDL-C target	Yes	N/A	No	No
Can require apheresis	Yes	Yes	No	No
Lipid targets often achieved with standard drugs and dietary intervention	Yes	No	Yes	Yes

Abbreviations: CAD, coronary artery disease; FCH, familial combined hyperlipidemia; HTN, hypertension; Lp(a), lipoprotein(a); T2DM, type 2 diabetes mellitus.
Adapted from Ellis KL, Hooper AJ, Burnett JR, Watts GF. Progress in the care of common inherited atherogenic disorders of apolipoprotein B metabolism. Nat Rev Endocrinol. 2016 Aug;12(8):467-84.

not lower Lp(a), healthy diet and exercise should be advocated, because a healthy lifestyle may significantly reduce cardiovascular risk in patients with high Lp(a) levels,[112] illustrating the principle of environmental modification of genetically mediated risk of ASCVD.

Treatment

It is estimated that the reduction of high plasma Lp(a) concentration by 80% to 90% is needed to achieve a clinically meaningful reduction in ASCVD risk, that is approximately 20% which is equivalent to a 1 mmol/L reduction in LDL-cholesterol.[90] Currently, no medication is approved specifically for hyper-Lp(a). Statins can increase Lp(a) by almost 50% in patients with small apo(a) isoforms, but mechanisms are unclear.[85] PCSK9 monoclonal antibodies can lower Lp(a) by 20% to 30%,[32,113] suggesting enhanced clearance of Lp(a) via LDL receptors. However, Lp(a) reduction may also be seen with PCSK9 inhibitors in true HoFH,[114] pointing to a mechanism involving LDL receptor-independent pathways. Post hoc analyses of PSCK9 inhibitor clinical outcome trials that reductions in Lp(a) may contribute to the lowering ASCVD events.[32,113] Niacin can lower Lp(a) by 20% to 30%,[115] but this agent did not reduce ASCVD risk in large clinical trials.[103,104] Lipoprotein apheresis lowers plasma Lp(a) levels acutely by 60% to 65%, but the postapheresis rebound is rapid and the mean inter-apheresis reduction of Lp(a) is approximately 30%.[116] The ASCVD benefits of the reduction in Lp(a) with apheresis may entail anti-atherosclerotic, anti-inflammatory, and antithrombotic effect.[116] Other agents that lower Lp(a) include mipomersen (c. 20%–30%),[117] and the CETP inhibitor anacetrapib (c. 38%),[118] but these agents are not in clinical use. Hormone replacement therapy in postmenopausal women[81] and thyroxine replacement in hypothyroidism[80] also lower Lp(a) concentrations. Less potent Lp(a) lowering agents (<10%) include fibrates, ascorbic acid, aspirin, angiotensin-converting enzyme inhibitor, and calcium antagonist.[76]

Novel therapies

APO(a)-L$_{RX}$, a GalNac$_3$-conjugated ASO targeted at *LPA* mRNA (Pelacarsen), that is selectively taken up by hepatocytes lower Lp(a) by 80% with 98% of patients achieving plasma concentrations less than 50 mg/dL (125 nmol/L).[119] Inhibiting apo(a) synthesis in the liver decreases the assembly of Lp(a) and the hepatic secretion of Lp(a) particles.[119] The randomized controlled trial HORIZON is currently investigating the effect of APO(a)-L$_{RX}$ (TQJ230), 80 mg s.c. monthly, (NCT04023552) in patients with established CAD on maximally treated statin and ezetimibe. Following the successful results reported in a phase 1 clinical trial,[120] a phase 2 study of the Gal-Nac$_3$-conjugated-siRNA (Olpasiran) targeting apo(a) and thus Lp(a) production is also currently undergoing (NCT04270760).

Gaps in Care

Major gaps include: (1) lack of data showing ASCVD risk reduction with specific lowering of Lp(a), (2) lack of availability of isoform-independent and well standardized assays for measuring Lp(a) molar concentrations, (3) inadequate information on ethnic-specific risk thresholds,[99] (4) the need for justification of screening programs for high Lp(a), and (5) lack of awareness of Lp(a) at patient, family, health care professional, organizational, and population levels.

SITOSTEROLEMIA

Sitosterolemia (or phytosterolemia) is an autosomal recessive disorder characterized by high plasma levels of plant sterols, particularly sitosterol, and to a lesser extent stigmasterol and campesterol.[121] The primary genetic defects involve two ATP-binding cassette subfamily G members, ABCG5 and ABCG8.[122,123] These genes encode the sterol efflux transporters that output plant sterols into the intestinal lumen, and transport plant sterols into bile.[122] This leads to an increase in gastrointestinal absorption of plant sterols from less than 5% in normal individual to 15% to 60% in patients with sitosterolemia.[123] This causes a phenotypic spectrum from asymptomatic, normocholesterolemia to severe hypercholesterolemia with tendon xanthoma, hematological abnormalities and premature atherosclerosis.[121,124,125] Homozygous sitosterolemia is estimated to occur in 1 per 200,000 in the population.[125] Sudden cardiac death has been reported in 5 years old and teenagers with sitosterolemia.[126] Heterozygotes are usually asymptomatic with normal to slightly increased plasma plant sterol concentrations, with a possible 2-fold increase in risk of CAD.[127] Sitosterolemia has been reported in breastfed infants, presumably due to increased cholesterol absorption from breast milk.[128]

Plasma concentrations of plant sterols should be measured in hypercholesterolemic patients with xanthomata that do not have FH, are poor responders to statins, are hyper-responsive to ezetimibe, or have unexplained hemolytic anemia. Management of sitosterolemia involves restricting dietary plant sterol and cholesterol intake, use of a sterol absorption inhibitor (ezetimibe), and BAS. Food rich in plant sterols including vegetable oil, nuts, avocado, seeds, margarine, shellfish, and seaweed should be avoided. Ezetimibe, which inhibits Niemann-Pick C1-Like 1 (NPCL1) efficiently lowers gastrointestinal absorption and thus of plasma sterols by 40% to 50% in homozygous sitosterolemia.[129] The BAS cholestyramine has been reported to reduce plasma sterols level by 20%.[130]

Cerebrotendinous Xanthomatosis

CTX is a rare autosomal recessive disorder of bile acid synthesis involving a deficiency in sterol 27-hydroxylase (cytochrome P450 CYP27A1) causing accumulation of cholestanol and cholesterol in plasma, tendons, lenses, and brain.[131] The prevalence is 3 to 5 per 100,000 in Caucasians but varies with ethnicity.[131] The presence of 2 of 4 hallmark criteria (premature cataract, chronic diarrhea, neurologic signs, tendon xanthomata) is a clue to the diagnosis of CTX.[132] Tendon xanthomata, which generally present by age 30, is seen in 70% of patients.[133] Neurologic abnormalities, seen in 48% to 74% of cases,[134] include impaired intellect, dementia, seizures, and psychiatric issues.[131,133] CTX can present in neonates as liver failure, but more commonly as nonspecific symptoms initially.[133] Approximately 7% to 20% of patients with CTX have premature CAD.[133,134] Diagnosis is confirmed by extremely elevated plasma cholestanol concentrations.[133] Patients with CTX have low/normal plasma levels of LDL-C with elevated plant sterols.[131] Treatment is with chenodeoxycholic acid (CDCA) 250 mg 3 times a day for adults and 15 mg/kg per day for children.[133] Early initiation of treatment prevents neurologic deficits, whereas late treatment may not reverse complications.[133,134] Statins may also be useful by decreasing synthesis of cholesterol and cholestanol, but this may potentially be offset by increased hepatic cholesterol uptake by the liver, so their use is not established in CTX other than for co-existent hypercholesterolemia.

SUMMARY

FH, PH, FCH, and hyper-Lp(a) are common inherited disorders of the metabolism of apo B-100 frequently seen in patients and families with premature ASCVD.

Sitosterolemia and CTX should be considered in the differential diagnosis of severe hypercholesterolemia or HoFH, but otherwise are exceptionally rare monogenic defects and best cared for in highly specialized clinics.

Lifetime risk of CAD is highest with FH, the most common Tier 1 genomic condition that requires early detection, preferably with genetic testing, and treatment with lifestyle and multiple cholesterol-lowering therapies. The case for screening for high Lp(a) is weakened by lack of effective therapies, but testing may be justified to risk-stratify people at intermediate absolute risk of ASCVD or those at low risk with a positive family history of ASCVD, thereby leading to risk-reduction treatments, such as statins. Cardiovascular outcome trials with RNA-based therapeutics targeted at apo(a) synthesis may change perceptions about the value of screening for high Lp(a) in secondary prevention. PH and FCH are polygenic conditions that should be treated according to general lipid guidelines with lifestyle modifications and pharmacotherapies primarily targeted at LDL-C and apoB-100, followed possibly by therapies for residual hypertriglyceridemia; FCH may be viewed as a forerunner of diabetes and managed accordingly by treating and preventing obesity. Knowledge of polygenic risk scores in FH and FCH may enable risk stratification but has no role at present in genetic cascade testing of family members, who should nevertheless be offered a nonfasting lipid profile in the first instance. All four disorders may coexist within an individual, placing them at particularly high lipoprotein-mediated risk of ASCVD.

Models of care are most developed for FH. These may be adapted, as indicated by new evidence, for managing hyper-Lp(a) and FCH. As new evidence accrues, the measurement of polygenic lipid and CAD risk scores may be incorporated into evolving models for care for FH, hyper-Lp(a), and FCH. Implementation of evidence-informed best clinical practice remains a major challenge, even for conditions like FH. Gaps in implementation need to be addressed at patient, population, health care professional, organizational, and government levels.

CLINICS CARE POINTS

- Secondary causes of raised plasma concentrations of LDL-cholesterol, such as hypothyroidism, use of corticosteroids, extreme cholesterol-raising diets, nephrotic syndrome, and obstructive liver disease, should always be excluded before making a diagnosis of FH.

- A well-curated family history is an essential component of the diagnosis of FH and guides the efficient use of genetic cascade testing.

- Risk stratification should only be carried out using ASCVD algorithms specific to FH (eg, SAFEHEART risk equation and FH-Risk-Score); coronary artery calcium scoring may be particularly useful when combined with the SAFEHEART equation.

- Lp(a) is a risk-enhancer that may be useful in improving ASCVD risk prediction in both primary and secondary prevention, particularly in patients with FH; elevated Lp(a) may be useful in risk re-stratification of people at intermediate absolute risk of ASCVD and low-risk people with a family history of ASCVD.

- Secondary causes of hyper-Lp(a) should be excluded and corrected for example, hypothyroidism and nephrotic range proteinuria. Currently available lipid regulating drugs do not effectively lower elevated Lp(a) levels; this will require the use of RNA therapeutics, currently in clinical trials.

- Plasma concentrations of plant sterols should be measured to exclude sitosterolemia in hypercholesterolemic patients with xanthomata that do not have FH, are poor responders to statins, are hyper-responsive to ezetimibe, or have unexplained hemolytic anemia.
- Polygenic hypercholesterolemia (PH) and familial combined hyperlipidemia (FCH) can mimic FH and are important differential diagnoses when genetic testing does not confirm a pathogenic variant for FH. However, patients with a frank phenotypic diagnosis of FH in whom a gene variant has not been identified should still be considered to have FH.
- The care of patients with PH and FCH should be based on guidelines for general lipid management. Lifestyle modifications are essential, and all modifiable causes of elevated cholesterol and other ASCVD risk factors must be corrected.
- Polygenic lipid and cardiovascular risk scores may identify patients particularly susceptible to ASCVD in all the 3 conditions (FCH, PH, and hyper-Lp(a)), but these scores are not yet ready for prime time.
- Evidence-informed guidelines should be followed regarding LDL-cholesterol treatment targets and the sequential use of statins, ezetimibe (or bempedoic acid), and a PCSK9 inhibitor; in very high-risk patients, such as those with FH and ASCVD, early use of combination therapy should be considered.

DISCLOSURE

GFW has received honoraria for advisory boards and research grants from Amgen, Arrowhead, Esperion, AstraZenca, Kowa, Novartis, Pfizer, Sanofi and Regeneron.

REFERENCES

1. Elder SJ, Lichtenstein AH, Pittas AG, et al. Genetic and environmental influences on factors associated with cardiovascular disease and the metabolic syndrome. J Lipid Res 2009;50(9):1917–26.
2. Nordestgaard BG, Chapman MJ, Humphries SE, et al. Familial hypercholesterolaemia is underdiagnosed and undertreated in the general population: guidance for clinicians to prevent coronary heart disease: consensus statement of the European Atherosclerosis Society. Eur Heart J 2013;34(45):3478–3490a.
3. Watts GF, Shaw JE, Pang J, et al. Prevalence and treatment of familial hypercholesterolaemia in Australian communities. Int J Cardiol 2015;185:69–71.
4. Akioyamen LE, Genest J, Shan SD, et al. Estimating the prevalence of heterozygous familial hypercholesterolaemia: a systematic review and meta-analysis. BMJ Open 2017;7(9):e016461.
5. Berberich AJ, Hegele RA. The complex molecular genetics of familial hypercholesterolaemia. Nat Rev Cardiol 2019;16(1):9–20.
6. De Backer G, Besseling J, Chapman J, et al. Prevalence and management of familial hypercholesterolaemia in coronary patients: an analysis of EUROASPIRE IV, a study of the European Society of Cardiology. Atherosclerosis 2015; 241(1):169–75.
7. Ellis KL, Hooper AJ, Burnett JR, et al. Progress in the care of common inherited atherogenic disorders of apolipoprotein B metabolism. Nat Rev Endocrinol 2016;12(8):467–84.
8. Watts GF, Gidding SS, Mata P, et al. Familial hypercholesterolaemia: evolving knowledge for designing adaptive models of care. Nat Rev Cardiol 2020; 17(6):360–77.

9. Usifo E, Leigh SE, Whittall RA, et al. Low-density lipoprotein receptor gene familial hypercholesterolemia variant database: update and pathological assessment. Ann Hum Genet 2012;76(5):387–401.

10. Fellin R, Arca M, Zuliani G, et al. The history of Autosomal Recessive Hypercholesterolemia (ARH). From clinical observations to gene identification. Gene 2015;555(1):23–32.

11. Risk of fatal coronary heart disease in familial hypercholesterolaemia. Scientific Steering Committee on behalf of the Simon Broome Register Group. BMJ 1991; 303(6807):893–6.

12. Gidding SS, Champagne MA, de Ferranti SD, et al. The Agenda for Familial Hypercholesterolemia: a Scientific Statement From the American Heart Association. Circulation 2015;132(22):2167–92.

13. Shi Z, Yuan B, Zhao D, et al. Familial hypercholesterolemia in China: prevalence and evidence of underdetection and undertreatment in a community population. Int J Cardiol 2014;174(3):834–6.

14. Harada-Shiba M, Arai H, Ishigaki Y, et al. Guidelines for diagnosis and treatment of familial hypercholesterolemia 2017. J Atheroscler Thromb 2018;25(8):751–70.

15. Watts GF, Sullivan DR, Hare DL, et al. Integrated guidance for enhancing the care of familial hypercholesterolaemia in Australia. Heart Lung Circ 2021; 30(3):324–49.

16. Brunham LR, Ruel I, Aljenedil S, et al. Canadian Cardiovascular Society Position Statement on Familial Hypercholesterolemia: Update 2018. Can J Cardiol 2018; 34(12):1553–63.

17. Khera AV, Won HH, Peloso GM, et al. Diagnostic Yield and Clinical Utility of Sequencing Familial Hypercholesterolemia Genes in Patients With Severe Hypercholesterolemia. J Am Coll Cardiol 2016;67(22):2578–89.

18. Perez de Isla L, Alonso R, Watts GF, et al. Attainment of LDL-Cholesterol treatment goals in patients with familial hypercholesterolemia: 5-Year SAFEHEART Registry Follow-Up. J Am Coll Cardiol 2016;67(11):1278–85.

19. Sturm AC, Knowles JW, Gidding SS, et al. Clinical Genetic Testing for Familial Hypercholesterolemia: JACC Scientific Expert Panel. J Am Coll Cardiol 2018; 72(6):662–80.

20. Perez-Calahorra S, Laclaustra M, Marco-Benedi V, et al. Effect of lipid-lowering treatment in cardiovascular disease prevalence in familial hypercholesterolemia. Atherosclerosis 2019;284:245–52.

21. Hopkins PN. Putting into perspective the hazards of untreated familial hypercholesterolemia. J Am Heart Assoc 2017;6(6):e006553.

22. Catapano AL, Lautsch D, Tokgozoglu L, et al. Prevalence of potential familial hypercholesteremia (FH) in 54,811 statin-treated patients in clinical practice. Atherosclerosis 2016;252:1–8.

23. Mundal LJ, Hovland A, Igland J, et al. Association of low-density lipoprotein cholesterol with risk of aortic valve stenosis in familial hypercholesterolemia. JAMA Cardiol 2019;4(11):1156–9.

24.. Hovland A, Mundal LJ, Igland J, et al. Risk of ischemic stroke and total cerebrovascular disease in familial hypercholesterolemia. Stroke 2019;50:172–4. STROKEAHA118023456.

25. Emanuelsson F, Nordestgaard BG, Benn M. Familial hypercholesterolemia and risk of peripheral arterial disease and chronic kidney disease. J Clin Endocrinol Metab 2018;103(12):4491–500.

26. Santos RD, Gidding SS, Hegele RA, et al. Defining severe familial hypercholesterolaemia and the implications for clinical management: a consensus statement

from the International Atherosclerosis Society Severe Familial Hypercholesterolemia Panel. Lancet Diabetes Endocrinol 2016;4(10):850–61.

27. Perez de Isla L, Alonso R, Mata N, et al. Predicting cardiovascular events in familial hypercholesterolemia: the SAFEHEART Registry (Spanish Familial Hypercholesterolemia Cohort Study). Circulation 2017;135(22):2133–44.

28. Paquette M, Bernard S, Cariou B, et al. Familial hypercholesterolemia-risk-
score: a new score predicting cardiovascular events and cardiovascular mortality in familial hypercholesterolemia. Arterioscler Thromb Vasc Biol 2021;41(10):
2632–40.

29. Gallo A, Perez de Isla L, Charriere S, et al. The added value of coronary calcium
score in predicting cardiovascular events in familial hypercholesterolemia.
JACC Cardiovasc Imaging 2021;14(12):2414–24.

30. Mach F, Baigent C, Catapano AL, et al. 2019 ESC/EAS Guidelines for the management of dyslipidaemias: lipid modification to reduce cardiovascular risk. Eur
Heart J 2020;41(1):111–88.

31. Averna M, Banach M, Bruckert E, et al. Practical guidance for combination lipid-
modifying therapy in high- and very-high-risk patients: A statement from a European Atherosclerosis Society Task Force. Atherosclerosis 2021;325:99–109.

32. O'Donoghue ML, Fazio S, Giugliano RP, et al. Lipoprotein(a), PCSK9 inhibition,
and cardiovascular risk. Circulation 2019;139(12):1483–92.

33. Raal FJ, Kallend D, Ray KK, et al. Inclisiran for the treatment of heterozygous
familial hypercholesterolemia. N Engl J Med 2020;382(16):1520–30.

34. Visek J, Blaha M, Blaha V, et al. Monitoring of up to 15 years effects of lipoprotein apheresis on lipids, biomarkers of inflammation, and soluble endoglin in familial hypercholesterolemia patients. Orphanet J Rare Dis 2021;16(1):110.

35. Cuchel M, Meagher EA, du Toit Theron H, et al. Efficacy and safety of a microsomal triglyceride transfer protein inhibitor in patients with homozygous familial
hypercholesterolaemia: a single-arm, open-label, phase 3 study. Lancet 2013;
381(9860):40–6.

36. Raal FJ, Rosenson RS, Reeskamp LF, et al. Evinacumab for Homozygous Familial Hypercholesterolemia. N Engl J Med 2020;383(8):711–20.

37. Musunuru K, Chadwick AC, Mizoguchi T, et al. In vivo CRISPR base editing of
PCSK9 durably lowers cholesterol in primates. Nature 2021;593(7859):429–34.

38. Shapiro MD, Tavori H, Fazio S. PCSK9: from basic science discoveries to clinical
trials. Circ Res 2018;122(10):1420–38.

39. Wang X, Musunuru K. Angiopoietin-Like 3: from discovery to therapeutic gene
editing. JACC Basic Transl Sci 2019;4(6):755–62.

40. Graham DF, Raal FJ. Management of familial hypercholesterolemia in pregnancy. Curr Opin Lipidol 2021;32(6):370–7.

41. Ofori B, Rey E, Berard A. Risk of congenital anomalies in pregnant users of
statin drugs. Br J Clin Pharmacol 2007;64(4):496–509.

42. Luirink IK, Wiegman A, Kusters DM, et al. 20-year follow-up of statins in children
with familial hypercholesterolemia. N Engl J Med 2019;381(16):1547–56.

43. Wiegman A, Gidding SS, Watts GF, et al. Familial hypercholesterolaemia in children and adolescents: gaining decades of life by optimizing detection and treatment. Eur Heart J 2015;36(36):2425–37.

44. Khera AV, Chaffin M, Zekavat SM, et al. Whole-Genome Sequencing to Characterize Monogenic and Polygenic Contributions in Patients Hospitalized With
Early-Onset Myocardial Infarction. Circulation 2019;139(13):1593–602.

45. Saadatagah S, Jose M, Dikilitas O, et al. Genetic basis of hypercholesterolemia
in adults. NPJ Genom Med 2021;6(1):28.

46. Trinder M, Brunham LR. Polygenic scores for dyslipidemia: the emerging genomic model of plasma lipoprotein trait inheritance. Curr Opin Lipidol 2021; 32(2):103–11.

47. Brouwers MC, van Greevenbroek MM, Stehouwer CD, et al. The genetics of familial combined hyperlipidaemia. Nat Rev Endocrinol 2012;8(6):352–62.

48. Brahm, Amanda J, and Robert A Hegele. Combined hyperlipidemia: familial but not (usually) monogenic.Current opinion in lipidology vol. 27,2 (2016): 131-40.

49. Jarvik GP, Brunzell JD, Austin MA, et al. Genetic predictors of FCHL in four large pedigrees. Influence of ApoB level major locus predicted genotype and LDL subclass phenotype. Arterioscler Thromb 1994;14(11):1687–94.

50. Venkatesan S, Cullen P, Pacy P, et al. Stable isotopes show a direct relation between VLDL apoB overproduction and serum triglyceride levels and indicate a metabolically and biochemically coherent basis for familial combined hyperlipidemia. Arterioscler Thromb 1993;13(7):1110–8.

51. Babirak SP, Brown BG, Brunzell JD. Familial combined hyperlipidemia and abnormal lipoprotein lipase. Arterioscler Thromb 1992;12(10):1176–83.

52. Gaddi A, Cicero AF, Odoo FO, et al. Practical guidelines for familial combined hyperlipidemia diagnosis: an up-date. Vasc Health Risk Manag 2007;3(6): 877–86.

53. Veerkamp MJ, de Graaf J, Hendriks JC, et al. Nomogram to diagnose familial combined hyperlipidemia on the basis of results of a 5-year follow-up study. Circulation 2004;109(24):2980–5.

54. Veerkamp MJ, de Graaf J, Bredie SJ, et al. Diagnosis of familial combined hyperlipidemia based on lipid phenotype expression in 32 families: results of a 5-year follow-up study. Arterioscler Thromb Vasc Biol 2002;22(2):274–82.

55. Mata P, Alonso R, Ruiz-Garcia A, et al. [Familial combined hyperlipidemia: consensus document]. Aten Primaria 2014;46(8):440–6.

56. Kwiterovich PO Jr, Coresh J, Bachorik PS. Prevalence of hyperapobetalipoproteinemia and other lipoprotein phenotypes in men (aged < or = 50 years) and women (< or = 60 years) with coronary artery disease. Am J Cardiol 1993;71(8): 631–9.

57. Hopkins PN, Heiss G, Ellison RC, et al. Coronary artery disease risk in familial combined hyperlipidemia and familial hypertriglyceridemia: a case-control comparison from the National Heart, Lung, and Blood Institute Family Heart Study. Circulation 2003;108(5):519–23.

58. Brouwers M, de Graaf J, Simons N, et al. Incidence of type 2 diabetes in familial combined hyperlipidemia. BMJ Open Diabetes Res Care 2020;8(1).

59. Mahley RW, Huang Y, Rall SC Jr. Pathogenesis of type III hyperlipoproteinemia (dysbetalipoproteinemia). Questions, quandaries, and paradoxes. J Lipid Res 1999;40(11):1933–49.

60. Austin MA, McKnight B, Edwards KL, et al. Cardiovascular disease mortality in familial forms of hypertriglyceridemia: a 20-year prospective study. Circulation 2000;101(24):2777–82.

61. Luijten J, van Greevenbroek MMJ, Schaper NC, et al. Incidence of cardiovascular disease in familial combined hyperlipidemia: a 15-year follow-up study. Atherosclerosis 2019;280:1–6.

62. Wang Y, Wang BF, Tong J, et al. USF-1 genetic polymorphisms confer a high risk of nonalcoholic fatty liver disease in Chinese population. Int J Clin Exp Med 2015;8(2):2545–53.

63. Virani SS, Morris PB, Agarwala A, et al. 2021 ACC Expert Consensus Decision Pathway on the Management of ASCVD Risk Reduction in Patients With

Persistent Hypertriglyceridemia: A Report of the American College of Cardiology Solution Set Oversight Committee. J Am Coll Cardiol 2021;78(9):960–93.

64. Grundy SM, Stone NJ, Bailey AL, et al. 2018 AHA/ACC/AACVPR/AAPA/ABC/ACPM/ADA/AGS/APhA/ASPC/NLA/PCNA Guideline on the Management of Blood Cholesterol: A Report of the American College of Cardiology/American Heart Association Task Force on Clinical Practice Guidelines. Circulation 2019;139(25):e1082–143.

65. Arca M, Montali A, Pigna G, et al. Comparison of atorvastatin versus fenofibrate in reaching lipid targets and influencing biomarkers of endothelial damage in patients with familial combined hyperlipidemia. Metabolism 2007;56(11):1534–41.

66. Saeed A, Virani SS. Lipoprotein(a) and cardiovascular disease: current state and future directions for an enigmatic lipoprotein. Front Biosci (Landmark Ed) 2018;23:1099–112.

67. Clarke R, Peden JF, Hopewell JC, et al. Genetic variants associated with Lp(a) lipoprotein level and coronary disease. N Engl J Med 2009;361(26):2518–28.

68. Kamstrup PR, Tybjaerg-Hansen A, Nordestgaard BG. Elevated lipoprotein(a) and risk of aortic valve stenosis in the general population. J Am Coll Cardiol 2014;63(5):470–7.

69. Emerging Risk Factors C, Erqou S, Kaptoge S, et al. Lipoprotein(a) concentration and the risk of coronary heart disease, stroke, and nonvascular mortality. JAMA 2009;302(4):412–23.

70. Kamstrup PR, Benn M, Tybjaerg-Hansen A, et al. Extreme lipoprotein(a) levels and risk of myocardial infarction in the general population: the Copenhagen City Heart Study. Circulation 2008;117(2):176–84.

71. Langsted A, Nordestgaard BG, Kamstrup PR. Elevated Lipoprotein(a) and Risk of Ischemic Stroke. J Am Coll Cardiol 2019;74(1):54–66.

72. Kamstrup PR, Tybjaerg-Hansen A, Steffensen R, et al. Genetically elevated lipoprotein(a) and increased risk of myocardial infarction. JAMA 2009;301(22):2331–9.

73. Patel AP, Wang M, Pirruccello JP, et al. Lp(a) (Lipoprotein[a]) concentrations and incident atherosclerotic cardiovascular disease: new insights from a large National Biobank. Arterioscler Thromb Vasc Biol 2021;41(1):465–74.

74.. Loh WJ, Chang X, Aw TC, et al. Lipoprotein(a) as predictor of coronary artery disease and myocardial infarction in a multi-ethnic Asian population. Atherosclerosis 2021. https://doi.org/10.1016/j.atherosclerosis.2021.11.018.

75. Boffa MB, Koschinsky ML. Oxidized phospholipids as a unifying theory for lipoprotein(a) and cardiovascular disease. Nat Rev Cardiol 2019;16(5):305–18.

76. Nordestgaard BG, Chapman MJ, Ray K, et al. Lipoprotein(a) as a cardiovascular risk factor: current status. Eur Heart J 2010;31(23):2844–53.

77. Ellis KL, Perez de Isla L, Alonso R, et al. Value of measuring lipoprotein(a) during cascade testing for familial hypercholesterolemia. J Am Coll Cardiol 2019;73(9):1029–39.

78. Chan DC, Watts GF, Coll B, et al. Lipoprotein(a) particle production as a determinant of plasma lipoprotein(a) concentration across varying apolipoprotein(a) isoform sizes and background cholesterol-lowering therapy. J Am Heart Assoc 2019;8(7):e011781.

79. Kronenberg F. Causes and consequences of lipoprotein(a) abnormalities in kidney disease. Clin Exp Nephrol 2014;18(2):234–7.

80. Murase T, Arimoto S, Okubo M, et al. Significant reduction of elevated serum lipoprotein(a) concentrations during levo-thyroxine-replacement therapy in a hypothyroid patient. J Clin Lipidol 2012;6(4):388–91.
81. Kostner KM, Marz W, Kostner GM. When should we measure lipoprotein (a)? Eur Heart J 2013;34(42):3268–76.
82. Chennamsetty I, Claudel T, Kostner KM, et al. Farnesoid X receptor represses hepatic human APOA gene expression. J Clin Invest 2011;121(9):3724–34.
83. Bittner VA, Szarek M, Aylward PE, et al. Effect of Alirocumab on Lipoprotein(a) and cardiovascular risk after acute coronary syndrome. J Am Coll Cardiol 2020;75(2):133–44.
84. Tsimikas S, Stroes ESG. The dedicated "Lp(a) clinic": A concept whose time has arrived? Atherosclerosis 2020;300:1–9.
85. Yahya R, Berk K, Verhoeven A, et al. Statin treatment increases lipoprotein(a) levels in subjects with low molecular weight apolipoprotein(a) phenotype. Atherosclerosis 2019;289:201–5.
86. Utermann G, Menzel HJ, Kraft HG, et al. Lp(a) glycoprotein phenotypes. Inheritance and relation to Lp(a)-lipoprotein concentrations in plasma. J Clin Invest 1987;80(2):458–65.
87. Lackner C, Boerwinkle E, Leffert CC, et al. Molecular basis of apolipoprotein (a) isoform size heterogeneity as revealed by pulsed-field gel electrophoresis. J Clin Invest 1991;87(6):2153–61.
88. Hoekstra M, Chen HY, Rong J, et al. Genome-Wide Association Study Highlights APOH as a Novel Locus for Lipoprotein(a) Levels-Brief Report. Arterioscler Thromb Vasc Biol 2021;41(1):458–64.
89. Said MA, Yeung MW, van de Vegte YJ, et al. Genome-Wide Association Study and Identification of a Protective Missense Variant on Lipoprotein(a) concentration: protective missense variant on lipoprotein(a) concentration-brief report. Arterioscler Thromb Vasc Biol 2021;41(5):1792–800.
90. Burgess S, Ference BA, Staley JR, et al. Association of LPA Variants With risk of coronary disease and the implications for lipoprotein(a)-lowering therapies: a mendelian randomization analysis. JAMA Cardiol 2018;3(7):619–27.
91. Trinder M, Uddin MM, Finneran P, et al. Clinical Utility of Lipoprotein(a) and LPA genetic risk score in risk prediction of incident atherosclerotic cardiovascular disease. JAMA Cardiol 2020;6(3):1–9.
92. Consortium CAD, Deloukas P, Kanoni S, et al. Large-scale association analysis identifies new risk loci for coronary artery disease. Nat Genet 2013;45(1):25–33.
93. Reyes-Soffer G, Ginsberg HN, Berglund L, et al. Lipoprotein(a): A Genetically Determined, Causal, and Prevalent Risk Factor for Atherosclerotic Cardiovascular Disease: A Scientific Statement From the American Heart Association. Arterioscler Thromb Vasc Biol 2021;42(1):e48–60. ATV0000000000000147.
94. Pare G, Caku A, McQueen M, et al. Lipoprotein(a) Levels and the Risk of Myocardial Infarction Among 7 Ethnic Groups. Circulation 2019;139(12):1472–82.
95. Lee SR, Prasad A, Choi YS, et al. LPA gene, ethnicity, and cardiovascular events. Circulation 2017;135(3):251–63.
96. Liu Y, Ma H, Zhu Q, et al. A genome-wide association study on lipoprotein (a) levels and coronary artery disease severity in a Chinese population. J Lipid Res 2019;60(8):1440–8.
97. Khalifa M, Noureen A, Ertelthalner K, et al. Lack of association of rs3798220 with small apolipoprotein(a) isoforms and high lipoprotein(a) levels in East and Southeast Asians. Atherosclerosis 2015;242(2):521–8.

98. White AL, Hixson JE, Rainwater DL, et al. Molecular basis for "null" lipoprotein(a) phenotypes and the influence of apolipoprotein(a) size on plasma lipoprotein(a) level in the baboon. J Biol Chem 1994;269(12):9060–6.

99. Tsimikas S, Fazio S, Ferdinand KC, et al. NHLBI Working Group Recommendations to Reduce Lipoprotein(a)-Mediated Risk of Cardiovascular Disease and Aortic Stenosis. J Am Coll Cardiol 2018;71(2):177–92.

100. Scharnagl H, Stojakovic T, Dieplinger B, et al. Comparison of lipoprotein (a) serum concentrations measured by six commercially available immunoassays. Atherosclerosis 2019;289:206–13.

101. Marcovina SM, Albers JJ. Lipoprotein (a) measurements for clinical application. J Lipid Res 2016;57(4):526–37.

102. McConnell JP, Guadagno PA, Dayspring TD, et al. Lipoprotein(a) mass: a massively misunderstood metric. J Clin Lipidol 2014;8(6):550–3.

103. Cegla J, Neely RDG, France M, et al. HEART UK consensus statement on Lipoprotein(a): a call to action. Atherosclerosis 2019;291:62–70.

104. Wilson DP, Jacobson TA, Jones PH, et al. Use of Lipoprotein(a) in clinical practice: A biomarker whose time has come. A scientific statement from the National Lipid Association. J Clin Lipidol 2019;13(3):374–92.

105. Viney NJ, Yeang C, Yang X, et al. Relationship between "LDL-C", estimated true LDL-C, apolipoprotein B-100, and PCSK9 levels following lipoprotein(a) lowering with an antisense oligonucleotide. J Clin Lipidol 2018;12(3):702–10.

106. Yeang C, Witztum JL, Tsimikas S. Novel method for quantification of lipoprotein(a)-cholesterol: implications for improving accuracy of LDL-C measurements. J Lipid Res 2021;62:100053.

107. Grundy SM, Stone NJ, Bailey AL, et al. 2018 AHA/ACC/AACVPR/AAPA/ABC/ACPM/ADA/AGS/APhA/ASPC/NLA/PCNA Guideline on the Management of Blood Cholesterol: Executive Summary: A Report of the American College of Cardiology/American Heart Association Task Force on Clinical Practice Guidelines. J Am Coll Cardiol 2019;73(24):3168–209.

108.. Pearson GJ, Thanassoulis G, Anderson TJ, et al. 2021 Canadian Cardiovascular Society Guidelines for the Management of Dyslipidemia for the Prevention of Cardiovascular Disease in the Adult. Can J Cardiol 2021;37(8):1129–50.

109. Wilson DP, Koschinsky ML, Moriarty PM. Expert position statements: comparison of recommendations for the care of adults and youth with elevated lipoprotein(a). Curr Opin Endocrinol Diabetes Obes 2021;28(2):159–73.

110. Kohn B, Ashraf AP, Wilson DP. Should Lipoprotein(a) be Measured in Youth? J Pediatr 2021;228:285–9.

111. Anderson TJ, Gregoire J, Pearson GJ, et al. 2016 Canadian Cardiovascular Society Guidelines for the Management of Dyslipidemia for the Prevention of Cardiovascular Disease in the Adult. Can J Cardiol 2016;32(11):1263–82.

112. Perrot N, Verbeek R, Sandhu M, et al. Ideal cardiovascular health influences cardiovascular disease risk associated with high lipoprotein(a) levels and genotype: The EPIC-Norfolk prospective population study. Atherosclerosis 2017; 256:47–52.

113. Ray KK, Vallejo-Vaz AJ, Ginsberg HN, et al. Lipoprotein(a) reductions from PCSK9 inhibition and major adverse cardiovascular events: pooled analysis of alirocumab phase 3 trials. Atherosclerosis 2019;288:194–202.

114. Stein EA, Honarpour N, Wasserman SM, et al. Effect of the proprotein convertase subtilisin/kexin 9 monoclonal antibody, AMG 145, in homozygous familial hypercholesterolemia. Circulation 2013;128(19):2113–20.

115. Sahebkar A, Reiner Z, Simental-Mendia LE, et al. Effect of extended-release niacin on plasma lipoprotein(a) levels: a systematic review and meta-analysis of randomized placebo-controlled trials. Metabolism 2016;65(11):1664–78.

116. Waldmann E, Parhofer KG. Apheresis for severe hypercholesterolaemia and elevated lipoprotein(a). Pathology 2019;51(2):227–32.

117. Santos RD, Raal FJ, Catapano AL, et al. Mipomersen, an antisense oligonucleotide to apolipoprotein B-100, reduces lipoprotein(a) in various populations with hypercholesterolemia: results of 4 phase III trials. Arterioscler Thromb Vasc Biol 2015;35(3):689–99.

118. Cannon CP, Shah S, Dansky HM, et al. Safety of anacetrapib in patients with or at high risk for coronary heart disease. N Engl J Med 2010;363(25):2406–15.

119. Tsimikas S, Karwatowska-Prokopczuk E, Gouni-Berthold I, et al. Lipoprotein(a) reduction in persons with cardiovascular disease. N Engl J Med 2020;382(3):244–55.

120. Koren M, Moriarty P, Neutel J, et al. Abstract 13951: Safety, Tolerability and Efficacy of Single-dose Amg 890, a Novel Sirna Targeting Lp(a), in Healthy Subjects and Subjects With Elevated Lp(a). Circulation 2020;142.

121. Bhattacharyya AK, Connor WE. Beta-sitosterolemia and xanthomatosis. A newly described lipid storage disease in two sisters. J Clin Invest 1974;53(4):1033–43.

122. Hubacek JA, Berge KE, Cohen JC, et al. Mutations in ATP-cassette binding proteins G5 (ABCG5) and G8 (ABCG8) causing sitosterolemia. Hum Mutat 2001;18(4):359–60.

123. Berge KE, Tian H, Graf GA, et al. Accumulation of dietary cholesterol in sitosterolemia caused by mutations in adjacent ABC transporters. Science 2000;290(5497):1771–5.

124. Bastida JM, Benito R, Janusz K, et al. Two novel variants of the ABCG5 gene cause xanthelasmas and macrothrombocytopenia: a brief review of hematologic abnormalities of sitosterolemia. J Thromb Haemost 2017;15(9):1859–66.

125. Tada H, Nohara A, Inazu A, et al. Sitosterolemia, hypercholesterolemia, and coronary artery disease. J Atheroscler Thromb 2018;25(9):783–9.

126. Yoo EG. Sitosterolemia: a review and update of pathophysiology, clinical spectrum, diagnosis, and management. Ann Pediatr Endocrinol Metab 2016;21(1):7–14.

127. Nomura A, Emdin CA, Won HH, et al. Heterozygous ABCG5 Gene deficiency and risk of coronary artery disease. Circ Genom Precis Med 2020;13(5):417–23.

128. Park JH, Chung IH, Kim DH, et al. Sitosterolemia presenting with severe hypercholesterolemia and intertriginous xanthomas in a breastfed infant: case report and brief review. J Clin Endocrinol Metab 2014;99(5):1512–8.

129. Lutjohann D, von Bergmann K, Sirah W, et al. Long-term efficacy and safety of ezetimibe 10 mg in patients with homozygous sitosterolemia: a 2-year, open-label extension study. Int J Clin Pract 2008;62(10):1499–510.

130. Belamarich PF, Deckelbaum RJ, Starc TJ, et al. Response to diet and cholestyramine in a patient with sitosterolemia. Pediatrics 1990;86(6):977–81.

131. Salen G, Steiner RD. Epidemiology, diagnosis, and treatment of cerebrotendinous xanthomatosis (CTX). J Inherit Metab Dis 2017;40(6):771–81.

132. Verrips A, van Engelen BG, Wevers RA, et al. Presence of diarrhea and absence of tendon xanthomas in patients with cerebrotendinous xanthomatosis. Arch Neurol 2000;57(4):520–4.

133. Duell PB, Salen G, Eichler FS, et al. Diagnosis, treatment, and clinical outcomes in 43 cases with cerebrotendinous xanthomatosis. J Clin Lipidol 2018;12(5):1169–78.

134. Koyama S, Sekijima Y, Ogura M, et al. Cerebrotendinous xanthomatosis: molecular pathogenesis, clinical spectrum, diagnosis, and disease-modifying treatments. J Atheroscler Thromb 2021;28(9):905–25.
135. Handelsman Y, Jellinger PS, Guerin CK, et al. Consensus Statement by the American Association of Clinical Endocrinologists and American College of Endocrinology on the Management of Dyslipidemia and Prevention of Cardiovascular Disease Algorithm - 2020 Executive Summary. Endocr Pract 2020; 26(10):1196–224.
136. Stefanutti C, Julius U, Watts GF, et al. Toward an international consensus-Integrating lipoprotein apheresis and new lipid-lowering drugs. J Clin Lipidol 2017;11(4):858–71.e3.
137. Puri R, Mehta V, Iyengar SS, et al. Lipid Association of India Expert Consensus Statement on Management of Dyslipidemia in Indians 2020: Part III. J Assoc Physicians India 2020;68(11 Special):8–9.

Hypertriglyceridemia

Alan Chait, MD

KEYWORDS

- Hypertriglyceridemia • Cardiovascular disease • Chylomicronemia
- Acute pancreatitis • Lipoprotein lipase • Apolipoprotein C3
- Angiopoietin-like protein 3

KEY POINTS

- Hypertriglyceridemia can be either genetic, usually due to multiple small variants in genes affecting triglyceride metabolism, or secondary to several conditions or medications, including the metabolic syndrome.
- Severe hypertriglyceridemia (triglycerides levels <1000–1500 mg/dL) is most commonly due to the multifactorial chylomicronemia syndrome, which usually results from the coexistence of genetic and secondary forms of hypertriglyceridemia, much less commonly due to familial partial lipodystrophy, and very rarely due to nonfunctioning mutations in lipoprotein lipase or related proteins.
- The main consequences of hypertriglyceridemia are increased risk of cardiovascular disease and acute pancreatitis when triglyceride levels are severely elevated.
- Prevention of cardiovascular disease in hypertriglyceridemia requires attention to treatable cardiovascular risk factors and the addition of a statin.
- Triglyceride-induced pancreatitis can be prevented by keeping triglyceride levels less than 500 mg/dL.

INTRODUCTION

During the past several decades, the major focus on lipids has been on low-density lipoproteins (LDL), largely as a result of LDL-lowering therapeutic advances that have led to a reduction in cardiovascular disease (CVD). During much of this time hypertriglyceridemia has been considered a putative risk factor and has taken somewhat of a backseat. However, with the current evidence indicating that hypertriglyceridemia clearly is a CVD risk factor, and as a result of LDL-lowering medications, there has been a renewed interest in this group of disorders.

Brief Overview of Triglyceride Metabolism

Triglyceride metabolism has been extensively reviewed elsewhere.[1,2] However, a brief review is included here as a preamble to disorders of triglyceride metabolism.

Division of Metabolism, Endocrinology and Nutrition, Department of Medicine, University of Washington, 850 Republican, Box 358062, Seattle, WA 98109, USA
E-mail address: achait@uw.edu

Endocrinol Metab Clin N Am 51 (2022) 539–555
https://doi.org/10.1016/j.ecl.2022.02.010
0889-8529/22/© 2022 Elsevier Inc. All rights reserved.

endo.theclinics.com

Abbreviations	
LPL	lipoprotein lipase
APOC3	apolipoprotein C3
ANGPTL3	angiopoeitin-like protein 3
CVD	cardiovascular disease
FCS	familial chylomicronemia syndrome
MFCS	multifactorial chylomicronemia syndrome
FPLD	familial partial lipodystrophy

Triglyceride-rich lipoproteins (TRLs) enter plasma either as chylomicrons following the ingestion of dietary fat (exogenous pathway) or after synthesis of very-low-density lipoproteins (VLDL) by the liver (endogenous pathway). A large portion of the triglyceride component of these lipoproteins is hydrolyzed by lipoprotein lipase (LPL), an enzyme that is synthesized by several tissues, including adipose tissue and skeletal and cardiac muscle, after which it is transported by glycosylphosphatidylinositol-anchored high-density lipoprotein (HDL)–binding protein 1 (GPIHBP1) to the luminal side of the endothelium, where it is available to hydrolyze triglycerides.[3] Several other proteins regulate LPL activity.[4] LPL is activated by apolipoprotein (APO)C2 and inhibited by APOC3. Other LPL activators include APOA4[5] and APOA5,[6,7] whereas angiopoietin-like protein 3 (ANGPTL3) and ANGPTL4 inhibit LPL. Triglyceride-depleted remnants of chylomicrons and VLDL are enriched in APOE and are taken up by the liver by the interaction of APOE on remnant particles with the LDL receptor, LDL receptor-related protein 1,[8] and syndecan 1, a heparin sulfate proteoglycan,[9] after which some of the VLDL but not chylomicron remnants are converted to LDL.

The clearance of triglycerides from plasma is saturable. When plasma triglyceride levels exceed approximately 500 to 700 mg/dL, additional chylomicrons and VLDL entering plasma cannot readily be removed and hence accumulate.[10]

Hypertriglyceridemia

Cut points for the diagnosis of hypertriglyceridemia are provided in most major guidelines related to hyperlipidemia. However, the biological basis for these cut points is often not supported by a strong rationale. Guidelines such as those from the American Heart Association/American College of Cardiology (AHA/ACC) and National Lipid Association regard values of less than 150 mg/dL as normal, 150 to 199 mg/dL as borderline elevated, 200 to 499 mg/dL as high, and greater than 500 mg/dL as very high. Roughly similar cut points are provided by societies such as the Endocrine Society, although they regard values of 1000 to 1999 mg/dL as severe and greater than 2000 mg/dL as very severe. Summaries of the definitions for the various grades of hypertriglyceridemia are reviewed in Refs.[2,11,12] However, a more rational approach might consider the upper limit of normal as values greater than which complications of hypertriglyceridemia occur, which may differ depending on the specific complication. For example, the value at which the risk of CVD increases is much lower than the level for the development of pancreatitis. As regards CVD risk, the associated lipid and lipoprotein abnormalities, and other CVD risk factors, may be more important determinants of CVD risk than the triglyceride level per se. Thus, establishing a normal range is actually more complicated than simply applying statistical approaches or arbitrary cut points.

Causes of Hypertriglyceridemia

Mild to moderate hypertriglyceridemia occurs commonly as part of the metabolic syndrome, can result from multiple small-effect genetic variants, and can be secondary to several diseases and drugs. Severe hypertriglyceridemia with plasma triglyceride levels greater than 1000 to 1500 mg/dL can result from 3 groups of conditions: (1) rare mutations in the LPL complex, which is termed the familial chylomicronemia syndrome (FCS); (2) the coexistence of genetic and secondary forms of hypertriglyceridemia, termed the multifactorial chylomicronemia syndrome (MFCS), which is a much more common cause of severe hypertriglyceridemia; and (3) familial partial lipodystrophy (FPLD). Each of these is discussed in more detail in later sections.

Genetic causes

Studies in the 1970s suggested that a variable pattern of lipid abnormalities was present in families of survivors of myocardial infarction that was termed familial combined hyperlipidemia (FCHL)[13] or multiple-type familial hyperlipoproteinemia.[14] These disorders were originally believed to be monogenic.[13] However, genome-wide association studies (GWAS) have identified single-nucleotide polymorphisms in at least 45 loci associated with plasma triglyceride levels, affecting triglycerides alone or in combination with other lipoproteins,[15,16] with some common variants in several genes being strongly associated with susceptibility to hypertriglyceridemia. It is now believed that most clinically relevant genetic abnormalities that result in mild to moderate elevations of plasma triglyceride levels are due to the presence of multiple common gene variants,[17,18] each with small effects. These gene variants also can interact with lifestyle measures and secondary forms of hypertriglyceridemia (see later). These minor gene variants, each having small phenotypic effects, can be quantified using a polygenic score,[19–21] but such gene scores are not yet in widespread clinical use. Monogenic causes of severe hypertriglyceridemia are discussed later.

Although FCHL is no longer believed to be a monogenic disorder,[20] there is some utility in making a *clinical* diagnosis of "FCHL" based on elevated APOB levels in combination with elevated triglycerides in subjects with premature CVD and lipoprotein abnormalities in their families,[22] because it identifies individuals and families at markedly increased risk for developing premature CVD who likely would benefit from lipid-lowering therapy.[23] Such individuals often also have features such as visceral obesity and insulin resistance, that is, features of the metabolic syndrome. In other words, some patients with FCHL have the metabolic syndrome, and vice versa (see later).

Genetic forms of hypertriglyceridemia often result from increased VLDL secretion, which can be associated with increased levels of APOB.[24] Increased residence time of VLDL in plasma favors the accumulation of small dense LDL particles,[25] which frequently are found in the presence of hypertriglyceridemia.

Remnant removal disease

Remnant removal disease, dysbetalipoproteinemia or type III hyperlipoproteinemia, is a rare autosomal recessive genetic form of hypertriglyceridemia in which remnants of chylomicrons and VLDL accumulate in plasma, resulting in mild to moderate elevations of triglyceride levels together with elevated cholesterol levels. This disease usually results from homozygosity for the APOE2 genotype plus a disorder resulting in VLDL overproduction,[26] which results in impaired hepatic uptake of APOE-containing lipoproteins[27] and impaired conversion of VLDL remnants to LDL.[28]

Hypertriglyceridemia as a component of the metabolic syndrome

Hypertriglyceridemia is a component of the metabolic syndrome. Some consider this to be a secondary form of hypertriglyceridemia. Because up to one-quarter to one-third of the US population have been estimated to have the metabolic syndrome,[29] it is worth considering the hypertriglyceridemia that occurs as a component of this syndrome as a separate category. Although the term "hypertriglyceridemic waist" has been used to describe patients with hypertriglyceridemia and central obesity who are at increased risk of developing CVD,[30] there is likely to be considerable overlap between these individuals and those classified as having the hypertriglyceridemia as part of the metabolic syndrome.

Secondary forms of hypertriglyceridemia

Hypertriglyceridemia can be present secondary to many other diseases and drugs. The most common of these is diabetes, particularly type 2 diabetes, in which up to 20% to 25% have increased triglyceride levels.[31] Hypertriglyceridemia in type 1 diabetes occurs mainly in those in poor glycemic control and in those who also have features of the metabolic syndrome.[32,33] As mentioned earlier, hypertriglyceridemia is a feature of the metabolic syndrome even in the absence of diabetes. Other common conditions that are associated with increased triglyceride levels include alcohol excess, chronic kidney disease, nephrotic syndrome, and hypothyroidism. These and rarer secondary causes are shown in **Box 1**. The most common medications that cause hypertriglyceridemia are beta-adrenergic blockers and diuretics. Other medications include drugs such as oral estrogen and estrogen receptor agonists, glucocorticoids, protease inhibitors, some antipsychotics, and antidepressants and retinoids. A more complete list is given in **Box 1**.

Treatment of some but not all these secondary causes of hypertriglyceridemia can result in normalization of the elevated triglyceride levels. Examples include treatment of diabetes and hypothyroidism, whereas hypertriglyceridemia secondary to chronic renal disease is not easily reversed. Discontinuation of drugs leading to hypertriglyceridemia often results in reduction in triglyceride levels. Substitution of lipid-neutral antihypertensive agents for beta-blockers or diuretics can lead to normalization of triglyceride levels.

The coexistence of secondary forms of hypertriglyceridemia with genetic forms of hypertriglyceridemia can result in saturation of triglyceride removal mechanisms, leading to severe hypertriglyceridemia and features of the chylomicronemia syndrome, which is discussed next.

Severe hypertriglyceridemia and the chylomicronemia syndrome

As noted earlier, hypertriglyceridemia is designated as being severe when values exceed 1000 to 1500 mg/dL, depending on which guidelines are used. If left untreated, triglyceride levels of this magnitude can result in recurrent episodes of acute pancreatitis. Such high levels are usually due to one of the following 3 conditions.

Familial chylomicronemia syndrome

FCS, originally termed type I hyperlipoproteinemia[34] and later, primary LPL deficiency,[35] is by far the least common cause of severe hypertriglyceridemia and results from rare mutations in LPL or associated proteins. Causes include nonfunctioning mutations of LPL itself,[36–38] loss-of-function mutations in APOC2[39,40] and APOA5,[39,41,42] and mutations leading to defective or absent GPIHBP1[39,43] or LMF1,[5] a protein responsible for maturation of LPL. These mutations result in impaired clearance of TRLs from plasma, and accumulation of chylomicrons and VLDL in plasma.

Multifactorial chylomicronemia syndrome

MFCS is by far the most common cause of severe hypertriglyceridemia (reviewed in Ref.[44]) and likely describes the same conditions that have previously been termed type V hyperlipoproteinemia[34] and polygenic late-onset chylomicronemia.[18,42] MFCS nearly always is the result of the coexistence of a genetic predisposition to hypertriglyceridemia with one or more of the secondary forms of hypertriglyceridemia

---

Box 1
Secondary causes of hypertriglyceridemia

- Common conditions
  - Hypothyroidism
  - Uncontrolled diabetes
  - Pregnancy
  - Nephrotic syndrome
  - Chronic renal failure
  - Acute hepatitis
  - Weight regain after weight loss
  - Sepsis
  - Autoimmune chylomicronemia
    - Systemic lupus erythematosus
    - Anti-LPL antibodies
    - Anti-GPIHPD1 antibodies

- Rare genetic causes
  - Glycogen storage disorders
  - Lipodystrophies
    - Congenital generalized or partial
    - Acquired: HIV or autoimmune

- Drugs
  - Alcohol
  - Beta-blockers
  - Diuretics
  - Oral estrogens
  - Selective estrogen reuptake modulators: tamoxifen, raloxifene
  - Androgens
  - Glucocorticoids
  - Atypical antipsychotics
  - Sertraline
  - Bile acid resins
  - Sirolimus, tacrolimus
  - Cyclosporine
  - RXR agonists: bexarotene, isotretinoin
  - HIV protease inhibitors
  - L-Asparaginase
  - Alpha-interferon
  - Propofol
  - Lipid emulsions

HIV, human immunodeficiency virus; RXR, retinoid X receptor.

Adapted from Chait A, Subramanian S. Hypertriglyceridemia: pathophysiology, role of genetics, consequences, and treatment. [Updated 2019 April 23]. In: Feingold KR, Anawalt B, Boyce A, et al., editors. Endotext [Internet]. South Dartmouth (MA): MDText.com, Inc.; 2000-. Available from: https://www.ncbi.nlm.nih.gov/books/NBK326743/.

---

shown in **Box 1**.[12,45] The coexistence of these disorders leads to saturation of triglyceride removal systems, such that additional input of chylomicrons from the diet or endogenously synthesized triglycerides from the liver are unable to be removed and hence accumulate in plasma (**Fig. 1**).

Familial partial lipodystrophy
Several forms of FPLD can be associated with severe hypertriglyceridemia and severe insulin-resistant diabetes.[46] The 2 most common forms are the Köbberling variety, in

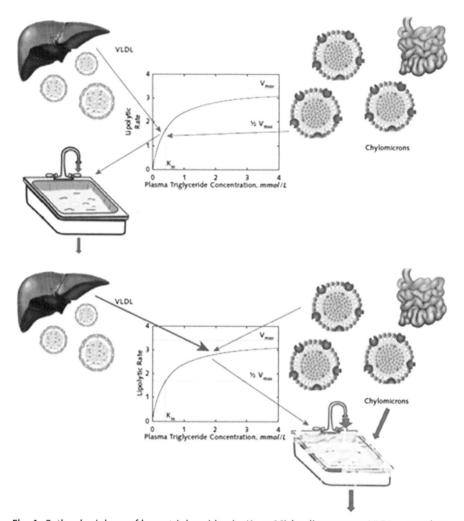

Fig. 1. Pathophysiology of hypertriglyceridemia. K_m = Michaelis constant; VLDL = very-low-density lipoprotein; V_{max} = maximum velocity. Top. When triglyceride removal mechanisms are not saturated (central graph), outflow from plasma equals inflow and plasma triglyceride levels are stable, as depicted by the level in the sink. Bottom. When increased hepatic input of VLDL leads to saturation of triglyceride removal mechanisms, inflow from VLDL and chylomicrons exceeds outflow, leading to a marked increase in the plasma triglyceride pool, depicted as the overflowing sink. (*From* Chait A, Eckel RH. The chylomicronemia syndrome is most often multifactorial: a narrative review of causes and treatment. Ann Intern Med 2019;170(9):626–34.)

which subcutaneous adipose tissue is absent in the limbs but not the trunk, and the Dunnigan variety, in which adipose tissues also are reduced in the visceral compartment. Mutations in LMNA gene (encoding A-type lamins) is commonly seen with the Dunnigan phenotype, whereas no single-gene mutations have been found to date with the Köbberling variety. The Köbberling form of FPLD is likely vastly underdiagnosed, due to its phenotypic resemblance to the metabolic syndrome, including the presence of central obesity, diabetes, hypertension, and hypertriglyceridemia.

However, a classical shelf above which subcutaneous fat is present and below which it is absent is observed by careful clinical examination of the buttocks.[44,47]

Consequences of Hypertriglyceridemia

Atherosclerotic cardiovascular disease

There has been a longstanding acceptance of the causal relationship between LDL and CVD. However, although hypertriglyceridemia has long been considered a CVD risk factor by some, recent studies have put this beyond doubt. Epidemiologic studies were the first to suggest that hypertriglyceridemia is a CVD risk factor,[48–52] which has been reconfirmed in a meta-analyses.[53] Although the association of triglycerides with CVD risk is attenuated when adjusted for HDL and non-HDL cholesterol, it, nonetheless, remains significant.[53] Moreover, a strong relationship also exists between non-fasting triglyceride levels and CVD.[52]

GWAS have shown that some genetic variants that influence triglyceride levels are also associated with increased CVD risk,[54–56] even after adjusting for their effects on other lipid traits.[57] Heterozygous deletion and other types of mutations of LPL also have been associated with increased CVD risk.[58] Variants in APOC3[59,60] and ANGPTL4[61,62] that are associated with reduced triglyceride levels are associated with reduced CVD risk, whereas variants in APOA5 that are associated with increased triglyceride levels are associated with increased CVD risk.[63,64] These genetic studies strongly support a role for triglycerides in CVD risk. However, the strongest evidence for triglycerides playing a causal role in the development of CVD comes from Mendelian randomization studies that focus on variants in genes encoding triglyceride-related proteins such as LPL, APOC2, APOA5, and ANGPTL3 and 4.[58,61,64,65] Confounding variables are equally distributed in such studies. When 185 common variants for plasma lipids were mapped, loci with a strong association with triglycerides also were associated with CAD, even after adjusting for LDL and HDL cholesterol levels.[57] Collectively these studies provide convincing evidence that triglycerides play a causal role in atherosclerotic CVD.

The exact mechanism by with TRLs cause CVD is not known. It is noteworthy that atherosclerotic plaques are not rich in triglycerides. Moreover, chylomicrons are too large to traverse the endothelial barrier and enter the subendothelial space. However, the cholesterol-enriched remnants of chylomicrons and VLDL are small enough to enter the arterial intima, where they can be retained by arterial wall proteoglycans and undergo various modifications that render them proinflammatory and atherogenic.[2,66–70] Chylomicrons also can enter endothelial cells in an SRB1-dependent manner, after which lysosomal hydrolysis generates lipid-rich exosomes, which might contain toxic and proinflammatory lipids.[71] Hypertriglyceridemia also often is accompanied by the presence of small, dense LDL particles and low levels of dysfunctional HDL,[2] both of which may play a role in the atherogenesis.

CVD risk in those with severe hypertriglyceridemia and the chylomicronemia syndrome depends on the cause of the syndrome and is discussed in more detail later.

Acute pancreatitis and other features of the chylomicronemia syndrome

The chylomicronemia syndrome describes a constellation of findings that occur with severe elevations of plasma triglyceride levels, usually greater than 1500 mg/dL. The most serious complication of severe hypertriglyceridemia is acute pancreatitis, which has a mortality rate of about 2% to 5%.[72,73] The mechanisms by which severe hypertriglyceridemia leads to acute pancreatitis remains somewhat speculative. Local liberation of lysolecithin and free fatty acids by the hydrolysis of lecithin and triglycerides by lipases in the pancreas are believed to play a role, because lysolecithin and free fatty acids result in chemically induced pancreatitis in animal models.[74,75] Inflammation in the pancreas liberates more pancreatic lipases, thereby establishing a vicious cycle.[74,75] Triglyceride-induced hyperviscosity leading to ischemic damage to the pancreas also is believed to play a role.[75]

Severe hypertriglyceridemia is the third most common cause of acute pancreatitis after alcohol and gallstones, and often is recurrent if triglyceride levels remain markedly elevated. Moreover, triglyceride-induced pancreatitis has a worse prognosis than other forms of pancreatitis, with an approximate doubling of renal and respiratory failure, a nearly 4-fold increase in shock, and a near doubling of mortality.[76]

Other features of the chylomicronemia syndrome include eruptive xanthomas, characterized by yellow-red papules on the buttocks, back, and extensor surfaces of the upper limbs; fatty liver, which is associated with an increased risk of CVD; and a whitish appearance of the optic fundus and retinal vessels termed lipemia retinalis, which is a curiosity and of no pathophysiological consequence. Acute memory loss for recent events and mental fogginess also have been reported.[77] These features are obviously of much less importance than acute pancreatitis but can help in the diagnosis of the chylomicronemia syndrome.

The chylomicronemia syndrome can be associated with an increased risk of CVD, depending on the cause. CVD risk usually is not increased in FCS unless there are other CVD risk factors such as cigarette smoking and diabetes.[78,79] However, individuals with the MFCS, the commonest cause of the chylomicronemia syndrome, often have polygenic mutations of triglyceride-raising genes that are associated with CVD, as well as other CVD risk factors, such as diabetes and hypertension. FPLD also is associated with increased CVD risk.[47,80,81]

Treatment of Hypertriglyceridemia

The approach to treating hypertriglyceridemia depends to a large extent on the cause and what the goals of treatment are. The major goal of treating mild to moderate hypertriglyceridemia is to prevent CVD, whereas the goal of management of individuals with severe hypertriglyceridemia is prevention of pancreatitis, as well as prevention of CVD in susceptible individuals.

Treatment of secondary forms of hypertriglyceridemia

Before instituting lifelong therapy for hypertriglyceridemia, it is essential to rule out and treat reversible secondary disorders that can elevate plasma triglyceride levels, including appropriate management of diabetes and hypothyroidism and substituting drugs that can elevate triglyceride levels with lipid-neutral alternatives, particularly with respect to the management of hypertension where beta-adrenergic blocking agents and diuretics should be replaced by agents such as calcium channel blockers, angiotensin-converting enzyme inhibitors, angiotensin receptor blockers, and alpha-adrenergic blockers. If triglyceride levels fall and remain normal after such strategies, no additional therapy may be needed, other than statins to reduce CVD risk in appropriate individuals, such as those with diabetes.

Approach to the prevention of cardiovascular disease in individuals with hypertriglyceridemia

Lifestyle measures are an important starting point for the prevention of CVD. Many individuals with hypertriglyceridemia are overweight or obese, and there is good evidence that triglyceride levels decrease with weight loss. However, weight loss has proved difficult to maintain. When triglyceride levels remain elevated, CVD risk should be assessed using one of the several risk calculators, such as that from the AHA/ACC. Statins are the initial drug therapy to reduce CVD risk in all high-risk individuals independent of triglyceride levels. However, their effect in reducing triglycerides is moderate.

There remains some controversy as to how to approach the patient on statins with residual triglycerides greater than 150 mg/dL, who have either CVD or diabetes plus 2 additional risk factors. Fibrates are peroxisome proliferator-activated receptor (PPAR) alpha agonists that are effective in reducing triglyceride levels. However, their effect on reducing CVD risk remains controversial. Early studies such as the Helsinki Heart Study and VA HDL Intervention Trial (VA-HIT) showed a reduction in CVD events with the use of gemfibrozil,[82,83] but these studies were performed before the widespread use of statins. Several subsequent studies such as BIP (bezafibrate infarction prevention study), FIELD (Fenofibrate Intervention and Event Lowering in Diabetes), and ACCORD (Action to Control Cardiovascular Risk in Diabetes, also with fenofibrate) have failed to show a significant overall CVD benefit of fibrates in the entire cohort studied, possibly because hypertriglyceridemia was not a prespecified inclusion criterion. However, subgroup analyses, which were not prespecified with the exception of the ACCORD trial, did show benefit in patients with triglyceride levels greater than 200 mg/dL and low levels of HDL.[84] A PPAR alpha polymorphism had been shown to influence the benefit of fenofibrate in the ACCORD study.[85] However, a cardiovascular outcome study of a novel PPAR alpha agonist added to a statin in individuals with hypertriglyceridemia and low HDL-C,[86] Pemafibrate to Reduce Cardiovascular Outcomes by Reducing Triglycerides in Patients With Diabetes (PROMINENT), recently was discontinued due to a low likelihood of the primary endpoint being met, thereby essentially ending the debate about potential cardiovascular benefits of adding a fibrate to a statin in individuals with hypertriglyceridemia.

Fish oils also reduce plasma triglyceride levels. Multiple studies and a meta-analysis have failed to show a CVD benefit of mixed eicosapentaenoic acid (EPA) and docosahexaenoic acid (DHA).[87] However, a landmark randomized controlled trial, Reduction of Cardiovascular Events with Icosapent Ethyl–Intervention Trial (REDUCE-IT), showed significant benefit of adding EPA ethyl ester to statins in reducing the risk of CVD in patients with residual high triglyceride levels and CVD or diabetes and 2 or more risk factors.[88] The risk reduction was unrelated to either the baseline triglyceride level or to the magnitude of triglyceride reduction. This study confirmed an earlier study from Japan, which was open label and termed Japan EPA Lipid Intervention Study (JELIS), which showed that a lower dose of EPA also reduced CVD events.[89] However, a subsequent study, Outcomes Study to Assess Statin Residual Risk Reduction With Epanova in High CV Risk Patients With Hypertriglyceridemia (STRENGTH), which used a combined EPA/DHA preparation, was stopped earlier due to futility.[90] Thus, despite a wide range of formulations and doses of omega-3-fatty acids in various trials, the current consensus is that EPA, but not DHA, affects CVD events. Potential mechanisms for the beneficial outcome of the REDUCE-IT study have been proposed.[91] In addition, proresolving mediators generated from EPA may also be playing a role (see Goldberg and colleagues' article, "Big Fish or No Fish; EPA and Cardiovascular Disease," in this issue on omega-3 fatty acids). Therefore, although some have suggested that the benefit seen in the REDUCE-IT trial might be attributable to adverse effects of the mineral oil control used, the current American Diabetes Association's recommendation is to consider adding EPA ethyl ester to a statin in patients with diabetes who have atherosclerotic CVD or other CV risk factors and have controlled LDL cholesterol levels but persistently elevated triglyceride levels. The role of fish oils in the prevention of atherosclerosis and CVD is discussed in more detail in Goldberg and colleagues' article, "Big Fish or No Fish; EPA and Cardiovascular Disease," in this issue.

A similar approach to CVD prevention should be applied to individuals with the MFCS and FPLD after their triglyceride levels have been lowered sufficiently to reduce their risk of pancreatitis (see later).

Several other protein targets that affect triglyceride metabolism are being evaluated in ongoing clinical trials. The rationale for these targets is based on genetic studies that indicate that individuals with genetically low levels of APOC3 and ANGPTL3 have protection against CVD. Antisense oligonucleotide (ASO) inhibitors of APOC3 and both ASO and monoclonal antibody inhibitors of ANGPTL3 have been shown to reduce plasma triglyceride levels,[92–94] but their effect on CVD events remains to be determined; these are discussed in more detail in Zambon and colleagues' article, "New and Emerging Therapies for Dyslipidemia," in this issue. However, the development of Vupanorsen, an ANGPTL3 ASO inhibitor that was being tested for CVD risk reduction and treatment of severe hypertriglyceridemia, recently was discontinued due to insufficient magnitude of triglyceride reduction.

Approach to the prevention of pancreatitis in individuals with severe hypertriglyceridemia

The best way to prevent the onset of triglyceride-induced pancreatitis is to keep triglyceride levels less than 500 mg/dL.[95–97] The approach to so doing will depend to a large extent on the cause of the severe hypertriglyceridemia, as reviewed in Ref.[44] Although FCS is very rare, it is extremely difficult to keep levels this low. The mainstay of therapy to date has been the use of a very-fat-restricted diet (<5% of calories from fat). However, this degree of fat restriction is a major burden on patients. A promising approach is the use of an APOC3 ASO, which has been shown to lower triglyceride levels in these patients by actions of APOC3 that are independent of LPL.[98,99]

The approach to triglyceride lowering in MFCS requires diagnosis and treatment of any of the reversible secondary forms of hypertriglyceridemia discussed earlier. Cessation of alcohol intake, appropriate treatment of diabetes, or substitution of beta-adrenergic blockers and diuretics for lipid-neutral antihypertensive agents often reduces triglyceride values sufficiently to reduce the risk of pancreatitis. As these individuals almost always have a genetic component to their hypertriglyceridemia, triglyceride values seldom fall to within the normal range with this approach. Residual hypertriglyceridemia should be treated with fibrates,[97] which will prevent recurrent episodes of acute pancreatitis. As APOC3 ASOs reduce triglyceride levels over a wide range of triglyceride levels,[93] with time this approach might prove to be of value in this difficult-to-treat group of patients.

The hypertriglyceridemia that can be seen with FPLD is often very severe and difficult to treat; it sometimes responds to fibrates, but levels often remain sufficiently high to put the patient at risk of recurrent pancreatitis. Thiazolidinediones and glucagonlike peptide-1–receptor analogs help reduce triglycerides in some patients with the Köbberling variety of FPLD, and leptin administration can be useful in congenital total lipodystrophy and in some cases of FPLD in patients with low leptin levels.[100] Because leptin levels are normal in Köbberling FPLD[47], there is little rationale for its use in this condition. The role of APOC3 and ANGPTL3 inhibition in the treatment of these difficult-to-treat disorders may prove to be of use with time.

Once triglyceride levels have been lowered sufficiently to prevent acute or recurrent pancreatitis, strategies to prevent CVD need to be undertaken in individuals with MFCS and FPLD. A statin should be added for CVD prevention, as well as lifestyle measures and appropriate treatment of other CVD risk factors. Because ANGPTL3 inhibition lowers LDL and HDL cholesterol levels in addition to triglycerides, and loss-of-function mutations of ANGPTL3 are associated with a reduced risk for CVD,[65]

ANGPTL3 inhibition might prove valuable in preventing CVD in addition to pancreatitis in these patients.

SUMMARY

The recent focus on hypertriglyceridemia, in large part prompted by genetic studies confirming its role as a CVD risk factor and by newer drug targets, offers lots of promise for the management of patients with hypertriglyceridemia, both from the standpoint of CVD prevention and also for the prevention of triglyceride-induced pancreatitis in severe hypertriglyceridemia.

CLINICS CARE POINTS

- Consider and exclude secondary causes of hypertriglyceridemia
- Mild to moderate hypertriglyceridemia is an established risk factor for CVD, so a careful family history is useful
- Use lifestyle measures and statins as the first-line therapy for the prevention of CVD
- Add EPA ethyl esters for residual hypertriglyceridemia with diabetes or 2 or more risk factors
- With triglyceride levels greater than 1000 mg/dL, distinguish between the 3 main causes, MFCS, FPLD, and the rare cases of FCS. Careful examination of the buttocks for a ledge above which fat is present and below which it is absent is helpful in making the diagnosis of the Köbberling form of FPLD.
- Treatment of severe hypertriglyceridemia depends on the cause. Maintaining triglyceride levels less than 500 mg/dL is necessary for pancreatitis prevention

DISCLOSURE

The author has nothing to disclose.

REFERENCES

1. Feingold KR. Introduction to Lipids and Lipoproteins. In: Feingold KR, Anawalt B, Boyce A, et al., eds. Endotext. South Dartmouth (MA)2000.
2. Ginsberg HN, Packard CJ, Chapman MJ, et al. Triglyceride-rich lipoproteins and their remnants: metabolic insights, role in atherosclerotic cardiovascular disease, and emerging therapeutic strategies-a consensus statement from the European Atherosclerosis Society. Eur Heart J 2021;42(47):4791–806.
3. Beigneux AP, Davies BS, Bensadoun A, et al. GPIHBP1, a GPI-anchored protein required for the lipolytic processing of triglyceride-rich lipoproteins. J Lipid Res 2009;50(Suppl):S57–62.
4. Kersten S. Physiological regulation of lipoprotein lipase. Biochim Biophys Acta 2014;1841(7):919–33.
5. Lamiquiz-Moneo I, Bea AM, Mateo-Gallego R, et al. [Identification of variants in LMF1 gene associated with primary hypertriglyceridemia]. Clin Investig Arterioscler 2015;27(5):246–52.
6. Nilsson SK, Heeren J, Olivecrona G, et al. Apolipoprotein A-V; a potent triglyceride reducer. Atherosclerosis 2011;219(1):15–21.
7. Priore Oliva C, Pisciotta L, Li Volti G, et al. Inherited apolipoprotein A-V deficiency in severe hypertriglyceridemia. Arterioscler Thromb Vasc Biol 2005;25(2):411–7.

8. Gordts PL, Nock R, Son NH, et al. ApoC-III inhibits clearance of triglyceride-rich lipoproteins through LDL family receptors. J Clin Invest 2016;126(8): 2855–66.

9. Foley EM, Gordts PL, Stanford KI, et al. Hepatic remnant lipoprotein clearance by heparan sulfate proteoglycans and low-density lipoprotein receptors depend on dietary conditions in mice. Arterioscler Thromb Vasc Biol 2013;33(9): 2065–74.

10. Brunzell JD, Hazzard WR, Porte D Jr, et al. Evidence for a common saturable triglyceride removal mechanism for chylomicrons and very low density lipoproteins in man. J Clin Invest 1973;52:1578–85.

11. Newman CB, Blaha MJ, Boord JB, et al. Lipid management in patients with endocrine disorders: an endocrine society clinical practice guideline. J Clin Endocrinol Metab 2020;105(12).

12. Chait A, Subramanian S. Hypertriglyceridemia: pathophysiology, role of genetics, consequences, and treatment. In: Feingold KR, Anawalt B, Boyce A, et al., eds. Endotext. South Dartmouth (MA)2000.

13. Goldstein JL, Schrott HG, Hazzard WR, et al. Hyperlipidemia in coronary heart disease. II. Genetic analysis of lipid levels in 176 families and delineation of a new inherited disorder, combined hyperlipidemia. J Clin Invest 1973;52: 1544–68.

14. Nikkila EA, Aro A. Family study of serum lipids and lipoproteins in coronary heart-disease. Lancet 1973;1(7810):954–9.

15. Willer CJ, Schmidt EM, Sengupta S, et al. Discovery and refinement of loci associated with lipid levels. Nat Genet 2013;45(11):1274–83.

16. Ripatti P, Ramo JT, Soderlund S, et al. The contribution of GWAS loci in familial dyslipidemias. PLoS Genet 2016;12(5):e1006078.

17. Berglund L, Brunzell J, Sacks FM. Patient information page from the hormone foundations. patient guide to the assessment and treatment of hypertriglyceridemia (high triglycerides). J Clin Endocrinol Metab 2012;97(9):31A–2A.

18. Hegele RA, Ginsberg HN, Chapman MJ, et al. The polygenic nature of hypertriglyceridaemia: implications for definition, diagnosis, and management. Lancet Diabetes Endocrinol 2014;2(8):655–66.

19. Hubacek JA, Dlouha D, Adamkova V, et al. The gene score for predicting hypertriglyceridemia: new insights from a czech case-control study. Mol Diagn Ther 2019;23(4):555–62.

20. Carrasquilla GD, Christiansen MR, Kilpelainen TO. The genetic basis of hypertriglyceridemia. Curr Atheroscler Rep 2021;23(8):39.

21. Dron JS, Hegele RA. Genetics of hypertriglyceridemia. Front Endocrinol 2020; 11:455.

22. Veerkamp MJ, de Graaf J, Hendriks JC, et al. Nomogram to diagnose familial combined hyperlipidemia on the basis of results of a 5-year follow-up study. Circulation 2004;109(24):2980–5.

23. Luijten J, van Greevenbroek MMJ, Schaper NC, et al. Incidence of cardiovascular disease in familial combined hyperlipidemia: a 15-year follow-up study. Atherosclerosis 2019;280:1–6.

24. Venkatesan S, Cullen P, Pacy P, et al. Stable isotopes show a direct relation between VLDL apoB overproduction and serum triglyceride levels and indicate a metabolically and biochemically coherent basis for familial combined hyperlipidemia. Arterioscler Thromb 1993;13:1110–8.

25. Berneis KK, Krauss RM. Metabolic origins and clinical significance of LDL heterogeneity. J Lipid Res 2002;43(9):1363–79.

26. Chait A, Ginsberg HN, Vaisar T, et al. Remnants of the triglyceride-rich lipoproteins, diabetes, and cardiovascular disease. Diabetes 2020;69(4):508–16.
27. Johansen CT, Wang J, Lanktree MB, et al. An increased burden of common and rare lipid-associated risk alleles contributes to the phenotypic spectrum of hypertriglyceridemia. Arterioscler Thromb Vasc Biol 2011;31(8):1916–26.
28. Chait A, Brunzell JD, Albers JJ, et al. Type-III Hyperlipoproteinaemia ("remnant removal disease"). Insight into the pathogenetic mechanism. Lancet 1977; 1(8023):1176–8.
29. Alberti KG, Eckel RH, Grundy SM, et al. Harmonizing the metabolic syndrome: a joint interim statement of the international diabetes federation task force on epidemiology and prevention; national heart, lung, and blood institute; american heart association; world heart federation; international atherosclerosis society; and international association for the study of obesity. Circulation 2009; 120(16):1640–5.
30. Lemieux I, Pascot A, Couillard C, et al. Hypertriglyceridemic waist : a marker of the atherogenic metabolic triad (hyperinsulinemia; hyperapolipoprotein b; small, dense LDL) in men? Circulation 2000;102:179–84.
31. Fan W, Philip S, Granowitz C, et al. Residual hypertriglyceridemia and estimated atherosclerotic cardiovascular disease risk by statin use in U.S. adults with diabetes: national health and nutrition examination survey 2007-2014. Diabetes Care 2019;42(12):2307–14.
32. Purnell JQ, Hokanson JE, Marcovina SM, et al. Effect of excessive weight gain with intensive therapy of type 1 diabetes on lipid levels and blood pressure: results from the DCCT. Diabetes Control and Complications Trial. JAMA 1998; 280(2):140–6.
33. Purnell JQ, Hokanson JE, Marcovina SM, et al. Weight gain accompanying intensive diabetes therapy in type 1 diabetes is associated with higher levels of dense LDL cholesterol. J Investig Med 1996;44:180A.
34. Fredrickson D, Levy R, Lees R. Fat transport and lipoproteins - an integrated approach to mechanisms and disorders. N Engl J Med 1967;276:32, 94,148,215,273.
35. Brunzell JD, Iverius P-H, Scheibel MS, et al. Primary lipoprotein lipase deficiency. In: Angel A, Frohlich J, editors. Lipoprotein deficiency syndromes. New York: Plenum Press; 1986. p. 227–39.
36. Brunzell JDDS. Familial lipoprotein lipase deficiency, apo CII deficiency and hepatic lipase deficiency. The metabolic and molecular basis of inherited disease. 8th edition. New York: McGraw-Hill Book Co.; 2001. p. 2789–816.
37. Rahalkar AR, Giffen F, Har B, et al. Novel LPL mutations associated with lipoprotein lipase deficiency: two case reports and a literature review. Can J Physiol Pharmacol 2009;87(3):151–60.
38. Nickerson DA, Taylor SL, Weiss KM, et al. DNA sequence diversity in a 9.7-kb region of the human lipoprotein lipase gene. Nat Genet 1998;19(3):233–40.
39. Surendran RP, Visser ME, Heemelaar S, et al. Mutations in LPL, APOC2, APOA5, GPIHBP1 and LMF1 in patients with severe hypertriglyceridaemia. J Intern Med 2012;272(2):185–96.
40. Fojo SS, Brewer HB. Hypertriglyceridaemia due to genetic defects in lipoprotein lipase and apolipoprotein C-II. J Intern Med 1992;231(6):669–77.
41. Calandra S, Priore Oliva C, Tarugi P, et al. APOA5 and triglyceride metabolism, lesson from human APOA5 deficiency. Curr Opin Lipidol 2006;17(2):122–7.
42. Brahm AJ, Hegele RA. Chylomicronaemia-current diagnosis and future therapies. Nat Rev Endocrinol 2015;11(6):352–62.

43. Rios JJ, Shastry S, Jasso J, et al. Deletion of GPIHBP1 causing severe chylomicronemia. J Inherit Metab Dis 2012;35(3):531–40.
44. Chait A, Eckel RH. The chylomicronemia syndrome is most often multifactorial: a narrative review of causes and treatment. Ann Intern Med 2019;170(9):626–34.
45. Chait A, Brunzell JD. Severe hypertriglyceridemia: role of familial and acquired disorders. Metabolism 1983;32:209–14.
46. Garg A. Clinical review#: Lipodystrophies: genetic and acquired body fat disorders. J Clin Endocrinol Metab 2011;96(11):3313–25.
47. Herbst KL, Tannock LR, Deeb SS, et al. Kobberling type of familial partial lipodystrophy: an underrecognized syndrome. Diabetes Care 2003;26(6):1819–24.
48. Miller M, Stone NJ, Ballantyne C, et al. Triglycerides and cardiovascular disease: a scientific statement from the American Heart Association. Circulation 2011;123(20):2292–333.
49. Castelli WP. The triglyceride issue: a view from framingham. Am Heart J 1986;112(2):432–7.
50. Harchaoui KE, Visser ME, Kastelein JJ, et al. Triglycerides and cardiovascular risk. Curr Cardiol Rev 2009;5(3):216–22.
51. Langsted A, Freiberg JJ, Tybjaerg-Hansen A, et al. Nonfasting cholesterol and triglycerides and association with risk of myocardial infarction and total mortality: the Copenhagen City Heart Study with 31 years of follow-up. J Intern Med 2011;270(1):65–75.
52. Nordestgaard BG, Varbo A. Triglycerides and cardiovascular disease. Lancet 2014;384(9943):626–35.
53. Hokanson JE, Austin MA. Plasma triglyceride level is a risk factor for cardiovascular disease independent of high-density lipoprotein cholesterol level: a meta-analysis of population-based prospective studies. J Cardiovasc Risk 1996;3(2):213–9.
54. Waterworth DM, Ricketts SL, Song K, et al. Genetic variants influencing circulating lipid levels and risk of coronary artery disease. Arterioscler Thromb Vasc Biol 2010;30(11):2264–76.
55. Teslovich TM, Musunuru K, Smith AV, et al. Biological, clinical and population relevance of 95 loci for blood lipids. Nature 2010;466(7307):707–13.
56. Rip J, Nierman MC, Ross CJ, et al. Lipoprotein lipase S447X: a naturally occurring gain-of-function mutation. Arterioscler Thromb Vasc Biol 2006;26(6):1236–45.
57. Do R, Willer CJ, Schmidt EM, et al. Common variants associated with plasma triglycerides and risk for coronary artery disease. Nat Genet 2013;45(11):1345–52.
58. Khera AV, Won HH, Peloso GM, et al. Association of rare and common variation in the lipoprotein lipase gene with coronary artery disease. JAMA 2017;317(9):937–46.
59. Tg, Hdl Working Group of the Exome Sequencing Project NHL, Blood I, et al. Loss-of-function mutations in APOC3, triglycerides, and coronary disease. N Engl J Med 2014;371(1):22–31.
60. Jorgensen AB, Frikke-Schmidt R, Nordestgaard BG, et al. Loss-of-function mutations in APOC3 and risk of ischemic vascular disease. N Engl J Med 2014;371(1):32–41.
61. Dewey FE, Gusarova V, O'Dushlaine C, et al. Inactivating variants in ANGPTL4 and risk of coronary artery disease. N Engl J Med 2016;374(12):1123–33.

62. Myocardial Infarction G, Investigators CAEC, Stitziel NO, et al. Coding Variation in ANGPTL4, LPL, and SVEP1 and the Risk of Coronary Disease. N Engl J Med 2016;374(12):1134-44.

63. Soufi M, Sattler AM, Kurt B, et al. Mutation screening of the APOA5 gene in subjects with coronary artery disease. J Investig Med 2012;60(7):1015-9.

64. Do R, Stitziel NO, Won HH, et al. Exome sequencing identifies rare LDLR and APOA5 alleles conferring risk for myocardial infarction. Nature 2015; 518(7537):102-6.

65. Stitziel NO, Khera AV, Wang X, et al. ANGPTL3 deficiency and protection against coronary artery disease. J Am Coll Cardiol 2017;69(16):2054-63.

66. Mangat R, Warnakula S, Borthwick F, et al. Arterial retention of remnant lipoproteins ex vivo is increased in insulin resistance because of increased arterial biglycan and production of cholesterol-rich atherogenic particles that can be improved by ezetimibe in the JCR:LA-cp rat. J Am Heart Assoc 2012;1(5): e003434.

67. Zilversmit DB. Atherogenic nature of triglycerides, postprandial lipidemia, and triglyceride-rich remnant lipoproteins. Clin Chem 1995;41(1):153-8.

68. Skalen K, Gustafsson M, Rydberg E, et al. Subendothelial retention of atherogenic lipoproteins in early atherosclerosis. Nature 2002;417:750-4.

69. Nordestgaard BG, Wootton R, Lewis B. Selective retention of VLDL, IDL, and LDL in the arterial intima of genetically hyperlipidemic rabbits in vivo. Molecular size as a determinant of fractional loss from the intima-inner media. Arterioscler Thromb Vasc Biol 1995;15(4):534-42.

70. Goldberg IJ, Eckel RH, McPherson R. Triglycerides and heart disease: still a hypothesis? Arterioscler Thromb Vasc Biol 2011;31(8):1716-25.

71. Cabodevilla AG, Tang S, Lee S, et al. Eruptive xanthoma model reveals endothelial cells internalize and metabolize chylomicrons, leading to extravascular triglyceride accumulation. J Clin Invest 2021;131(12).

72. Omdal T, Dale J, Lie SA, et al. Time trends in incidence, etiology, and case fatality rate of the first attack of acute pancreatitis. Scand J Gastroenterol 2011; 46(11):1389-98.

73. Lowenfels AB, Maisonneuve P, Sullivan T. The changing character of acute pancreatitis: epidemiology, etiology, and prognosis. Curr Gastroenterol Rep 2009;11(2):97-103.

74. Yang F, Wang Y, Sternfeld L, et al. The role of free fatty acids, pancreatic lipase and Ca+ signalling in injury of isolated acinar cells and pancreatitis model in lipoprotein lipase-deficient mice. Acta Physiol (Oxf) 2009;195(1):13-28.

75. Valdivielso P, Ramirez-Bueno A, Ewald N. Current knowledge of hypertriglyceridemic pancreatitis. Eur J Intern Med 2014;25(8):689-94.

76. Wang Q, Wang G, Qiu Z, et al. Elevated serum triglycerides in the prognostic assessment of acute pancreatitis: a systematic review and meta-analysis of observational studies. J Clin Gastroenterol 2017;51(7):586-93.

77. Chait A, Robertson HT, Brunzell JD. Chylomicronemia syndrome in diabetes mellitus. Diabetes Care 1981;4:343-8.

78. Benlian P, De Gennes JL, Foubert L, et al. Premature atherosclerosis in patients with familial chylomicronemia caused by mutations in the lipoprotein lipase gene. N Engl J Med 1996;335(12):848-54.

79. Saika Y, Sakai N, Takahashi M, et al. Novel LPL mutation (L303F) found in a patient associated with coronary artery disease and severe systemic atherosclerosis. Eur J Clin Invest 2003;33(3):216-22.

80. Bruder-Nascimento T, Kress TC, Belin de Chantemele EJ. Recent advances in understanding lipodystrophy: a focus on lipodystrophy-associated cardiovascular disease and potential effects of leptin therapy on cardiovascular function. F1000Res 2019;8.
81. Hussain I, Patni N, Garg A. Lipodystrophies, dyslipidaemias and atherosclerotic cardiovascular disease. Pathology 2019;51(2):202–12.
82. Manninen V, Huttunen JK, Heinonen OP, et al. Relation between baseline lipid and lipoprotein values and the incidence of coronary heart disease in the Helsinki Heart Study. Am J Cardiol 1989;63(16):42H–7H.
83. Rubins HB, Robins SJ, Collins D, et al. Gemfibrozil for the secondary prevention of coronary heart disease in men with low levels of high-density lipoprotein cholesterol. veterans affairs high-density lipoprotein cholesterol intervention trial study group. N Engl J Med 1999;341(6):410–8.
84. Maki KC, Guyton JR, Orringer CE, et al. Triglyceride-lowering therapies reduce cardiovascular disease event risk in subjects with hypertriglyceridemia. J Clin Lipidol 2016;10(4):905–14.
85. Morieri ML, Shah HS, Sjaarda J, et al. PPARA polymorphism influences the cardiovascular benefit of fenofibrate in type 2 diabetes: findings from ACCORD-lipid. Diabetes 2020;69(4):771–83.
86. Pradhan AD, Paynter NP, Everett BM, et al. Rationale and design of the pemafibrate to reduce cardiovascular outcomes by reducing triglycerides in patients with diabetes (PROMINENT) study. Am Heart J 2018;206:80–93.
87. Hu Y, Hu FB, Manson JE. Marine omega-3 supplementation and cardiovascular disease: an updated meta-analysis of 13 randomized controlled trials involving 127 477 participants. J Am Heart Assoc 2019;8(19):e013543.
88. Bhatt DL, Steg PG, Miller M, et al. Cardiovascular risk reduction with icosapent ethyl for hypertriglyceridemia. N Engl J Med 2018;380(1):11–22.
89. Yokoyama M, Origasa H, Matsuzaki M, et al. Effects of eicosapentaenoic acid on major coronary events in hypercholesterolaemic patients (JELIS): a randomised open-label, blinded endpoint analysis. Lancet 2007;369(9567):1090–8.
90. Nicholls SJ, Lincoff AM, Garcia M, et al. Effect of high-dose omega-3 fatty acids vs corn oil on major adverse cardiovascular events in patients at high cardiovascular risk: the strength randomized clinical trial. JAMA 2020;324(22):2268–80.
91. Mason RP, Libby P, Bhatt DL. Emerging mechanisms of cardiovascular protection for the Omega-3 fatty acid eicosapentaenoic acid. Arterioscler Thromb Vasc Biol 2020;40(5):1135–47.
92. Schmitz J, Gouni-Berthold I. APOC-III antisense oligonucleotides: a new option for the treatment of hypertriglyceridemia. Curr Med Chem 2018;25(13):1567–76.
93. Gaudet D, Alexander VJ, Baker BF, et al. Antisense inhibition of apolipoprotein C-III in patients with hypertriglyceridemia. N Engl J Med 2015;373(5):438–47.
94. Graham MJ, Lee RG, Brandt TA, et al. Cardiovascular and metabolic effects of ANGPTL3 antisense oligonucleotides. N Engl J Med 2017;377(3):222–32.
95. Brown WV, Brunzell JD, Eckel RH, et al. Severe hypertriglyceridemia. J Clin Lipidol 2012;6(5):397–408.
96. Chaudhry R, Viljoen A, Wierzbicki AS. Pharmacological treatment options for severe hypertriglyceridemia and familial chylomicronemia syndrome. Expert Rev Clin Pharmacol 2018;11(6):589–98.
97. Capell WH, Eckel RH. Treatment of hypertriglyceridemia. Curr Diab Rep 2006;6(3):230–40.

98. Gaudet D, Brisson D, Tremblay K, et al. Targeting APOC3 in the familial chylomicronemia syndrome. N Engl J Med 2014;371(23):2200–6.

99. Witztum JL, Gaudet D, Freedman SD, et al. Volanesorsen and triglyceride levels in familial chylomicronemia syndrome. N Engl J Med 2019;381(6):531–42.

100. Diker-Cohen T, Cochran E, Gorden P, et al. Partial and generalized lipodystrophy: comparison of baseline characteristics and response to metreleptin. J Clin Endocrinol Metab 2015;100(5):1802–10.

High-Density Lipoprotein and Cardiovascular Disease—Where do We Stand?

Iulia Iatan, PhD, MD, Hong Y Choi, PhD, Jacques Genest, MD*

KEYWORDS

- High-density lipoproteins • ATP-binding cassette transporters • Cholesterol
- Atherosclerosis • Genetics

KEY POINTS

- The epidemiologic association between high-density lipoprotein cholesterol (HDL-C) and cardiovascular disease is strong and coherent.
- Strong biological plausibility for HDL as a therapeutic target.
- Mendelian randomization does not support HDL-C as a causal risk factor.
- Severe HDL deficiency can be associated with atherosclerosis.
- The clinical trial data on HDL-C raising drugs is neutral.

Abbreviations	
ATP	Adenosine triphosphate
ABCA1	ATP binding cassette transporter A1
HDL	Hidh density lipoproteins
ASCVD	Atheroscelrosit cardiovascular disease
DSC1	Desmocollin 1
RCT	Reverse cholesterol transport
LCAT	Lecithin:cholesterol acyltransferase
CETP	Cholesteryl ester transfer protein
SR-B1	Scavenger receptor B1
S1P	Sphingosine-1-phosphate
GWAS	Genome-wide association studies

INTRODUCTION. BRIEF HISTORY OF HIGH-DENSITY LIPOPROTEIN DISCOVERY, NOMENCLATURE, AND COMPLEXITY

High-density lipoproteins (HDL) were described over 50 years ago following the identification of lipoproteins by thin layer chromatography and density ultracentrifugation.

Research Institute of the McGill University Health Center, 1001 Decarie Boulevard, Bloc E, EM12212, Montreal, Quebec H4A 3J1, Canada
* Corresponding author. Research Institute of the McGill University Health Center, 1001 Decarie Boulevard, Bloc E, EM12212, Montreal, Quebec H4A 3J1, Canada.
E-mail address: jacques.genest@mcgill.ca

Endocrinol Metab Clin N Am 51 (2022) 557–572
https://doi.org/10.1016/j.ecl.2022.01.003
0889-8529/22/© 2022 Elsevier Inc. All rights reserved.

An inverse link between coronary artery disease (CAD)—myocardial infarctions (MI)—and the cholesterol content of HDL was soon established, and the strength of this association was confirmed in multiple, independent studies. The Emerging Risk Factor Collaborative Studies firmly established HDL cholesterol (HDL-C) as a strong, coherent, and independent cardiovascular risk factor.[1] Basic research into the putative protective effects of HDL revealed pleiotropic effects in cellular and plasma membrane cholesterol homeostasis, modulation of inflammation and oxidative stress, arterial endothelial function, endothelial progenitor cell proliferation, and apoptosis. These data markedly strengthened the role of HDL in preventing atherosclerosis. Drugs were soon developed to increase HDL-C.

Yet, these findings have not translated into clinical benefit. Here, the authors review the epidemiology of HDL and cardiovascular disease (CVD), discuss the effects of HDL on the pathogenesis of atherosclerosis, review the genetic disorders of HDL and their relation to CVD, and the clinical trials conducted thus far. They finally discuss future directions for translational research into the biology of HDL and potential clinical applications.

Refinements in analytical techniques signifies that HDL particles have become increasingly complex. It is important to understand the extraordinary diversity of HDL particles, their content, and dynamic interactions in plasma, lymph, and vascular wall environments. As such, defining HDL requires a deeper look at measurement and analytical techniques. Clinicians and epidemiologists have focused on the cholesterol content (free cholesterol and cholesteryl esters) within HDL. Measurement techniques for HDL particles have evolved considerably since the days of ultracentrifugation and the measurement of cholesterol and triglycerides.[2] Briefly, preparative and analytical techniques examine HDL by size and density in a salt solution, by chromatography or magnetic resonance, and by charge and size in 2-dimensional electrophoresis (**Fig. 1**).

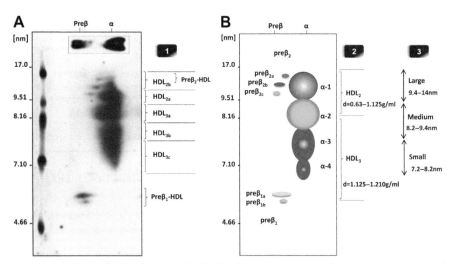

Fig. 1. Analytical techniques for HDL lipids. (*A-1*) Representative 2-dimensional gradient gel electrophoresis where HDL particles are separated by charge (horizontal dimension) and by size (vertical dimension). HDL particle size varies between 7 and 17 nm; lipid-poor (nascent) HDL particles comprising mostly apoA-I and some phospholipids are termed pre-ß HDL. (*B*) Stylized diagram showing discrete HDL particles separated in HDL2 and HDL3 (*B-2*) or by large, medium, and small HDL particles when analyzed by nuclear magnetic resonance (NMR) (*B-3*). (*Modified from* Hafiane A, Genest J. High density lipoproteins: Measurement techniques and potential biomarkers of cardiovascular risk. BBA Clin. 2015 Jan 31;3:175–88.)

Although the time-honored definition includes a specific density range with respect to plasma (1.063<d < 1.210 g/mL), size (5–20 nm), and the presence of apolipoprotein A-I (apoA-I), HDL particles carry a very complex proteome with at least 90 separate proteins that are generally recognized by most research laboratories and perhaps as many as greater than 800 different proteins thus far identified.[3] The HDL proteome may shift toward an inflammatory phenotype, depending on the milieu created by such circumstances such as acute coronary syndromes and inflammatory diseases.[4–6] The HDL lipidome is also very complex. Although cholesterol and cholesteryl esters are a major source of lipids, comprising ~50% of lipids, sphingolipids, especially sphingomyelin and several species of phospholipids (phosphatidyl serine and phosphatidyl choline), lysophospholipids, and sulfatides are found.[7] Serna and colleagues identified 172 lipid species within HDL particles.[8] Lastly, the identification of circulating small and circular RNAs that are carried within HDL particles and influence their metabolic fate expands their potential physiologic roles[9,10] (**Table 1**). Cellular export of microRNAs (miRNAs) to HDL is regulated, at least in part, by sphingomyelinase. Interestingly, the miRNA profile varies distinctly according to specific physiologic states such as atherosclerosis, inflammation and hyperlipidemia.

It must be noted that "Reconstituted" HDL particles used in clinical trials are composed of a fixed molar (or mass) ratio of apoA-I, phosphatidyl choline, and free cholesterol. These particles may exhibit some of the characteristics of HDL particles in terms of density and electrophoretic mobility, but likely do not exist in nature, nor are they likely to present the 3-dimensional configuration of its protein, apoA-I, essential for various cellular interactions.

HIGH-DENSITY LIPOPROTEIN METABOLISM

The liver and small intestine are the principal sites for the generation of HDL particles. The HDL metabolic pathway may be the major route by which cholesterol is delivered to cells that require the sterol nucleus for hormone synthesis (adrenals, mammary glands, ovaries, testicles) and rapidly dividing tissues requiring cholesterol for membrane integrity (**Fig. 2**)[11]. This pathway is distinct from the triglyceride transport pathway that uses chylomicrons and very-low-density lipoprotein (VLDL), respectively, and delivers fatty acids to muscle and adipose tissues. The HDL pathway is intricately linked to plasma VLDL metabolism. During lipolysis of VLDL triglycerides via lipoprotein lipase, there is exchange of apolipoproteins (especially apo-I, apo E, and apo CII) between VLDL and HDL particles, and it is thought that some of the phospholipids are also transferred onto nascent HDL particles. Importantly, there is an equimolar exchange of cholesteryl esters from HDL onto VLDL and IDL mediated by cholesteryl ester transfer protein (CETP) such that HDL can transfer cholesterol back to the liver, in exchange for triglycerides. This leads to the formation of HDL particles, depleted in cholesterol and enriched in triglycerides, which are then degraded by hepatic lipase (HL). These lipid-depleted HDL particles can continue their cycle of cellular cholesterol uptake.

A second pathway, that of "reverse cholesterol transport (RCT)" is a mechanism by which excess cellular cholesterol from peripheral cells (including lipid laden macrophages and smooth muscle cells in the arterial wall) is transferred onto lipid-poor nascent HDL particles containing apoA-I and delivered to the liver for secretion as bile acids.

HDL biogenesis, or the formation of HDL particles, occurs when lipid-free or lipid-poor apoA-I comes in contact with the ATP-binding cassette transporter A-1 (ABCA1). The transfer of plasma membrane phospholipids onto apoA-I alters its 3-

Table 1
Characteristics and components of high-density lipoprotein

Origin	Density (g/mL)	Size (nm)
Major: liver, intestine Minor: macrophage foam cells	1.063–1.210	5–20
PROTEIN	LIPIDS	RNA
40%–55% weight	[Chol] 0.9–1.6 mmol/L (35–62 mg/dL) [Trig] 0.1–0.2 (mmol/L) (9–18 mg/dL)	miRNA, circular RNA
Major: ApoA-I, A-II	• Cholesteryl esters • Triglycerides • Free cholesterolphosphatidyletanolamine • Phosphatidylinositol • Sulfatides • Phosphatidylcholine • Lysophosphatidylcholine sphingomyelin	From multiple cell types
At least 90 proteins reliably identified in HDL particles[3]	At least 171 lipid species identified in HDL[8]	>100[10]

dimensional structure; cholesterol lipidation seems to occur by lateral transfer on the plasma membrane.[12] These particles become substrate for the ABCG1 transporter present on many cell types including hepatic, macrophages, and vascular endothelial cells. Circulating HDL particles undergo multiple changes, especially the enzymatic conversion of free cholesterol into cholesteryl esters by lecithin:cholesterol acyltransferase (LCAT), the transfer of these cholesteryl esters onto VLDL particles in exchange for triglycerides by CETP. Multiple enzymes, such as sphingomyelinase and other phospholipases, alter the phospholipid moiety of HDL, thus altering some functional aspect. The scavenger receptor B1 (SR-B1) mediates the bidirectional movement of cholesterol between HDL and cells. Here, the authors review the pleiotropic effects of HDL particles on pathologic processes such as atherosclerosis, inflammation, and infections, thus providing biological plausibility for targeting this pathway. Casting doubt on the protective role of HDL, Frikke-Schmidt and colleagues published the first of many reports using Mendelian randomization, showing that the relationship between genetic variants of the ABCA1 gene associated with decreased HDL-C levels and atherosclerosis ASCVD is not robust.[13] Clinical trials aimed at raising HDL-C and further described later also failed to change relevant clinical outcomes such as major adverse cardiovascular events. A more granular picture thus emerges that HDL-C might be a biomarker of cardiovascular health that does not reflect the many biological functions of HDL particles. The future in HDL research and translational medicine will therefore consist in identifying reproducible and upscalable biomarkers of HDL function, novel pharmacologic agents that promote the beneficial effects of HDL function and alter clinical outcomes.

MECHANISMS BY WHICH HIGH-DENSITY LIPOPROTEIN MIGHT BE ATHEROPROTECTIVE

HDL plays key roles in pathways related to the development of atherosclerotic disease including RCT, antioxidation and antiinflammation, endothelial function, as well as in

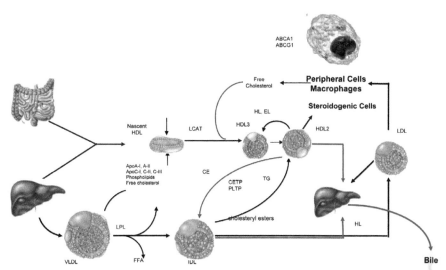

Fig. 2. HDL metabolism in plasma. The intestine and the liver are the main source of HDL particles (*blue arrows*). Nascent HDL particles (lipid-poor apoA-I phospholipid complexes) come in contact with cells expressing the ABCA1 transporter, which acts predominantly as a phospholipid transfer protein from the plasma membrane onto nascent HDL. Cholesterol efflux requires ABCA1 but seems to occur in distinct lipid rafts within the membrane. Further lipidation is mediated via ABCG1. In plasma, several lipases, including LCAT, mediate the conversion of cholesterol into cholesteryl esters, increasing the size of HDL. HDL cholesterol can be transferred via CETP onto triglyceride-rich lipoproteins in exchange for triglyceride. HDL can also bind to hepatocytes via the SR-B1 receptor. Hepatic cholesterol can then be converted to bile acids. The reverse cholesterol transport pathway (*red arrows*) proposes that HDL particles can also remove cholesterol from cells such as macrophages or smooth muscle cells within arterial wall and return it to the liver for disposal. (*Modified from* Genest J, Libby P. Chapter 48: Lipoprotein Disorders and Cardiovascular Disease. In: Zipes DP, Libby P, Bonow RO, Mann DL, Tomaselli GF, and Braunwald E. eds. Braunwald's Heart Diseas: A Textbook if Cardiovascular Medicine. 11th[th] ed. Elsevier; 2019:960-982.)

other physiologic systems including immune system modulation, cellular apoptosis, and endothelial progenitor cell homeostasis (**Fig. 3**). It must be kept in mind that many physiologic effects described here have been studied in in-vitro systems and the physiologic relevance is, for the most part, not fully understood.

The RCT pathway is thought to be the major pathway by which HDL prevents atherosclerosis; this might be because it is the most extensively studied. It must be noted that HDL-mediated cellular cholesterol efflux is only weakly correlated with the cholesterol mass of HDL and depends more on the HDL proteome and lipidome. To exert antiatherosclerosis effects, plasma circulating HDL must cross the endothelium, to mediate cholesterol efflux from macrophages and smooth muscle cells and exert antioxidant and antiinflammatory functions. Transendothelial HDL transport is a highly regulated process involving several receptor and enzymes, including SR-B1, ABCA1, and ABCG1 transporters, as well as endothelial lipase. Furthermore, HDL helps maintain endothelial barrier integrity by stimulating the proliferation and migration of endothelial progenitor and endothelial cells, by promoting intercellular junction closure to prevent transmigration of inflammatory cells, and by enhancing nitric oxide and prostacyclin production.[14–17]

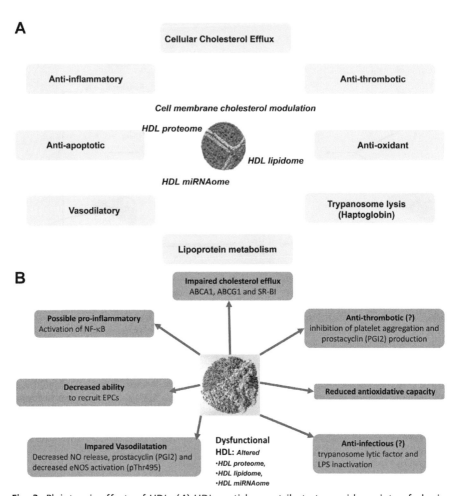

Fig. 3. Pleiotropic effects of HDL. (*A*) HDL particles contribute to a wide variety of physiologic processes. Individual components of HDL (proteins, lipids and RNA), as well as the ability to modulate plasma membrane cholesterol content mediate these effects. (*B*) Dysfunctional HDL are encountered in acute and chronic inflammatory states, diabetes, and metabolic syndrome and may contribute to the pathogenesis of atherosclerosis. (*Modified from* Schwertani A, Choi HY, Genest J. HDLs and the pathogenesis of atherosclerosis. Curr Opin Cardiol. 2018 May;33(3):311-316.)

From large population studies, the potential role of HDL as an important modulator of inflammation is emerging. Madsen and colleagues examined the incidence of autoimmune disease in 117,341 subjects from the general population of the Copenhagen Heart study and concluded that a low HDL-C level is associated with a high risk of autoimmune disease.[18] Although causality cannot be inferred, this finding suggests that HDL may modulate the emergence of inflammatory diseases. Studies of patients with systemic inflammation, including acute coronary syndromes, have revealed a shift of HDL proteins toward an inflammatory phenotype. It follows that these "altered HDL" may become dysfunctional and thus contribute to atherosclerosis disease progression, rather than its prevention (see **Fig. 3**B).[4–6,18,19]

Plasma from patients with acute inflammatory conditions (eg, acute coronary syndromes) or chronic inflammatory conditions reveal a striking shift in the proteome and lipidome of HDL particles, especially oxidized phospholipids, and these lead to dysfunctional HDL particles that cause—rather than prevent—atherosclerosis. ApoA-I and nascent HDL modulate plasma membrane function and may alter the composition of membrane microdomains, such as lipid rafts. Most cells contain these domains, including immune cells that express key receptors involved in their activation. However, dysfunctional HDL particles may lead to the disruption of B- and T-cell receptors and Toll-like receptors and subsequent activation of monocytes and macrophages and cytokine production.[20,21]

HDL-associated sphingosine-1-phosphate (S1P) has also multiple roles in regulating the immune response. S1P seems to have an immunoregulatory role during infection by reducing proinflammatory cytokine secretion by dendritic cells and favoring the production of regulatory cytokines such as interleukin-10. S1P was further shown to inhibit macrophage activation in response to TLR2 ligation and nitric oxide–induced damage and to influence dendritic cell trafficking, lymphocyte trafficking, and antigen presentation.[20] Deficient or dysfunctional HDL might lose its immunomodulatory properties or participate in inflammatory reactions, thus tipping the balance toward autoimmunity in susceptible individuals.

EPIDEMIOLOGY AND GENETICS OF HIGH-DENSITY LIPOPROTEIN IN RELATION TO CARDIOVASCULAR DISEASE

To date, HDL-C has been evaluated as a risk marker in multiple studies, including 68 long-term population-based studies involving more than 302,430 individuals from Europe and North America.[1] In multivariate models adjusted for both nonlipid and lipid risk factors, HDL-C was shown to be inversely correlated with CAD events. For every 0.39 mmol/L increase in HDL-C concentration, the risk of a CAD event was reduced by 22% (95% confidence interval [CI], 18%–26%).[15] Despite this, after decades of belief that HDL protected from atherosclerosis, the "HDL hypothesis" has been put into question, as there still lacks unequivocal evidence of a beneficial effect of HDL-raising treatments on cardiovascular end points.[22,23] This was demonstrated in several studies, including a meta-analysis of 95 clinical trials involving greater than 300,000 individuals, suggested that on-trial HDL-C concentrations were not significantly related to CAD events.[24] Investigations using statins also showed that by aggressively lowering LDL-C (<2.0 mmol/L), HDL-C levels no longer predicted residual cardiovascular risk.[25] These findings, combined with Mendelian randomization data on genetic HDL deficiency states, stirs controversy on the validity of HDL-C as a therapeutic target.[13] Mendelian randomization principles assume that the existence of a causal relationship between HDL-C and CAD would imply that association between a gene variant and HDL-C levels will translate into the CAD risk expected from the effect on HDL-C. Using this approach, however, several genetic studies[26–28] have casted doubt on a direct protective effect of HDL-C on atherosclerotic risk, as gene variants affecting HDL-C levels do not necessarily correlate with a corresponding effect on heart disease. For example, subjects with genetic forms of HDL deficiency, such as apoA-I Milano, or some mutations at ABCA1 and LCAT, are not necessarily associated with premature CAD, whereas mutations in the HL or the CETP genes—leading to high HDL-C—may not be protective.[29] In some cases, elevated HDL-C levels are paradoxically associated with increased cardiovascular and overall mortality, suggesting a U-shaped relationship between mortality and HDL-C concentrations.[30] As such, these observations indicate that the relationship between CAD and HDL-C remains more complex than originally thought.

INHERITED DISORDERS OF HIGH-DENSITY LIPOPROTEIN METABOLISM AND THEIR RELATIONSHIP TO ATHEROSCLEROSIS

It must be emphasized that plasma levels of HDL-C are highly related to lifestyle. Yet, HDL-C concentrations are also under strong genetic control, with heritability estimates ranging between 40% and 80% across multiple populations. Genetic determinants include both rare large-effect variants and common small-effect variants.[28,31] As such, several monogenic disorders have been described, with very low (<5th percentile age-sex matched) or high (>90th percentile age-sex matched) HDL-C levels. Genes implicated in monogenic disorders associated with these low HDL-C concentrations include *APOA1*, *LCAT*, and *ABCA1*, whereas those associated with elevated HDL-C levels include *CETP*, *SCARB1*, and *LIPC*.[28,32,33,55]

Low High-Density Lipoprotein Cholesterol States

Apolipoprotein A-I deficiency

ApoA-I is the main apolipoprotein of HDL, accounting for 70% of the protein mass. Primary defects affecting the production of HDL particles can be caused by variants in the apoAI-apoCIII-apoAIV-apoAV gene complex. Complete apoA-I deficiency resulting from homozygous or compound heterozygous mutations is a rare condition leading to undetectable plasma apoA-I levels accompanied by tuberoeruptive xanthomas, marked decrease in HDL-C, and an increased risk of premature ASCVD. Heterozygous mutations within apoA-I have also been described, with at least 47 variants affecting apoA-I structure, some leading to a marked reduction in apoA-I and HDL-C levels, and concomitant coronary artery disease, whereas others with low HDL but no incidence of heart disease. In line with these observations, some rare variants of apoA-I, such as apoA-I Milano and apoA-I Paris, are paradoxically associated with low HDL-C concentrations and reduced risk of ASCVD and longevity.[34]

ATP-binding cassette transporter A-1 deficiency

The identification of ABCA1 as the rate-limiting step in HDL biogenesis and the first step of the RCT pathway has triggered a great deal of investigation into its role as a genetic factor in atherosclerosis. Tangier disease (TD) is a rare form of severe HDL deficiency due to homozygous or compound heterozygous mutations at the *ABCA1* gene. The major biochemical abnormality is a near-absence of HDL-C due to impaired cholesterol efflux to lipid-free Apo-I, mild to moderate increased triglyceride levels, and a marked decrease in LDL-C. The association of TD and premature CAD is however tenuous and has been subject to considerable debate over the years, as ABCA1 deficiency is not clearly associated with an increased risk of CVD, possibly due to low LDL-C levels. In individuals with heterozygous ABCA1 mutations, however, the association with CAD seems less ambiguous.[35] Although the risk of heart disease in individuals with heterozygous ABCA1 mutations was increased 3-fold compared with unaffected controls, a more recent study also showed that carriers of 1 or 2 loss-of-function *ABCA1* mutations with significantly low HDL-C but similar LDL-C levels displayed a larger atherosclerotic burden compared with their unaffected relatives.[36] In contrast, additional insights into the effects of ABCA1 genetic variation on CAD have been described by Frikke-Schmidt in Mendelian randomization analyses of the Copenhagen City Heart Study; this revealed that lower plasma HDL-C levels owing to heterozygous, rare *ABCA1* loss-of-function mutations were not associated with increased risk of CVD end points.[13]

Lecithin:cholesterol acyltransferase deficiency
Naturally occurring mutations in LCAT are another rare cause of low HDL-C levels. Classic homozygous or familial LCAT deficiency results from a complete loss of LCAT activity, whereas Fish-eye disease (partial LCAT deficiency) is associated with a change in the substrate specificity of LCAT that retains its activity to esterify free cholesterol of apoB-containing lipoproteins but becomes inactive toward HDL. This property leads to higher LDL-C levels in Fish-eye disease and thus acceleration of atherosclerosis, relative to complete LCAT deficiency, where a decreased risk of CAD has been observed.[29] As such, the absence of an association between homozygous LCAT deficiency and increased risk of CVD has been attributed to concomitant low levels of serum LDL-C, as well as an increase in endothelial nitric oxide production. Of note however, in Mendelian randomization studies, Haase and colleagues investigated the effect of S208 T, a homozygous loss-of-function variant of LCAT, in 2 Danish cohorts. The investigators identified that a 13% decrease in plasma HDL-C levels predicts an 18% increased risk of MI but genetically decreased HDL-C concentrations, associated with the S208 T variant, did not.[26]

High High-Density Lipoprotein States

Cholesteryl ester transfer protein *deficiency*
  Complete loss of CETP activity associated with homozygous *CETP* gene variants leads to increased HDL-C and a reduction in LDL-C, due to impaired transfer of cholesteryl esters from HDL to LDL. Based on epidemiologic observations, this mechanism of action was expected to reduce atherosclerosis by generating antiatherogenic lipoprotein profiles. Yet, this promise has not been realized in clinical outcome trials of CETP inhibitors. In fact, a recent meta-analysis of 11 randomized controlled trials examined the effects of CETP inhibitors on major cardiovascular events and all-cause mortality, showing a nonsignificant reduction in the risk of nonfatal myocardial infarction (-7%) and death from cardiovascular causes (-8%).[37] As such, despite the limited cardiovascular benefits of CETP inhibitors and their off-target toxic effects, data from multiple large human genetic studies and animal investigations suggest that CETP deficiency is protective against atherosclerosis.[38,39] Moreover, several loss-of-function SNPs in the *CETP* gene that are associated with increased HDL-C and concomitant decreases in TG and LDL-C are also associated with corresponding risk reductions in CAD and MI.

Hepatic lipase and endothelial lipase deficiency
Complete HL deficiency due to rare loss-of-function variants in *LIPC* alleles is associated with 2- to 3-fold increase in HDL-C and ApoA-I concentrations.[29] Concurrently however, it is also associated with elevations in apoB-containing lipoproteins, as well as atherogenic remnant particles, explaining the increase in premature CHD in some families with HL deficiency. Similarly, endothelial lipase (EL) deficiency also induces hyperalphalipoproteinemia and increases HDL-C, but without decreasing MI risk. Voight and colleagues performed 2 Mendelian randomization analyses, using both an SNP in *EL* (LIPG Asn396Ser) and a genetic score consisting of 14 common SNPs known to exclusively associate with increased HDL-C. Both approaches failed to show any association with a reduced risk of MI.[27] These data challenge the concept that raising plasma HDL-C will uniformly translate into CVD risk reduction.

Scavenger receptor B1 deficiency
SR-B1 mediates the selective uptake of CE from HDL into hepatocytes and steroidogenic tissues. The atheroprotective effects of SR-BI are therefore primarily attributable to its role in cholesterol efflux from lipid-laden macrophages to HDL and in the delivery

of HDL CE to the liver. Interestingly though, SR-B1 knockout mice exhibit increased atherosclerosis despite having higher levels of HDL-C, a process that was attributed to a critical block in the RCT to the liver (see **Fig. 2**). In humans, several studies have described genetic *SCARB1* variants associated with HDL-C levels. In a kindred with the P297S missense variant in *SCARB1*, carriers showed an increase in HDL-C levels, although no differences in carotid intima-media thickness were observed. Similarly, a recent study showed that elevated HDL-C due to pathogenic variants in *SCARB1* carriers were not predictive of CAD.[40]

Genome-wide association studies and complex genetic determinants of high-density lipoprotein cholesterol

Genome-wide association studies (GWAS) have previously confirmed multiple loci that modulate HDL-C in man, as well as identified novel genomic regions for HDL-C.[29,41] The Global Lipid Genetics Consortium Collaboration GWAS initially identified 47 loci primarily associated with HDL-C levels in more than 100,000 individuals, with a subsequent additional 30 loci associated with HDL-C found in 196,000 individuals.[42] The strongest associations included common variants in *ABCA1*, *CETP*, *LCAT*, *LIPG*, and *LPL* genes and in the *apoAI–apoCIII–apoAIV– apoAV* gene cluster. These common variants can be present in up to 50% of the general population, in contrast with rare variants in the same genes underlying monogenic dyslipidemias, occurring in less than 1% of the population. Furthermore, despite statistical significant associations between these common genetic variants and HDL-C plasma concentrations, cumulatively, they only account for a small proportion (10%–15%) of the total variance in serum HDL-C levels.

Why have current clinical trials of high-density lipoprotein cholesterol raising failed?

The "HDL hypothesis" postulates that the association between low HDL-C and ASCVD should provide a therapeutic goal, namely, that raising HDL-C would be beneficial. However, the effects of a therapeutic modality that exclusively raises HDL-C (without affecting other lipoproteins of pathways) has proved elusive. To date, therefore, clinicians had to rely on inference from clinical trials to assess whether raising HDL-C decreases ASCVD outcomes.

FIBRATES

The fibric acid derivatives, or fibrates, activate peroxisome proliferator-activated receptor alpha (PPARα) and enhance lipoprotein lipase activity, in part, by decreasing the expression of its inhibitor, apoCIII. This, in turn, decreases plasma triglyceride levels and raises HDL-C. Early trials using bezafibrate or gemfibrozil yielded positive results on some components of major cardiac adverse events (MACE). However, in the statin era, the FIELD (Fenofibrate Intervention and Event Lowering in Diabetes) and ACCORD (Action to Control Cardiovascular Risk in Diabetes—also with fenofibrate) trials failed to reduce cardiovascular outcomes in diabetic patients, despite a significant increase in HDL-C.[38,39] Newer PPARα and γ, such as aleglitazar, also failed to change outcomes in diabetic patients. Pemafibrate is a selective PPARα modulator with quantitatively better triglyceride lowering and HDL-C raising than fenofibrate.[43] It remains to be determined however if, in combination with statin therapy, this will decrease MACE.

NIACIN

Niacin has been used for over 60 years to treat lipoprotein disorders and was used in early clinical trials. The AIM-HIGH (Atherothrombosis Intervention in Metabolic

Syndrome with Low HDL Cholesterol/High Triglyceride and Impact on Global Health Outcomes) was a relatively modest trial of 3300 patients with ASCVD and residual dyslipidemia that did not meet its primary outcome of reducing ASCVD risk. The large HPS2-THRIVE (Heart Protection Study-2 Treatment of HDL to Reduce the Incidence of Vascular Events) randomized 25,673 high-risk patients taking simvastatin to placebo or the combination of niacin and laropiprant (an inhibitor of prostaglandin D2), thought to mediate the cutaneous flushing reaction seen with niacin. Although no beneficial effects on ASCVD risk were observed, an increase in complications led to the withdrawal of the combination drug and a decrease in the use of niacin clinically.

CHOLESTERYL ESTER TRANSFER PROTEIN INHIBITORS

Inhibitors of CETP were developed to increase HDL-C, by interfering with the exchange of cholesteryl esters from HDL particles to triglyceride-rich lipoproteins in exchange for triglycerides in an equimolar ratio. Trials with torcetrapib, dalcetrapib, and evacetrapib ended because of toxicity or futility.[68] The REVEAL trial (Heart Protection-3 Randomized Evaluation of the Effects of Anacetrapib Through Lipid-modification) randomized 30,449 patients with ASCVD on atorvastatin with atherosclerotic vascular disease who were receiving intensive atorvastatin therapy to placebo or anacetrapib,100 mg/d. After a median follow-up of 4 years, the primary outcome was reduced by an absolute rate of 1.0% (rate ratio, 0.91; 95% CI 0.85–0.97; $P = .004$). HDL-C increased by 104% and non-HDL-C decreased by 18% (0,44 mmol/L or 17 mg/dL). Although there were no differences in the risk of death, cancer, or serious adverse events, this very modest benefit was likely explained by the slight reduction in non-HDL-C.[37,44,45] Obicetrapib is currently investigated as a lipid-modifying drug, mostly for patients intolerant to statins.

APOLIPOPROTEIN A-I INFUSIONS

Based on animal models, it was proposed that the intravenous injection of proteolipo-somes containing apoA-I combined with a fixed molar ratio of phospholipids—usually phosphatidylcholine (lecithin) and free cholesterol ("reconstituted" HDL particle)—would either stabilize atherosclerotic plaques in acute coronary syndromes or promote the regression of established plaques. Unfortunately, this approach has not met clinical success. It is likely that the apoA-I provided in this fashion transiently enters the plasma apoA-I pool but this effect seems physiologically insufficient.[46–48]

APOLIPOPROTEIN A-I MIMETICS

Novel agents that increase apoA-I protein or function include apoA-I mimetics, HDL mimetics, and RVX 208 (Apabetalone), a bromodomain and extraterminal (BET) antagonist that raises the transcriptional regulation of apoA-I, showed promise in animal models and early phase clinical trials. However, in the BETonMACE trial, Apabetalone failed to meet its primary end point.[49]

Overall, this brief overview of clinical trials shows the futility of raising HDL-C as a therapeutic target. It is now time to put to rest the "HDL hypothesis" and consider plasma levels of HDL-C as a biomarker of cardiovascular health, rather than a goal of therapy.

WHERE DO WE GO FROM HERE?

There is agreement that modulation of HDL functions for therapeutic purposes shows considerable promise. The future lies in the identification of novel biomarkers of HDL function that predict outcomes and in that of new targets that act in the arterial *suben-dothelium*. It is well known that ApoA-I accumulates in the arterial subendothelial layer[50] and subsequently becomes trapped. Therefore, developing biomarkers of HDL biogenesis (the ability of apoA-I or lipid-poor HDL to remove cellular cholesterol) that can be scaled up to a clinical test will be essential.[51,52] There are however challenges to developing these biomarkers of HDL function, such as cell-based cholesterol efflux and inflammatory indices mediated by HDL, as compared with the current static biochemical measurements. The standardization, validation, and large-throughput commercialization can be considered important barriers to their implementation into clinical practice. As of now, the validity of these measurements and their commercial availability remain obstacles to a realistic transition to clinical medicine.[17]

The failure of translating the HDL hypothesis into clinical benefit has demonstrated that HDL-C does not necessarily reflect HDL function. This has led us to rethink of *the primary* HDL function contributing to cardiovascular health. ASCVD is a chronic inflammatory process initiated by cholesterol deposition in the subendothelial space of arteries; therefore, removal of cholesterol accumulated in the atherosclerotic plaque is believed to be the most beneficial effect of HDL. The formation and maturation of HDL particles are coupled with cellular cholesterol removal occurring through cholesterol efflux pathways, and thus the HDL biogenic process has been reviewed as the most clinically relevant therapeutic target for the development of HDL-directed therapies. There are 4 major cholesterol efflux pathways, and the one mediated by ABCA1 is responsible for the formation of nascent HDL particles (**Fig. 4**). Although ABCA1-and ABCG1-dependent cholesterol efflux are unidirectional in the removal of excess cellular cholesterol, SR-BI and aqueous diffusion are involved in both cholesterol influx as well as efflux (see **Fig. 4**). Although the ABCA1- and ABCG1-dependent unidirectional pathways have long been attractive targets to develop drugs promoting cholesterol efflux, it has been challenging to identify druggable molecular targets in the pathways. Recent efforts to characterize plasma membrane microdomains involved in ABCA1-dependent cholesterol efflux allowed us to identify desmocollin-1 (DSC1)

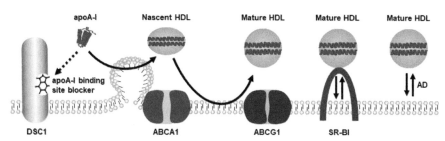

Fig. 4. The HDL biogenic process and four major cholesterol efflux pathways. ABCA1 creates a plasma membrane microdomain to facilitate efflux of cellular phospholipids and cholesterol to lipid-free or lipid-poor apolipoproteins such as apoA-I. The lipidated apoA-I is called a nascent HDL particle. An apoA-I binding protein DSC1 sequesters apoA-I to prevent the formation of nascent HDL; therefore, blocking of the apoA-I binding site in DSC1 promotes ABCA1-dependent HDL formation. Nascent HDL particles are matured by acquiring additional cholesterol via ABCG1-dependent cholesterol efflux. ABCG1 facilitates cholesterol efflux by increasing the pool of cholesterol available for efflux in the outer leaflet of the plasma membrane. Matured HDL particles are able to acquire more cholesterol via SR-BI–dependent cholesterol efflux and aqueous diffusion. These 2 pathways are however involved in both efflux and influx of cholesterol, and thus it is difficult to therapeutically modulate them.

as a negative regulator of the ABCA1 pathway.[53] The DSC1 action mechanism was to bind apoA-I so as to prevent apoA-I lipidation by ABCA1. The apoA-I binding site in DSC1 was highly druggable and was successfully targeted with small molecules.[54] The potency and efficacy of a small molecule, docetaxel, in promoting ABCA1-dependent cholesterol efflux have suggested that the ABCA1 pathway may be therapeutically modulated.[54] In addition to small molecules, peptides and antibodies may also be developed to inhibit apoA-I–DSC1 interactions, proposing DSC1 as a viable therapeutic target. As seen in **Fig. 4**, nascent HDL particles can acquire additional cholesterol via the other cholesterol efflux pathways, suggesting that identification of druggable molecular targets in the ABCA1 pathway may provide us with new opportunities to develop HDL-directed therapies.

Another issue of consideration with therapeutic strategies aimed at enhancing atheroprotective HDL function is the absence of methods to assess HDL function in clinical practice. Although cell-based cholesterol efflux assays are useful research tools, they are not only far from clinical practice but also different from measuring cholesterol efflux in the atherosclerotic plaque. It will be ideal to identify circulating biomarkers that directly reflect cholesterol efflux activity in the plaque, but such studies have not been reported due to lack of drugs with which such studies can be performed. DSC1 is abundantly expressed in the atherosclerotic plaque,[53] and docetaxel is an efficient DSC1-targeting agent, thus it will be interesting to investigate if administration of docetaxel reduces atherosclerosis and releases lipid and/or inflammatory biomarkers into the circulation.

In conclusion, the future lies in the identification of new druggable targets in cholesterol efflux pathways in the atherosclerotic plaque along with discovery of biomarkers that can accurately predict atheroprotective HDL function. Development of DSC1-targeting strategies may be a good starting point.

CLINICS CARE POINTS

- A low HDL-C should trigger the search for a suboptimal lifestyle (obesity, lack of exercise, poorly controlled diabetes).
- Patients should be counseled that their low HDL-C in itself is not a reason for treatment with medications.
- Rare forms of HDL deficiency should be evaluated in a specialized lipid clinic.
- Targeting HDL function remains a sound therapeutic avenue but will require rigorous clinical outcomes.

DISCLOSURE

J. Genest and H. Choi: funded by a project grant from the Canadian Institutes of Health Research on Desmocollin 1 (DSC1) and atherosclerosis (PJT-165924). J. Genest and H. Choi have filed Patent Cooperation Treaty (PCT) and United States patent applications entitled "Desmocollin 1 Inhibitors for the Prevention or Treatment of atherosclerosis" (PCT/CA2018/050,669 and US application no. 16/619,789). I. Iatan: no disclosures.

REFERENCES

1. Emerging Risk Factors Collaboration, Di Angelantonio E, Sarwar N, Perry P, et al. Major lipids, apolipoproteins, and risk of vascular disease. JAMA 2009;302: 1993–2000.

2. Hafiane A, Genest J. High Density Lipoproteins: Measurement Techniques and Potential Biomarkers of Cardiovascular Risk. BBA Clin 2015;3:175–88.
3. Davidson S. Available at: https://homepages.uc.edu/~davidswm/HDLproteome. html. Accessed October 2021.
4. Vaisar T, Pennathur S, Green PS, et al. Shotgun proteomics implicates protease inhibition and complement activation in the antiinflammatory properties of HDL. J Clin Invest 2007;117:746–56.
5. de la Llera Moya M, McGillicuddy FC, Hinkle CC, et al. Inflammation modulates human HDL composition and function in vivo. Atherosclerosis 2012;222:390–4.
6. Alwaili K, Bailey D, Awan Z, et al. The HDL proteome in acute coronary syndromes shifts to an inflammatory profile. Biochim Biophys Acta 2012;1821: 405–15.
7. Kontush A, Lhomme M, Chapman MJ. Unraveling the complexities of the HDL lipidome. J Lipid Res 2013;54:2950–63.
8. Serna J, García-Seisdedos D, Alcázar A, et al. Quantitative lipidomic analysis of plasma and plasma lipoproteins using MALDI-TOF mass spectrometry. Chem Phys Lipids 2015;189:7–18.
9. Rayner KJ, Esau CC, Hussain FN, et al. Inhibition of miR-33a/b in non-human primates raises plasma HDL and lowers VLDL triglycerides. Nature 2011;478(7369): 404–7.
10. Vickers KC, Michell DL. HDL-small RNA Export, Transport, and Functional Delivery in Atherosclerosis. Curr Atheroscler Rep 2021;23(7):38.
11. Genest J, Libby P. Chapter 48: Lipoprotein Disorders and CAD and Guidelines: Management of Lipid. In: Braunwald E, Libby P, Zipes D, et al, editors. Braunwald's heart disease 11th Edition. New York: Saunders; 2019.
12. Iatan I, Bailey D, Ruel I, et al. Membrane microdomains modulate oligomeric ABCA1 function: impact on apoAI-mediated lipid removal and phosphatidylcholine biosynthesis. J Lipid Res 2011;52(11):2043–55, 21846716.
13. Frikke-Schmidt R. Genetic variation in the ABCA1 gene, HDL cholesterol, and risk of ischemic heart disease in the general population. Atherosclerosis 2010;208(2): 305–16.
14. Jang E, Robert J, Rohrer L, et al. Transendothelial transport of lipoproteins. Atherosclerosis 2020;315:111–25.
15. Rosenson RS, Brewer HB, Ansell BJ, et al. Dysfunctional HDL and atherosclerotic cardiovascular disease. Sci Rep 2020;10(1):19223.
16. Robert J, Osto Elena, Arnold von Eckardstein. The Endothelium Is Both a Target and a Barrier of HDL's Protective Functions. Cells 2021;10(5):1041. PMID: 33924941.
17. Allard-Ratick MP, Kindya BR, Khambhati J, et al. HDL: Fact, fiction, or function? HDL cholesterol and cardiovascular risk. Eur J Prev Cardiol 2021;28(2):166–73.
18. Annema W, von Eckardstein A. Dysfunctional high-density lipoproteins in coronary heart disease: implications for diagnostics and therapy. Transl Res 2016; 173:30–57.
19. Madsen CM, Varbo A, Nordestgaard B. Low HDL cholesterol and high risk of autoimmune disease: two population-based cohort studies including 117341 individuals. Clin Chem 2019;65:644–52.
20. Schwertani A, Choi H, Genest J. High-density Lipoproteins and the Pathogenesis of Atherosclerosis. Curr Opin Cardiol 2018;33(3):311–6.
21. Gupta N, DeFranco AL. Lipid Rafts and B cell signaling. Semin Cell Dev Biol 2007;18:616–26.

22. Catapano AL, Pirillo A, Bonacina F, et al. HDL in innate and adaptive immunity. Cardiovasc Res 2014;103:372–83. 15.

23. Libby P. The changing landscape of atherosclerosis. Nature 2021;592(7855): 524–33.

24. Riaz H, Khan SU, Rahman H, et al. Effects of high-density lipoprotein targeting treatments on cardiovascular outcomes: A systematic review and meta-analysis. Eur J Prev Cardiol 2019;26(5):533–43.

25. Briel M, Ferreira-Gonzalez I, You JJ, et al. Association between change in high density lipoprotein cholesterol and cardiovascular disease morbidity and mortality: systematic review and meta-regression analysis. BMJ 2009;338:b92.

26. Mora S, Glynn RJ, Boekholdt SM, et al. On-treatment non-high-density lipoprotein cholesterol, apolipoprotein B, triglycerides, and lipid ratios in relation to residual vascular risk after treatment with potent statin therapy: JUPITER (justification for the use of statins in prevention: an intervention trial evaluating rosuvastatin). J Am Coll Cardiol 2012;59(17):1521–8.

27. Haase CL, Tybjærg-Hansen A, Qayyum AA, et al. LCAT, HDL cholesterol and ischemic cardiovascular disease: a Mendelian randomization study of HDL cholesterol in 54,500 individuals. J Clin Endocrinol Metab 2012;97(2):E248–56.

28. Voight BF, Peloso GM, Orho-Melander M, et al. Plasma HDL cholesterol and risk of myocardial infarction: a mendelian randomisation study. Lancet 2012;380: 572–80.

29. Brewer HB Jr, Barter PJ, Björkegren JLM, et al. HDL and atherosclerotic cardiovascular disease: genetic insights into complex biology. Nat Rev Cardiol 2018; 15(1):9–19.

30. Weissglas-Volkov D, Pajukanta P. Genetic causes of high and low serum HDL-cholesterol. J Lipid Res 2010;51(8):2032–57.

31. Ko DT, Alter DA, Guo H, et al. High-Density Lipoprotein Cholesterol and Cause-Specific Mortality in Individuals Without Previous Cardiovascular Conditions: The CANHEART Study. J Am Coll Cardiol 2016;68(19):2073–83.

32. Schaefer EJ, Anthanont P, Diffenderfer MR, et al. Diagnosis and treatment of high density lipoprotein deficiency. Prog Cardiovasc Dis 2016;59:97–106.

33. Geller AS, Polisecki EY, Diffenderfer MR, et al. Genetic and secondary causes of severe HDL deficiency and cardiovascular disease. J Lipid Res 2018;59: 2421–35.

34. Casula M, Colpani O, Xie S, et al. HDL in Atherosclerotic Cardiovascular Disease: In Search of a Role. Cells 2021;10(8):1869.

35. Chiesa G, Sirtori CR. Apolipoprotein A-I(Milano): current perspectives. Curr Opin Lipidol 2003;14(2):159–63.

36. Hooper AJ, Hegele RA, Burnett JR. Tangier disease: update for 2020. Curr Opin Lipidol 2020;31(2):80–4.

37. Westerterp M, Bochem AE, Yvan-Charvet L, et al. ATP-binding cassette transporters, atherosclerosis, and inflammation. Circ Res 2014;114(1):157–70.

38. Taheri H, Filion KB, Windle SB, et al. Cholesteryl Ester Transfer Protein Inhibitors and Cardiovascular Outcomes: A Systematic Review and Meta-Analysis of Randomized Controlled Trials. Cardiology 2020;145(4):236–50.

39. Rader DJ, Tall AR. The not-so-simple HDL story: Is it time to revise the HDL cholesterol hypothesis? Nat Med 2012;18(9):1344–6.

40. Tall AR, Dader DJ. Trials and Tribulations of CETP Inhibitors. Circ Res 2017;65: 607–8.

41. Helgadottir A, Gretarsdottir S, Thorleifsson G, et al. Variants with large effects on blood lipids and the role of cholesterol and triglycerides in coronary disease. Nat Genet 2016;48(6):634–9.

42. Helgadottir A, Sulem P, Thorgeirsson G, et al. Rare SCARB1 mutations associate with high-density lipoprotein cholesterol but not with coronary artery disease. Eur Heart J 2018;39(23):2172–8.

43. Willer CJ, Schmidt EM, Sengupta S, et al. Global Lipids Genetics Consortium. Discovery and refinement of loci associated with lipid levels. Nat Genet 2013; 45(11):1274–83.

44. Yamashita S, Masuda D, Matsuzawa Y. Pemafibrate, a New Selective PPARalpha Modulator: Drug Concept and Its Clinical Applications for Dyslipidemia and Metabolic Diseases. Curr Atheroscler Rep 2020;22(1):5.

45. Genest J, Choi HY. Novel Approaches for HDL-directed therapies. Curr Atheroscler Rep 2017;19(12):55.

46. Barter P, Genest J. HDL Cholesterol and ASCVD Risk Stratification – A Debate. Atheroscler 2019. https://doi.org/10.1016/j.atherosclerosis.2019.01.001.

47. Nicholls SJ, Andrews J, Kastelein JJP, et al. Effect of Serial Infusions of CER-001, a Pre-beta High-Density Lipoprotein Mimetic, on Coronary Atherosclerosis in Patients Following Acute Coronary Syndromes in the CER-001 Atherosclerosis Regression Acute Coronary Syndrome Trial: A Randomized Clinical Trial. JAMA Cardiol 2018;3(9):815–22.

48. Nicholls SJ, Puri R, Ballantyne CM, et al. Effect of Infusion of High-Density Lipoprotein Mimetic Containing Recombinant Apolipoprotein A-I Milano on Coronary Disease in Patients With an Acute Coronary Syndrome in the MILANO-PILOT Trial: A Randomized Clinical Trial. JAMA Cardiol 2018;3(9):806–14.

49. Gibson CM, Kastelein JJP, Phillips AT, et al. Rationale and design of ApoA-I Event Reducing in Ischemic Syndromes II (AEGIS-II): A phase 3, multicenter, double-blind, randomized, placebo-controlled, parallel-group study to investigate the efficacy and safety of CSL112 in subjects after acute myocardial infarction. Am Heart J 2021;231:121–7.

50. Neele AE, Willemsen L, Chen HJ, et al. Targeting epigenetics as atherosclerosis treatment: an updated view. Curr Opin Lipidol 2020;31(6):324–30.

51. DiDonato JA, Huang Y, Aulak KS, et al. Function and distribution of apolipoprotein A1 in the artery wall are markedly distinct from those in plasma. Circulation 2013; 128(15):1644–55.

52. Khera AV, Demler OV, Adelman SJ, et al. Cholesterol Efflux Capacity, HDL Particle Number, and Incident Cardiovascular Events. An Analysis from the JUPITER Trial. Circulation 2017;135(25):2494–504.

53. Wang N, Westerterp M. ABC Transporters, Cholesterol Efflux, and Implications for Cardiovascular Diseases. Adv Exp Med Biol 2020;1276:67–83.

54. Choi H, Ruel I, Malina A, et al. Desmocollin 1 is abundantly expressed in atherosclerosis and impairs HDL biogenesis. Eur Heart J 2018;39(14):1194–202.

55. Choi HY, Ruel I, Genest J. Chemical compounds targeting desmocollin 1: a new paradigm for HDL-directed therapies. Front Pharmacol 2021;12:679456, eCollection 2021.

Evaluation and Management of Lipids and Lipoproteins in Children and Adolescents

Amisha Patel, MD[a], Nivedita Patni, MD[b],*

KEYWORDS

- Pediatric dyslipidemia • Universal screening • CHILD-1 • CHILD-2 • Statin
- Bile acid sequestrants • Ezetimibe • PCSK9 inhibitor

KEY POINTS

- Universal lipid screening should be performed in all children aged 9 to 11 years and 17 to 21 years by measuring nonfasting non-HDL-C.
- Lifestyle modifications with the "Cardiovascular Health Integrated Lifestyle diet" and daily moderate-vigorous physical activity are the mainstay for pediatric dyslipidemia.
- Statins, or HMG-CoA reductase inhibitors, are the first-line pharmacologic therapy for children and adolescents with severe hypercholesterolemia that persists despite diet and exercise.
- Bile acid sequestrants, ezetimibe, and PCSK9 inhibitors are also available for treatment of persistent pediatric hypercholesterolemia.
- Fibrates are indicated in youth with severe hypertriglyceridemia that persists despite lifestyle changes.

INTRODUCTION

The National Heart, Blood, and Lung Institute (NHBLI) established acceptable, borderline high and high plasma lipid levels based on NHANES III (third National Health and Nutrition Examination Survey) data on cholesterol levels in more than 7000 children aged 0 to 19 years from 1988 to 1994 (**Table 1**). Borderline high values reflect the 75th percentile, except for the high-density lipoprotein cholesterol (HDL-C), for which they reflect the 25th percentile. Abnormal values reflect the 95th percentile except for HDL-C, for which they reflect the 10th percentile.

By studying patterns of lipoprotein levels throughout childhood, it is now known that levels may change based on age group. Mean low-density lipoprotein cholesterol (LDL-C) levels at birth have been reported to be 30.4 ± 10.3 mg/dL in the Bogalusa Heart

[a] Department of Pediatrics, UT Southwestern Medical Center, 5323 Harry Hines Boulevard, Dallas, TX 75390, USA; [b] Division of Pediatric Endocrinology, Department of Pediatrics, UT Southwestern Medical Center, 5323 Harry Hines Boulevard, Dallas, TX 75390-9063, USA
* Corresponding author.
E-mail address: nivedita.patni@utsouthwestern.edu

Endocrinol Metab Clin N Am 51 (2022) 573–588
https://doi.org/10.1016/j.ecl.2022.02.002
0889-8529/22/© 2022 Elsevier Inc. All rights reserved.

Table 1
Acceptable, borderline, and abnormal plasma lipid and lipoprotein concentrations (mg/dL) for children and adolescents

Category	Acceptable	Borderline High	Abnormal
Total cholesterol	< 170	170–199	≥ 200
LDL-C	< 110	110–129	≥ 130
Non-HDL-C	< 120	120–144	≥ 145
Triglycerides			
0–9 y	< 75	75–99	≥ 100
10–19 y	< 90	90–129	≥ 130
HDL-C	> 45	40–45	< 40

Abbreviations: HDL-C, high-density lipoprotein cholesterol; LDL-C, low-density lipoprotein cholesterol.
Adapted from Expert Panel on Integrated Guidelines for Cardiovascular Health and Risk Reduction in Children and Adolescents Summary Report. U.S. Department of Health and Human Services, National Institutes of Health. 2011.

Study; however, there are significant racial differences.[1] LDL-C levels increase in the first 6 months (mean change 43 mg/dL) but have small additional increments till age 7 years.[2] Then, until adolescence, lipoprotein levels will remain relatively stable. However, during puberty, total cholesterol (TC) and LDL-C levels will decrease until late adolescence when they begin to increase again.[3] Furthermore, it is well known that obtaining lipoprotein levels in childhood are good predictors of levels in young adulthood.[3]

SCREENING FOR PEDIATRIC DYSLIPIDEMIA

It has been well established that children with abnormal lipid levels have increased evidence of atherosclerosis, and early identification and control of dyslipidemia during youth and into adulthood will significantly reduce the risk of cardiovascular disease (CVD).[4,5] The goal of screening for pediatric dyslipidemia is to identify those children and adolescents at high risk for premature CVD, or those with an increased risk, due to dyslipidemia to intervene and provide appropriate treatment to lower these risks.

The first set of guidelines regarding dyslipidemia in the pediatric population was published in 1992 by the National Heart, Lung, and Blood Institute National Cholesterol Education Program.[6] These guidelines were largely based on the screening, diagnosis, and treatment guidelines for adults and were eventually adopted by the American Heart Association and the American Academy of Pediatrics (AAP). At that time, screening was largely based on family history of dyslipidemia or premature CVD, and further evaluation was conducted based almost exclusively on elevated LDL-C as a risk factor. These guidelines were updated by the AAP based on new evidence available in 1998 and again in 2008, but screening remained targeted to those children with certain risk factors. As new data became available, there was evidence indicating that 30% to 60% of children with moderate dyslipidemia (LDL level ≥160 mg/dL) likely secondary to familial hypercholesterolemia (FH) were missed using the selective screening approach.[7] Furthermore, more evidence was emerging suggesting that treatment of dyslipidemia in children resulted in regression of markers of atherosclerosis. A randomized controlled trial showed significant improvement in carotid intima-media thickness 5 years postinitiation of statins in the group aged 8 to 11 years compared with the group aged 12 to 18 years.[8] This finding led to the recommendations of considering a universal screening approach to identify those children with possible genetic dyslipidemia, intervening sooner to achieve improved outcomes, and identifying those children with dyslipidemia associated with lifestyle and obesity.

Universal Screening

In 2011, the NHLBI and the AAP published an updated set of evidence-based guidelines for pediatric dyslipidemia including updated guidelines for screening (**Table 2**). These guidelines recommend universal screening for all children aged between 9 and 11 years, and between 17 and 21 years, because the TC and LDL-C can decrease as much as 10% to 20% during puberty.[9] However, if new family history is available or if there are additional risk factors, the individual should be screened. Screening should be performed by obtaining nonfasting, non-high-density lipoprotein cholesterol (non-HDL-C) levels.

Selective Screening

Target screening refers to a strategy of identifying and screening individuals with certain risk factors. The NHLBI guidelines recommend selective screening for certain

Table 2
Lipid screening recommendations in children and adolescents

Age Group	Recommendation	Grade/Recommendation Level
Birth–12 mo	No lipid screening	Grade C/recommend
2–8 y	No routine lipid screening	Grade B/recommend
	Selective screening; FLP ×2[a] if:	Grade B/strongly recommend
	• First- or second-degree relative with premature CVD[b]	
	• Parent with TC ≥ 240 mg/dL or known dyslipidemia	
	• Child has diabetes, hypertension, BMI ≥ 95 percentile, or smokes cigarettes	
	• Child has a moderate- or high-risk medical condition (see **Table 3**)	
9–11 y	Universal screening	Grade B/strongly recommend
12–16 y	No routine lipid screening	Grade B/recommend
	Selective screening; measure FLP ×2 if new knowledge of:	Grade B/strongly recommend
	• First- or second-degree relative with premature CVD[b]	
	• Parent with TC ≥ 240 mg/dL or known dyslipidemia	
	• Child has diabetes, hypertension, BMI ≥ 85 percentile, or smokes cigarettes	
	• Patient has a moderate- or high-risk medical condition (see **Table 3**)	
17–21 y	Universal screening	Grade B/recommend

Abbreviations: BMI, body mass index; FLP, fasting lipid profile.
[a] Measure FLP twice at least 2 weeks apart but within 3 months and average values.
[b] Parent, grandparent, aunt/uncle, or sibling with myocardial infarction, angina, stroke, coronary artery bypass graft/stent/angioplasty at less than 55 years in males, less than 65 years in females
Adapted from Expert Panel on Integrated Guidelines for Cardiovascular Health and Risk Reduction in Children and Adolescents Summary Report. U.S. Department of Health and Human Services, National Institutes of Health. 2011.

risk groups for individuals older than 2 years (see **Table 2, Table 3**). Screening should be performed by obtaining a fasting lipid profile (FLP) twice within an interval of at least 2 weeks to 3 months. An FLP includes TC, HDL-C, and triglycerides (TGs). LDL-C is calculated using the Friedewald equation LDL-C = TC (HDL-C + TG/5). This equation cannot be used if TG levels are greater than 400 mg/dL. The 2 lipid profile values should be averaged to determine whether further workup or intervention is warranted.

EVALUATION OF PEDIATRIC DYSLIPIDEMIA

Children with abnormal universal screening should have 2 additional fasting lipid panels measured, separated by at least 2 weeks but within 3 months, and the results should be averaged and compared with normal lipid values per **Table 1**. If abnormal, the patient should be evaluated for the underlying cause of the dyslipidemia, which may be primary or secondary (**Table 4**). Primary or monogenic dyslipidemias are a group of single-gene defects with mendelian transmission, characterized by extremely elevated LDL-C or TG levels. These disorders include but are not limited to FH, sitosterolemia lysosomal acid lipase deficiency, cerebrotendinous xanthomatosis, and familial chylomicronemia syndrome (type 1 hyperlipoproteinemia). Secondary causes should be ruled out before initiating treatment (see **Table 4**).

Combined (mixed) dyslipidemia is a common cause of dyslipidemia in the pediatric population and is characterized by elevated levels of TGs and non-HDL-C and decreased levels of HDL-C. This pattern has been associated with childhood obesity and shown to be related to vascular dysfunction and cardiovascular events in adulthood.[10] Combined dyslipidemia has been shown to respond to lifestyle changes as described later.[11]

TREATMENT OF PEDIATRIC DYSLIPIDEMIA

Treatment options for dyslipidemia can be categorized into lifestyle changes (diet and exercise) and pharmacologic.

Lifestyle Modifications

Cardiovascular Health Integrated Lifestyle Diet-1
The NHLBI describes the Cardiovascular Health Integrated Lifestyle Diet-1 (CHILD-1) as the first-step nutritional guidelines for all children older than 2 years and for those

Table 3
Special risk conditions for selective lipid screening in children and adolescents

High Risk	Moderate Risk
Diabetes mellitus, types 1 and 2	Kawasaki disease with previous history of coronary aneurysms
Chronic renal disease, end-stage renal disease, or post–renal transplant	Chronic inflammatory disease[a]
Postorthotopic heart transplant	HIV
Kawasaki disease with current aneurysms	Nephrotic syndrome

Abbreviation: HIV, human immunodeficiency virus.
  [a] Systemic lupus erythematosus, juvenile rheumatoid arthritis.
  Adapted from Expert Panel on Integrated Guidelines for Cardiovascular Health and Risk Reduction in Children and Adolescents Summary Report. U.S. Department of Health and Human Services, National Institutes of Health. 2011.

Table 4
Secondary causes of dyslipidemia in pediatric patients

Endocrine/metabolic	Storage disease
Acute intermittent porphyria	Cystine storage disease
Diabetes mellitus (types 1 and 2)	Gaucher disease
Hypopituitarism	Glycogen storage disease
Hypothyroidism	Tay-Sachs disease
Lipodystrophy	Niemann-Pick disease
Pregnancy	Infectious
Renal	Acute viral/bacterial infection
Chronic renal failure	Human immunodeficiency virus infection
Hemolytic uremic syndrome	Hepatitis
Nephrotic syndrome	Inflammatory
Hepatic	Rheumatoid arthritis
Obstructive liver disease/cholestasis	Systemic lupus erythematosus
Congenital biliary atresia	Other
Alagille syndrome	Anorexia nervosa
Exogenous	Cancer survivor
Corticosteroids	Post–solid organ transplantation
Isoretinoin	Idiopathic hypercalcemia
Beta blockers	Kawasaki disease
Oral contraceptives	Klinefelter disease
Some chemotherapeutic agents	Progeria
Alcohol	Werner syndrome

children with dyslipidemias as the first-line treatment (**Table 5**). The guidelines state that fat intake in infants younger than 12 months should not be restricted without a specific medical indication. For older children, this diet limits calories from fat to 30%, calories from saturated fat to 10%, and cholesterol intake to less than 300 mg/d. The diet also includes recommendations for breastfeeding of infants as possible based on data showing decreased TC levels in adults who were breastfed as infants compared with those who were formula-fed.[12] In the Special Turku Coronary Risk Factor Intervention Project for Children (STRIP) study, families of infants starting at age 7 months were counseled on a low-saturated-fat, low-cholesterol diet similar to that of the CHILD-1 diet. This study showed that at age 3 years, those infants in the intervention group had serum cholesterol, non-HDL-C, and HDL-C concentrations 3% to 6% lower than those infants without the dietary intervention, without detrimental effects on growth and development.[13] The study further showed that serum TC and LDL-C were also lower at age 7 years.[14] A meta-analysis reviewing 37 studies between 1981 and 1997 on the effects of the dietary guidelines of the CHILD-1 diet showed a 12% decrease in the serum LDL-C concentration in all subjects.[15] These studies all show the benefits of the CHILD-1 diet on serum TC and LDL-C levels without harm to the growth and development of children. Further details regarding the guidelines of the CHILD-1 diet are listed in **Table 5**. At least 1 hour of moderate to vigorous physical activity daily should be encouraged for all children.

Cardiovascular Health Integrated Lifestyle Diet-2
If, after a 3-month trial of the CHILD-1 diet, a patient fails to reach a therapeutic goal, the patient and family should work with a dietician to implement the Cardiovascular Health Integrated Lifestyle Diet-2 (CHILD-2) diet. This more rigorous diet limits calories from fat to 30%, calories from saturated fat to 7%, and goal dietary cholesterol to 200 mg/dL or less. **Table 6** describes the CHILD-2 diet in greater detail including

Table 5
Cardiovascular Health Integrated Lifestyle Diet-1 (CHILD-1) dietary guidelines

Birth to 6 mo	Exclusively breastfeed; if unavailable or contraindicated, consider expressed breast milk or iron-fortified infant formula
6–12 mo	Continue breastfeeding until 12 mo of age (unless unavailable or contraindicated) Gradual addition of solids No restriction of fat intake unless medically indicated No sweetened beverages; encourage water
12–24 mo	Unflavored, reduced-fat milk (2% to fat free) Avoid sweetened beverages; encourage water Table foods with total fat 30% of daily kcal intake, saturated fat 8%–10% of daily kcal intake, monounsaturated and polyunsaturated fat up to 20% daily kcal intake, cholesterol <300 mg/d Avoid transfats, limit sodium intake
2–10 y	Unflavored, fat-free milk Limit/avoid sweetened beverages; encourage water Total fat 25%–30% of daily kcal intake, saturated fat 8%–10% of daily kcal intake, mono- and polyunsaturated fat up to 20% daily kcal intake, cholesterol <300 mg/d Avoid transfats, limit sodium intake Encourage high dietary fiber intake
11–21 y	Unflavored, fat-free milk Limit/avoid sweetened beverages; encourage water Total fat 25%–30% of daily kcal intake, saturated fat 8%–10% of daily kcal intake, monounsatirated and polyunsaturated fat up to 20% daily kcal intake, cholesterol <300 mg/d Avoid trans fats, limit sodium intake Encourage high dietary fiber intake

specific recommendations for both LDL-C- and TG-lowering modifications. Like CHILD-1, the CHILD-2 diet has been proved to be both safe and efficacious. The Dietary Intervention Study in Children (DISC) was a large randomized controlled trial initiated by the NHLBI in 1987 studying the long-term effects in LDL-C after initiating children on the DISC diet, which was similar to the CHILD-2 diet.[16] The trial found that the mean LDL-C was significantly lower in the intervention group without affecting growth during puberty. The same meta-analysis that reviewed the CHILD-1 dietary guidelines discussed earlier also reviewed the CHILD-2 dietary guidelines to assess for efficacy and found that LDL-C levels decreased by 16% in the intervention group.[15] The dietary guidelines for CHILD-2 include addition of plant sterols, dietary fiber, and/ or omega-3 fatty acid supplementation, which are described later.

Dietary supplement with plant sterols/stanols
There is evidence to support the use of plant sterols/stanols as a supplement to lower LDL-C levels. Plant sterols/stanols are cholesterollike substances found in plants and exist in our diet as vegetable oils or margarines, seeds, nuts, yogurt, milk, and legumes. Because they are more hydrophobic, when consumed, they inhibit intestinal absorption of cholesterol by preventing incorporation of cholesterol in the micelles, therefore reducing the bioavailability of cholesterol in the bloodstream. Several meta-analyses in the adult population have shown a 7% to 12% reduction in LDL-C with use of 1.5 to 3 g/d of plant sterols.[17] The STRIP study evaluated the effect of replacement of dietary fat with a stanol-enriched margarine in 6-year-old children

Table 6	
Lifestyle recommendations for persistent dyslipidemia after 3-month trial of the Cardiovascular Health Integrated Lifestyle Diet-1 diet	
LDL-C Lowering	
CHILD-2-LDL diet	Total fat: 25%–30% of total calories/d Saturated fat: ≤7% of total calories/d Avoid transfat Monounsaturated fat: 10% of total calories/d Cholesterol: <200 mg/d
Plant sterols	Can consider up to 2 g/d to replace usual dietary fat sources
Water-soluble fiber	Can consider 6 g/d (2–12 y) or 12 g/d (≥12 y)
Activity	≥ 1 h moderate-vigorous physical activity with 2-h limitation on sedentary screen time
TG lowering	
CHILD-2-TG diet	Total fat: 25%–30% of total calories/d Saturated fat: ≤7% of total calories/d Avoid transfat Monounsaturated fat: 10% of total calories/d Cholesterol: <200 mg/d Reduce sugar intake Replace simple carbohydrates with complex carbohydrates
Omega-3 fatty acid	Increase dietary fish Supplement omega-3 fatty acid 1–4 g/d for TG > 200–499 mg/dL

Abbreviation: TG, triglyceride.

and found a decrease in TC and LDL-C levels by 5.4% and 7.5%, respectively.[18] Multiple other studies have seen LDL-C level lowering by 9% to 16% with the addition of a plant sterol/stanol supplementation in the pediatric population; however, long-term effects have not yet been evaluated.[19–21]

Dietary supplement with water-soluble fiber
There is evidence to support the use of water-soluble fiber, such as psyllium, to lower LDL-C levels. Data from studies evaluating the effectiveness of fiber on serum LDL-C levels range from no change to 8% reduction in the group receiving fiber.[22–25] The NHBLI recommends that water-soluble fiber psyllium can be added to a CHILD-2 diet for those children with elevated LDL-C levels at a dose of 6 g/d for children aged 2 to 12 years and 12 g/d for those aged 12 years or older.

Considering Pharmacologic Treatment

Elevated levels of low-density lipoprotein-cholesterol
When considering further treatment options, it is important that at least 2 FLPs obtained at least 2 weeks but no further than 3 months apart have been collected. The NHBLI recommends considering pharmacologic therapy when the LDL-C level is greater than or equal to 190 mg/dL after a 6-month trial of lifestyle management for children at least 10 years of age, 160 to 189 mg/dL after a 6-month trial of lifestyle management for children at least 10 years of age with a family history of premature CVD, or 1 or more high-level risk factor or 2 or more moderate-level CVD risk factors (see **Table 3**). The goal of therapy should be to lower LDL-C levels to less than 130 mg/dL. The AAP and NHLBI recommend consideration of pharmacologic therapy at 8 years for children with an LDL-C level greater than or equal to 190 mg/dL after a trial of lifestyle management if there is a clinical suspicion or genetic confirmation of FH, or

there is at least 1 high-level risk factor or risk condition or at least 2 moderate-level risk factors or risk conditions.

Elevated triglyceride

The NHBLI recommends pharmacologic therapy for hypertriglyceridemia in patients with an average fasting TG level of greater than or equal to 500 mg/dL or any single measurement of 1000 mg/dL or more in the setting of a primary hypertriglyceridemia. Pharmacologic therapy in these patients should be done in addition to the CHILD-2-TG diet to help prevent the complication of pancreatitis.

HMG-CoA Reductase Inhibitors (Statins)

Statins are the first-line pharmacologic therapy for the treatment of elevated LDL-C levels that persists after diet and lifestyle changes (**Table 7**). Statins work by inhibiting 3-hydroxy-3-methyl-glutaryl-coenzyme A reductase (HMG-CoA reductase), which results in upregulation of LDL receptors therefore reducing plasma LDL-C levels. Large-scale evidence on the use of statins shows a significant reduction in coronary morbidity and mortality in high-risk populations.[26,27] Statin therapy in children with FH has been shown to slow the progression of carotid intima-media thickness,[28,29] and reduce the risk of CVD.[29–33] In children, LDL-C reduction ranges from 17% to 50% from baseline and TC reduction from 13% to 39% with different statins (see **Table 7**).[34–47] Pravastatin, pitavastatin, and rosuvastatin are approved by the US Food and Drug Administration (FDA) for children 8 years and older, and all statins listed in **Table 8** are approved for children 10 years and older. When initiating statin therapy, the lowest available dose should be started once daily. Medication should be titrated within the range detailed in **Table 7**, with the goal LDL-C level less than 130 mg/dL.[48] FLP, aspartate aminotransferase, alanine aminotransferase, and creatine kinase (CK) should be checked at baseline and then repeated 4 weeks, 8 weeks, and then every 3 to 6 months after initiation of therapy.[48] If the goal LDL-C level is not reached, addition of a second agent should be considered, under the direction of a lipid specialist.

Statins are usually well tolerated in children and have an excellent safety profile.[49] A systematic review by the US Preventive Services Task Force (2014) concluded that in children with FH treated with statins, adverse events did not significantly differ in those randomized to statins compared with placebo.[50] In a meta-analysis of statin use in children, there were no significant differences in hepatic enzyme elevation in children receiving statins compared with those receiving placebo.[30] Patients should be

Table 7
Statin (HMG-CoA reductase inhibitor) initiation age and approved pediatric doses per US Food and Drug Administration

Drug	Age (years)	Dose	Effect on LDL Reduction
Atorvastatin	≥10	10–20 mg/d	30%–38%[36]
Fluvastatin	≥10	20–80 mg/d	24%–33%[35,37,38]
Lovastatin	≥10	10–40 mg/d	38%–50%[39]
Pitavastatin	≥ 8	2-4 mg/d	38%–44%[40,41]
Pravastatin	≥ 8	20–40 mg/d	23%–34%[42]
Rosuvastatin	≥ 8	5–20 mg/d	17%–36%[43–45]
Simvastatin	≥10	5–40 mg/d	25%–41%[46,47]

Abbreviation: HMG-CoA, 3-hydroxy-3-methyl-glutaryl-coenzyme A.

Table 8
Pharmacologic therapy for pediatric dyslipidemia

Type of Medication	Examples	Mechanism of Action	Major Effects	Adverse Reactions
HMG-CoA reductase inhibitors	Atorvastatin Fluvastatin Lovastatin Pitavastatin Pravastatin Rosuvastatin Simvastatin	Upregulation of LDLR by inhibiting cholesterol synthesis	↓ LDL-C	Elevated hepatic enzymes, elevated CK
Bile acid sequestrants	Cholestyramine Colesevelam Colestipol	Upregulation of LDLR by binding bile acids and stimulating hepatic bile acid production from cholesterol	↓ LDL-C	Gastrointestinal side effects, folate deficiency, vitamin D deficiency
Cholesterol absorption inhibitors	Ezetimibe	Inhibiting cholesterol absorption resulting in upregulation of LDLR	↓ LDL-C	Gastrointestinal upset, myalgia
PCSK9 Inhibitor	Evolocumab	Binds PCSK9 causing increased LDLR availability	↓ LDL-C	Headache, flulike symptoms, oropharyngeal pain, constipation
Niacin	Niacin	Inhibit DGAT2 and release of FFA, decreasing triglyceride production	↓ LDL-C	Flushing, headache, gastrointestinal upset
Fibrates	Fenofibrate Gemfibrozil	Upregulation of PPARα, causing lipolysis and decrease in triglycerides	↓ TG	Gastrointestinal side effects, myositis when used with statins
Fish oil	Omega-3 acid ethyl esters	Decreases FA and TG synthesis, increases FA degradation	↓ TG ↑ HDL-C	Unpleasant taste, gastrointestinal upset

Abbreviations: CK, creatine kinase; DGAT2, diglycerol acyltransferase2; FA, fatty acid; FFA, free fatty acid; LDLR, LDL receptor; PCSK9, proprotein convertase subtilisin/kexin type 9; PPARα, peroxisome proliferator-activated receptor.

counseled on the development of myopathy while using statins; however, the pediatric trials did not show any significant difference in the development of muscle enzyme elevations (CK > 10-fold) between those children receiving statins and those receiving placebo. Statins should be discontinued if the liver enzyme levels are greater than 3 times the upper limit of normal, CK level is greater than 10 times the upper limit of normal, or if a patient develops adverse effects to therapy. If the patient reports symptoms of myopathy (muscle pain or weakness), consider checking the CK level to assess if the statin needs to be stopped. The use of statins has been contraindicated during pregnancy and while breastfeeding, and females should be informed about the need to avoid pregnancy and breastfeeding while using statins; however, FDA has recently requested removal of the strongest warning against using statins during pregnancy.[51]

Bile Acid Sequestrants

Bile acid sequestrants (BAS) such as colesevelam, cholestyramine, and colestipol decrease LDL-C levels in the serum by binding bile acids in the intestine and preventing their reabsorption through the ileal bile acid transporter therefore stimulating the conversion of cholesterol to bile acids. To achieve this, LDL-C receptors are upregulated resulting in decreased serum LDL-C levels; they can lower LDL-C levels by 10% to 15% and can be used as a monotherapy or combined with statins if statins alone do not help to achieve target LDL-C levels.[52] These were the only class of medications recommended by national cholesterol education program (NCEP) in 1992.[6] The first-generation BAS, cholestyramine and colestipol, cause significant gastrointestinal side effects, decreased serum folate levels, and 25-hydroxyvitamin D deficiency in addition to poor tolerability.[53,54] Second-generation BAS, colesevelam, is better tolerated and is FDA approved for children aged 10 years or older.[55] Caution should be taken when other medications are used with BAS because BAS may decrease absorption of some medications.

Cholesterol Absorption Inhibitor (Ezetimibe)

Ezetimibe, a cholesterol absorption inhibitor, works by inhibiting NPC1L1, an intestinal cholesterol transporter, which results in a compensatory upregulation of endogenous cholesterol biosynthesis, which increases LDL receptor activity and therefore decreases LDL-C levels in the serum. Ezetimibe is approved by the FDA in children aged 10 years and older with heterozygous FH, homozygous FH, and sitosterolemia.[56] Ezetimibe monotherapy, dose 10 mg/d, can cause LDL-C level reduction of about 28% to 30%.[57,58] Coadministration of ezetimibe and statin can cause an additional 20% decrease in LDL-C levels compared with the use of statin alone.[59] Ezetimibe is generally well tolerated with no significant side effects, although mild gastrointestinal upset and myalgia have been reported at the daily dose of 10 mg.[57,58]

Niacin

Niacin works by inhibiting hepatic diacylglycerol acyltransferase-2, an enzyme that converts diacylglycerol to TGs, and the release of free fatty acids from adipose tissue, thus decreasing very-low-density lipoprotein (VLDL) and LDL-C production and HDL-C degradation. Niacin is not routinely used in pediatric population due to the lack of published safety data. One retrospective review, in children aged 4 to 14 years, showed that niacin reduced levels of TC by 23% and LDL-C by 30%, with no significant effect on TGs.[60] Adverse effects were significant and included flushing, abdominal pain, vomiting, and headache.[60] These well-known side effects make niacin a poorly tolerated medication even in adults. Clinical trials of niacin in combination with a statin in adults have found serious adverse effects of infection, gastrointestinal bleeding, myopathy, and rare hepatotoxicity[61,62] (see Connie B. Newman's article, "Safety of Statins and Non-Statins for Treatment of Dyslipidemia," in this issue), and in 2015, the FDA removed the indication for the use of niacin in combination with a statin.

PCSK9 Inhibitor

Human proprotein convertase subtilisin/kexin type 9 (PCSK9) is an enzyme responsible for degrading LDL receptors. Evolocumab is a human monoclonal immunoglobulin that binds to PCSK9 in the liver thereby increasing the availability of LDL receptors resulting in decreased serum LDL-C levels. In adult studies, evolocumab has been shown to decrease LDL-C levels up to 60%.[63] A recent study on the efficacy and safety of evolocumab added to statin therapy in children aged 10 to 17 years with heterozygous FH showed an average decrease of LDL-C levels of about 38% compared with placebo.[64] The most common adverse events were nasopharyngitis, headache, upper respiratory tract infection, influenza, oropharyngeal pain, and gastroenteritis; however, the incidence of adverse events was similar in the evolocumab and the placebo groups.[64] Evolocumab is given as a subcutaneous injection once a month at a dose of 420 mg; it is now approved by the FDA for children older than 10 years with heterozygous and homozygous FH.

Fibrates

Fibric acid derivatives, fenofibrate and gemfibrozil, lower serum TG levels by acting as agonists of the peroxisome proliferator-activated receptor alpha (PPARα) causing upregulation of lipoprotein lipase in adipose tissue and muscle leading to decreased TG levels. These derivatives are not approved by the FDA for use in pediatric patients but may be used in adolescents with a fasting TG level of greater than 500 mg/dL with an increased risk of pancreatitis. Most common side effects include nausea, vomiting, and abdominal pain.[56] Fibrates should not be used with statins due to an increased incidence of myositis, myalgia, and rhabdomyolysis and are contraindicated in patients with gallbladder disease.[65]

Omega-3 Fish Oils

Omega-3 fish oils contain eicosapentaenoic acid (EPA) and docosahexaenoic acid (DHA) both of which lower TG levels by reducing circulating nonesterified fatty acids, the primary source of fatty acids for VLDL-TG production.[66] Evidence suggests that omega-3-fatty acids reduce apo-C III plasma levels via the PPARα pathway, decrease hepatic fatty acid and TG synthesis, and augment fatty acid degradation/oxidation, causing overall reduction in hepatic VLDL cholesterol synthesis and release. Omega-3 fish oil has been studied in the adult population and shown to reduce TG levels by 30% to 45% and increase HDL-C levels.[67] Adult studies show an increased reduction of TG levels with higher doses (4 g/d) compared with lower doses (1 g/d).[68] DHA has been shown to increase LDL-C levels and change LDL particle size, whereas both EPA and DHA lower TG levels and increase HDL-C levels.[69–71] Prescription fish oils have not been approved by the FDA for use in children; however, over-the-counter (OTC) preparations are commonly used in children to lower serum TG levels. OTC preparations may have varying amounts of EPA or DHA, whereas prescription fish oils contain specific amounts of these oils. Fish oils in adult studies have side effects including gastrointestinal upset and unpleasant taste or smell, and less frequently, atrial fibrillation.

CLINICS CARE POINTS

- Universal screening in all children aged 9 to 11 years and 17 to 21 year will aid in improving cardiovascular health of the US population.
- Targeted screening in children with high-risk factors, like diabetes mellitus, chronic renal disease, nephrotic syndrome or end-stage renal disease, Kawasaki disease, chronic inflammatory diseases, post–heart transplant, or human immunodeficiency virus, will significantly reduce their clinical CVD risk in adult life.
- Lifestyle modifications with heart-healthy diet and moderate-vigorous activity are fundamental in the management of pediatric dyslipidemia.
- Pharmacotherapy with statins, BASs, ezetimibe and PCSK9 inhibitors, fibrates, niacin, and omega-3 fish oils are available for use in the pediatric population.

DISCLOSURE

The authors have nothing to disclose.

REFERENCES

1. Frerichs RR, Srinivasan SR, Webber LS, et al. Serum lipids and lipoproteins at birth in a biracial population: the Bogalusa heart study. Pediatr Res 1978;12(8):858–63.
2. Freedman DS, Srinivasan SR, Cresanta JL, et al. Cardiovascular risk factors from birth to 7 years of age: the Bogalusa Heart Study. Serum lipids and lipoproteins. Pediatrics 1987;80(5 Pt 2):789–96.
3. Webber LS, Srinivasan SR, Wattigney WA, et al. Tracking of serum lipids and lipoproteins from childhood to adulthood. The Bogalusa Heart Study. Am J Epidemiol 1991;133(9):884–99.
4. Berenson GS, Srinivasan SR, Bao W, et al. Association between multiple cardiovascular risk factors and atherosclerosis in children and young adults. The Bogalusa Heart Study. N Engl J Med 1998;338(23):1650–6.
5. Lauer RM, Lee J, Clarke WR. Factors affecting the relationship between childhood and adult cholesterol levels: the Muscatine Study. Pediatrics 1988;82(3):309–18.
6. American Academy of Pediatrics. National cholesterol education program: report of the expert panel on blood cholesterol levels in children and adolescents. Pediatrics 1992;89(3 Pt 2):525–84.
7. Ritchie SK, Murphy EC, Ice C, et al. Universal versus targeted blood cholesterol screening among youth: the CARDIAC project. Pediatrics 2010;126(2):260–5.
8. Rodenburg J, Vissers MN, Wiegman A, et al. Statin treatment in children with familial hypercholesterolemia: the younger, the better. Circulation 2007;116(6):664–8.
9. Hickman TB, Briefel RR, Carroll MD, et al. Distributions and trends of serum lipid levels among United States children and adolescents ages 4-19 years: data from the Third National Health and Nutrition Examination Survey. Prev Med 1998;27(6):879–90.
10. Cook S, Kavey RE. Dyslipidemia and pediatric obesity. Pediatr Clin North Am 2011;58(6):1363–73, ix.
11. Epstein LH, Kuller LH, Wing RR, et al. The effect of weight control on lipid changes in obese children. Am J Dis Child 1989;143(4):454–7.
12. Owen CG, Whincup PH, Odoki K, et al. Infant feeding and blood cholesterol: a study in adolescents and a systematic review. Pediatrics 2002;110(3):597–608.

13. Simell O, Niinikoski H, Ronnemaa T, et al. Special turku coronary risk factor intervention project for babies (STRIP). Am J Clin Nutr 2000;72(5 Suppl):1316S–31S.
14. Kaitosaari T, Ronnemaa T, Raitakari O, et al. Effect of 7-year infancy-onset dietary intervention on serum lipoproteins and lipoprotein subclasses in healthy children in the prospective, randomized Special Turku Coronary Risk Factor Intervention Project for Children (STRIP) study. Circulation 2003;108(6):672–7.
15. Yu-Poth S, Zhao G, Etherton T, et al. Effects of the national cholesterol education program's step I and step II dietary intervention programs on cardiovascular disease risk factors: a meta-analysis. Am J Clin Nutr 1999;69(4):632–46.
16. Lauer RM, Obarzanek E, Hunsberger SA, et al. Efficacy and safety of lowering dietary intake of total fat, saturated fat, and cholesterol in children with elevated LDL cholesterol: the Dietary Intervention Study in Children. Am J Clin Nutr 2000; 72(5 Suppl):1332S–42S.
17. Trautwein EA, Vermeer MA, Hiemstra H, et al. LDL-cholesterol lowering of plant sterols and stanols-which factors influence their efficacy? Nutrients 2018;10(9): 1262.
18. Tammi A, Ronnemaa T, Gylling H, et al. Plant stanol ester margarine lowers serum total and low-density lipoprotein cholesterol concentrations of healthy children: the STRIP project. Special Turku Coronary Risk Factors Intervention Project. J Pediatr 2000;136(4):503–10.
19. Mantovani LM, Pugliese C. Phytosterol supplementation in the treatment of dyslipidemia in children and adolescents: a systematic review. Rev Paul Pediatr 2020; 39:e2019389.
20. de Jongh S, Vissers MN, Rol P, et al. Plant sterols lower LDL cholesterol without improving endothelial function in prepubertal children with familial hypercholesterolaemia. J Inherit Metab Dis 2003;26(4):343–51.
21. Guardamagna O, Abello F, Baracco V, et al. Primary hyperlipidemias in children: effect of plant sterol supplementation on plasma lipids and markers of cholesterol synthesis and absorption. Acta Diabetol 2011;48(2):127–33.
22. Davidson MH, Dugan LD, Burns JH, et al. A psyllium-enriched cereal for the treatment of hypercholesterolemia in children: a controlled, double-blind, crossover study. Am J Clin Nutr 1996;63(1):96–102.
23. Dennison BA, Levine DM. Randomized, double-blind, placebo-controlled, two-period crossover clinical trial of psyllium fiber in children with hypercholesterolemia. J Pediatr 1993;123(1):24–9.
24. Gold K, Wong N, Tong A, et al. Serum apolipoprotein and lipid profile effects of an oat-bran-supplemented, low-fat diet in children with elevated serum cholesterol. Ann N Y Acad Sci 1991;623:429–31.
25. Kwiterovich PO Jr. The role of fiber in the treatment of hypercholesterolemia in children and adolescents. Pediatrics 1995;96(5 Pt 2):1005–9.
26. Belay B, Belamarich PF, Tom-Revzon C. The use of statins in pediatrics: knowledge base, limitations, and future directions. Pediatrics 2007;119(2):370–80.
27. Collins R, Reith C, Emberson J, et al. Interpretation of the evidence for the efficacy and safety of statin therapy. Lancet 2016;388(10059):2532–61.
28. Wiegman A, Gidding S, Watts G, et al. European atherosclerosis society consensus panel. Familial hypercholesterolaemia in children and adolescents: gaining decades of life by optimizing detection and treatment. Eur Heart J 2015;36(36):2425–37.
29. Luirink IK, Wiegman A, Kusters DM, et al. 20-Year follow-up of statins in children with familial hypercholesterolemia. N Engl J Med 2019;381(16):1547–56.

30. Avis HJ, Vissers MN, Stein EA, et al. A systematic review and meta-analysis of statin therapy in children with familial hypercholesterolemia. Arterioscler Thromb Vasc Biol 2007;27(8):1803–10.

31. Saskia de Jongh M, Lilien MR, Jos op't Roodt M, et al. Early Statin therapy restores endothelial function in children with familial hypercholesterolemia. J Am Coll Cardiol 2002;40(12):2117–21.

32. Wiegman A, de Groot E, Hutten BA, et al. Arterial intima-media thickness in children heterozygous for familial hypercholesterolaemia. Lancet 2004;363(9406): 369–70.

33. Wiegman A. Lipid screening, action, and follow-up in children and adolescents. Curr Cardiol Rep 2018;20(9):80.

34. Eiland LS, Luttrell PK. Use of statins for dyslipidemia in the pediatric population. J Pediatr Pharmacol Ther 2010;15(3):160–72.

35. Wiegman A, Hutten BA, de Groot E, et al. Efficacy and safety of statin therapy in children with familial hypercholesterolemia: a randomized controlled trial. JAMA 2004;292(3):331–7.

36. Braamskamp MJ, Stefanutti C, Langslet G, et al. Efficacy and safety of pitavastatin in children and adolescents at high future cardiovascular risk. J Pediatr 2015; 167(2):338–343 e335.

37. Hedman M, Matikainen T, Fohr A, et al. Efficacy and safety of pravastatin in children and adolescents with heterozygous familial hypercholesterolemia: a prospective clinical follow-up study. J Clin Endocrinol Metab 2005;90(4):1942–52.

38. Knipscheer HC, Boelen CC, Kastelein JJ, et al. Short-term efficacy and safety of pravastatin in 72 children with familial hypercholesterolemia. Pediatr Res 1996; 39(5):867–71.

39. Avis HJ, Hutten BA, Gagne C, et al. Efficacy and safety of rosuvastatin therapy for children with familial hypercholesterolemia. J Am Coll Cardiol 2010;55(11): 1121–6.

40. Langslet G, Breazna A, Drogari E. A 3-year study of atorvastatin in children and adolescents with heterozygous familial hypercholesterolemia. J Clin Lipidol 2016; 10(5):1153–1162 e3.

41. McCrindle BW, Ose L, Marais AD. Efficacy and safety of atorvastatin in children and adolescents with familial hypercholesterolemia or severe hyperlipidemia: a multicenter, randomized, placebo-controlled trial. J Pediatr 2003;143(1):74–80.

42. van der Graaf A, Nierman MC, Firth JC, et al. Efficacy and safety of fluvastatin in children and adolescents with heterozygous familial hypercholesterolaemia. Acta Paediatr 2006;95(11):1461–6.

43. Stein EA, Illingworth DR, Kwiterovich PO Jr, et al. Efficacy and safety of lovastatin in adolescent males with heterozygous familial hypercholesterolemia: a randomized controlled trial. JAMA 1999;281(2):137–44.

44. Clauss SB, Holmes KW, Hopkins P, et al. Efficacy and safety of lovastatin therapy in adolescent girls with heterozygous familial hypercholesterolemia. Pediatrics 2005;116(3):682–8.

45. Lambert M, Lupien PJ, Gagne C, et al. Treatment of familial hypercholesterolemia in children and adolescents: effect of lovastatin. Canadian Lovastatin in Children Study Group. Pediatrics 1996;97(5):619–28.

46. Dirisamer A, Hachemian N, Bucek RA, et al. The effect of low-dose simvastatin in children with familial hypercholesterolaemia: a 1-year observation. Eur J Pediatr 2003;162(6):421–5.

47. de Jongh S, Ose L, Szamosi T, et al. Efficacy and safety of statin therapy in children with familial hypercholesterolemia: a randomized, double-blind, placebo-controlled trial with simvastatin. Circulation 2002;106(17):2231–7.

48. Expert panel on integrated guidelines for cardiovascular health and risk reduction in children and adolescents: summary report. Pediatrics 2011;128(Suppl 5): S213–56.

49. Newman CB, Preiss D, Tobert JA, et al. Statin safety and associated adverse events: a scientific statement from the american heart association. Arterioscler Thromb Vasc Biol 2019;39(2):e38–81.

50. Lozano P, Henrikson NB, Dunn J, et al. Lipid screening in childhood and adolescence for detection of familial hypercholesterolemia: evidence report and systematic review for the us preventive services task force. JAMA 2016;316(6): 645–55.

51. https://www.fda.gov/media/150774/download. 2021.

52. Augustine AH, Lowenstein LM, Harris WS, et al. Treatment with omega-3 fatty acid ethyl-ester alters fatty acid composition of lipoproteins in overweight or obese adults with insulin resistance. Prostaglandins Leukot Essent Fatty Acids 2014;90(2–3):69–75.

53. Tonstad S, Sivertsen M, Aksnes L, et al. Low dose colestipol in adolescents with familial hypercholesterolaemia. Arch Dis Child 1996;74(2):157–60.

54. Tonstad S, Knudtzon J, Sivertsen M, et al. Efficacy and safety of cholestyramine therapy in peripubertal and prepubertal children with familial hypercholesterolemia. J Pediatr 1996;129(1):42–9.

55. Stein EA, Marais AD, Szamosi T, et al. Colesevelam hydrochloride: efficacy and safety in pediatric subjects with heterozygous familial hypercholesterolemia. J Pediatr 2010;156(2):231–6.

56. Garg A. Dyslipidemias : pathophysiology, evaluation and management. Humana Press; 2015.

57. Clauss S, Wai KM, Kavey RE, et al. Ezetimibe treatment of pediatric patients with hypercholesterolemia. J Pediatr 2009;154(6):869–72.

58. Yeste D, Chacon P, Clemente M, et al. Ezetimibe as monotherapy in the treatment of hypercholesterolemia in children and adolescents. J Pediatr Endocrinol Metab 2009;22(6):487–92.

59. van der Graaf A, Cuffie-Jackson C, Vissers MN, et al. Efficacy and safety of coadministration of ezetimibe and simvastatin in adolescents with heterozygous familial hypercholesterolemia. J Am Coll Cardiol 2008;52(17):1421–9.

60. Colletti RB, Neufeld EJ, Roff NK, et al. Niacin treatment of hypercholesterolemia in children. Pediatrics 1993;92(1):78–82.

61. Anderson TJ, Boden WE, Desvigne-Nickens P, et al. Safety profile of extended-release niacin in the AIM-HIGH trial. N Engl J Med 2014;371(3):288–90.

62. HPS 2-THRIVE Collaborative Group, Landray MJ, Haynes R, et al. Effects of extended-release niacin with laropiprant in high-risk patients. N Engl J Med 2014;371(3):203–12.

63. Sabatine MS, Giugliano RP, Keech AC, et al. Evolocumab and clinical outcomes in patients with cardiovascular disease. N Engl J Med 2017;376(18):1713–22.

64. Santos RD, Ruzza A, Hovingh GK, et al. Evolocumab in pediatric heterozygous familial hypercholesterolemia. N Engl J Med 2020;383(14):1317–27.

65. Valaiyapathi B, Sunil B, Ashraf AP. Approach to hypertriglyceridemia in the pediatric population. Pediatr Rev 2017;38(9):424–34.

66. Shearer GC, Savinova OV, Harris WS. Fish oil – how does it reduce plasma triglycerides? Biochim Biophys Acta 2012;1821(5):843–51.

67. Goldberg RB, Sabharwal AK. Fish oil in the treatment of dyslipidemia. Curr Opin Endocrinol Diabetes Obes 2008;15(2):167–74.
68. Brinton EA, Ballantyne CM, Guyton JR, et al. Lipid Effects of icosapent ethyl in women with diabetes mellitus and persistent high triglycerides on statin treatment: ANCHOR trial subanalysis. J Womens Health (Larchmt) 2018;27(9): 1170–6.
69. Yang ZH, Amar M, Sampson M, et al. Comparison of omega-3 eicosapentaenoic acid versus docosahexaenoic acid-rich fish oil supplementation on plasma lipids and lipoproteins in normolipidemic adults. Nutrients 2020;12(3):749.
70. Jacobson TA, Glickstein SB, Rowe JD, et al. Effects of eicosapentaenoic acid and docosahexaenoic acid on low-density lipoprotein cholesterol and other lipids: a review. J Clin Lipidol 2012;6(1):5–18.
71. Engler MM, Engler MB, Malloy MJ, et al. Effect of docosahexaenoic acid on lipoprotein subclasses in hyperlipidemic children (the EARLY study). Am J Cardiol 2005;95(7):869–71.

Management of Dyslipidemia in Endocrine Diseases

Lisa R. Tannock, MD*

KEYWORDS

- Lipids • Cardiovascular • Endocrine • Dyslipidemia

KEY POINTS

- Treatment of dyslipidemia decreases cardiovascular risk.
- Many endocrine diseases are associated with dyslipidemia.
- Many endocrine diseases can affect cardiovascular risk, but are not considered when assessing risk.

INTRODUCTION/HISTORY/DEFINITIONS/BACKGROUND

Most lipid management guidelines recommend assessment of lipid levels and cardiovascular risk factors within an individual, then based on estimated cardiovascular disease (CVD) risk, suggest lipid-lowering therapy and/or lipid goals.[1] Overall, this approach works well. However, one of the limitations is that the cardiovascular risk factors typically included in risk calculators and guidelines are somewhat limited: smoking, hypertension, diabetes, age, sex, and race are the typical factors. In some guidelines additional factors, such as family history of premature CVD events, chronic inflammatory disorders, chronic kidney disease, and premature menopause (age <40 years), are often also noted as risk-enhancing factors. However, these factors are fairly difficult to turn into a quantitative risk, and thus often not included in risk calculators, and may be overlooked by providers.

Most endocrine disorders are chronic in nature, and thus even a minor effect to increase risk for CVD can lead to a significant impact when duration of exposure is considered. Although robust therapies exist for many endocrine disorders (whether it be suppression of excess hormone amounts, or replacement of hormone deficiencies), the therapies do not perfectly restore normal physiology. Thus, individuals with endocrine disorders are at potential increased CVD risk, and maximizing

Division of Endocrinology, Diabetes, and Metabolism, University of Kentucky, Department of Veterans Affairs, MN145, 780 Rose Street, Lexington, KY 40536, USA
* Corresponding author.
E-mail address: Lisa.Tannock@uky.edu

Endocrinol Metab Clin N Am 51 (2022) 589–602
https://doi.org/10.1016/j.ecl.2022.02.003
0889-8529/22/Published by Elsevier Inc.

strategies to reduce that risk are needed. The Endocrine Society recently published a guideline explicitly assessing the lipid profile and CVD risk and thus indications for lipid-lowering therapy in individuals with endocrine diseases.[2] This new guideline suggests that some endocrine diseases, including hyperthyroidism, hypothyroidism, Cushing disease, chronic glucocorticoid therapy with doses greater than physiologic needs, obesity, postmenopausal hormone-replacement therapy use, and premature menopause, should be included in the list of risk enhancing factors. This article reviews various endocrine conditions that can impact lipid levels and/or CVD risk.

CASE STUDY

A 47-year-old woman presents to clinic to establish care. She has recently moved to your region. She was diagnosed with autoimmune adrenal insufficiency at age 12, and takes glucocorticoid-replacement therapy. She currently takes 20 mg every morning and 5 to 10 mg in the afternoon. She tells you that her previous endocrinologist kept attempting to reduce her hydrocortisone dose, but every time she decreased the dose she suffered severe fatigue and would go back up to this dose. She states she was trained in sick day management, and doubles the dose for 2 to 4 days each time she has nausea, vomiting, fever, or severe fatigue. She estimates that she doubles her dose at least five times each year.

At age 22 she presented with Graves disease, was treated with radioactive iodine ablation, and subsequently became hypothyroid treated with levothyroxine. Her current dose is 150 μg daily. She was diagnosed with endometriosis in her teens. She had one pregnancy complicated by preeclampsia at age 32, and had hysterectomy and oophorectomy at age 37. She took estrogen for 2 to 3 years afterward, but then discontinued it because she did not see the need. She has struggled with her weight for years, but has recently put on about 10 lb (4.5 kg) with the stress of the move, and her current weight is 216 lb (98.2 kg). She reports her height as 5 ft, 6 inches (1.67 m); and her body mass index is 34.9 kg/m^2. She has long-standing depression controlled with citalopram 40 mg daily. She has never smoked.

Her current medications are:

Hydrocortisone, 25 to 30 mg daily
Levothyroxine, 150 μg daily
Multivitamin, one daily
Citalopram, 40 mg daily.

Her blood pressure is 132/74 mm Hg. Her pulse is 82 beats per minute. Her examination is notable for generalized obesity with numerous pale striae on her abdomen. Her thyroid is not palpable. The remainder of the examination is normal.

Fasting laboratory studies are as follows:

Metabolic panel normal, with fasting glucose 97 mg/dL and estimated glomerular filtration rate greater than 60 mL/min/m^2
Hemogram, normal
Thyroid-stimulating hormone 6.9 mIU/mL (normal range, 0.5–5.0 mIU/mL); free T4 0.6 ng/dL (normal range, 0.8–1.8 ng/dL)
Total cholesterol (TC) 234 mg/dL
Low-density lipoprotein cholesterol (LDL-c) 148 mg/dL
High-density lipoprotein cholesterol (HDL-c) 32 mg/dL
Triglycerides (TG) 268 mg/dL

The ASCVD risk calculator estimates her 10-year risk as 2.8%.

Clinical Questions

Does the ASCVD risk calculator 10-year risk estimate reassure you? Are there any other factors you need to consider?

DISCUSSION

On the surface, this patient seems to have several endocrine issues that need to be addressed, but cardiovascular risk does not seem to be one. She is obese, has premature menopause, inadequately treated hypothyroidism, and overtreated adrenal insufficiency. Managing these chronic conditions is important, and would likely be addressed by most endocrinologists. However, the 10-year CVD risk estimate may seem reassuring, and it would not be surprising if most providers did not consider CVD risk reduction and lipid-lowering therapy as high priorities. The recent guidelines published by the Endocrine Society suggest that her endocrine comorbidities may impact her cardiovascular risk, and should be considered.[2] In the following sections we address these (and others) one by one.

Changes in Lipids with Hyperthyroidism and Hypothyroidism

Altered thyroid hormone levels can have profound effects on lipoprotein metabolism and thus lipid levels. Thyroid hormone decreases intestinal absorption of cholesterol; increases biliary secretion leading to decreased hepatic cholesterol content and compensatory increase in LDL-receptors; increases HMG-CoA reductase activity; and increases enzymes involved in LDL metabolism including lipoprotein lipase, hepatic lipase, cholesteryl ester transfer protein and lecithin cholesterol acyltransferase.[3-7] Thus, hyperthyroidism tends to lead to accelerated metabolism of lipoprotein particles such that TC and LDL-c are often low, whereas TG and HDL-c are not usually affected. Conversely, hypothyroidism tends to lead to elevated TC, LDL-c, HDL-c, and TG. The Endocrine Society meta-analysis[8] found that treatment of hyperthyroidism (with surgery, radioactive iodine, or antithyroid medication) led to significant increases in TC and LDL-c and HDL-c with restoration of euthyroid state; however, this was only true in overt hyperthyroidism and not in subclinical hyperthyroidism. Treatment of overt hypothyroidism correspondingly led to significant decreases of TC, LDL-c, HDL-c, and TG.[8] Indeed, levothyroxine has been studied as a therapy for elevated lipid levels (**Table 1**).[9]

Whether hyperthyroidism or hypothyroidism directly influence CVD (rather than indirectly, via dyslipidemia) is unknown. Epidemiologic studies suggest that coronary disease prevalence is increased in hypothyroidism compared with euthyroid controls.[10,11] Hypothyroidism can affect cardiac contractility and exacerbate angina;

Table 1
Change in lipid parameters after treatment of thyroid disease

Mean % Change with Treatment	TC	LDL-c	HDL-c	TG
Overt hypothyroidism	↓22%	↓24%	↓7%	↓18%
Subclinical hypothyroidism	↓5%	↓8%	0%	↓4%
Overt hyperthyroidism	↑28%	↑35%	↑12%	↑7%
Subclinical hyperthyroidism	↑5%	↑6%	0%	↓30%

Data adapted from a meta-analysis of n=3-72 studies per parameter, with total patients from 104-4588 per parameter.[8]

however, it is not clear if there are direct pathophysiologic changes related to thyroid hormone abnormalities, or if the association is mediated through dyslipidemia.

Considerations for clinical management

The Endocrine Society guidelines recommend screening for hypothyroidism as a cause of dyslipidemia and deferring treatment decisions until after restoration of euthyroid status when a patient has either hyperthyroidism or hypothyroidism. These recommendations are prudent and will help avoid unnecessary lipid-lowering therapy in the setting of hypothyroidism (if the repeated lipid panel shows resolution of hyperlipidemia), and avoid a missed therapeutic opportunity in the setting of hyperthyroidism if the lipid panel is falsely reassuring when the patient is hyperthyroid.

Thus, for the case vignette presented, it would be prudent to adjust her levothyroxine dose, and repeat the lipid panel 6 to 8 weeks later when she would be expected to be euthyroid. Although her freeT4 is only marginally low, restoration of euthyroid state could lead to some improvement in her dyslipidemia.

Changes in Lipids with Glucocorticoid Excess or Therapy

Elevated glucocorticoid levels (whether endogenous, such as in Cushing syndrome, or exogenous, as in the case vignette) can lead to elevations in TC, LDL-c, and TG. Glucocorticoids stimulate preadipocyte differentiation and increased adipose tissue, especially visceral adipose, and also promote fatty acid and cholesterol synthesis in the liver, leading to hepatic steatosis.[12] Chronic elevations in glucocorticoids increase metabolic syndrome prevalence, with associated hypertension, insulin resistance, and prothrombotic state, all of which contribute to increased CVD risk. Patients cured of Cushing syndrome typically experience improvements in dyslipidemia, and reduced obesity, hypertension, and insulin resistance.[13] For patients using exogenous steroids the literature is conflicted, but at least one study indicates a glucocorticoid dose-dependent increase in TC, LDL-c, and TG levels.[14,15] Furthermore, several studies suggest increased CVD in patients using exogenous glucocorticoids, particularly for those with iatrogenic hypercortisolism and Cushing syndrome.[16–19]

Considerations for clinical management

The Endocrine Society guidelines address lipid screening and management in settings of excess endogenous or exogenous glucocorticoids. The guidelines recommend screening lipid levels in adults with Cushing syndrome and those on chronic glucocorticoid therapy greater than standard physiologic replacement doses. The guidelines go on to suggest statin therapy in addition to lifestyle modification in adults with persistent Cushing syndrome to reduce CVD risk, regardless of cardiovascular risk score. There is not any evidence to guide recommendation of lipid lowering therapies (statins) in individuals with exogenous glucocorticoids greater than physiologic doses, but certainly, there is accumulating evidence that supraphysiologic doses of glucocorticoids convey health risks. Thus, at a minimum it is prudent to recommend decreasing glucocorticoid doses, which may help decrease lipid levels and CVD risk.

Thus, for the case vignette presented, it would be prudent to taper her hydrocortisone dose down, review sick day rules to minimize excessive dosing, and repeat the lipid panel when stable on a lower dose. Collectively, her use of glucocorticoid therapy should be considered along with other risk factors when making a decision about lipid-lowering therapy.

Changes in Lipids with Obesity

Obesity prevalence is high and rising, and thus a common concern for health care providers. In particular, when obesity is mainly central it often exists as part of the metabolic syndrome (elevated TG, reduced HDL, increased waist circumference, hyperglycemia, increased blood pressure) where dyslipidemia is highly prevalent, and robust evidence indicates an increased risk for CVD. Even without metabolic syndrome, obesity is associated with elevations in TG and decreases in HDL-c, and although LDL-c may not be elevated, the particles are often small and dense, which are thought to be more atherogenic.[20–22] In addition, delayed lipoprotein metabolism leads to prolonged and exacerbated postprandial hyperglycemia.[23–25] Furthermore, elevated body mass index, or increased waist circumference or waist/hip ratio are predictors of CVD mortality.[24,26–28]

Considerations for clinical management

Weight loss, whether induced by caloric restriction, medications, or surgery, leads to improvements in the lipid profile. Five percent body weight reduction can lead to improvements in several comorbidities of obesity.[29] There is a corresponding improvement in lipids with increased weight loss, so that 3-kg weight loss is associated with a TG decrease of 15 mg/dL (0.17 mmol/L), but weight loss of 5 to 8 kg is associated with decreases in LDL-c of −5 mg/dL (−0.13 mmol/L) and increases in HDL-c of 2 to 3 mg/dL (0.5–0.8 mmol/L).[30] A meta-analysis showed that the most consistent and favorable effect of weight loss is a lowering of TG.[31] When patients are actively undergoing weight loss several changes in lipid levels can occur, including paradoxic drops in HDL-c during active weight loss[32,33]; thus, the Endocrine Society recommends reassessment of lipids after weight loss once weight has stabilized.

Lipid-lowering therapy with statins has been clearly shown to decrease CVD events in patients with and without obesity. Although LDL-c is not always high in obesity, statins (which target LDL-c) are highly efficacious in lowering CVD risk.[34,35] Conversely, fibrates (which target TG) have not been consistently shown to decrease CVD risk. Thus, if there are indications for lipid-lowering therapy then most guidelines recommend statins as the first-line therapy. Of note, when TG are elevated to the extent that pancreatitis is a risk there is uniform agreement of using fibrates to lower TG.

Thus, for the case vignette presented, it would be appropriate to screen her for metabolic syndrome (based on information provided she does have metabolic syndrome because she has high TG, low HDL-c, and high systolic blood pressure; even without knowing her fasting glucose or waist circumference), and counsel her on weight loss strategies. The Endocrine Society recommends use of a risk calculator to assess 10-year CVD risk, and initiation of lipid-lowering therapy if indicated by the calculator. In this vignette the 10-year CVD risk was 2.8%, and thus she does not clearly meet recommendations for lipid-lowering therapy. However, as discussed throughout this article, the risk calculator does not adjust for potential CVD impact of her combined metabolic disorders, and may underestimate her risk.

Changes in Lipids with Menopause

Although the changes in lipid levels from premenopause to postmenopause are fairly small, epidemiologic evidence consistently indicates an increase in CVD risk. Studies have yielded variable results, but in general the lipid panel shows decreases in HDL-c, increases in TC, and a shift in LDL particle size toward a small, dense phenotype; collectively these are proatherogenic changes. The mechanisms behind shifts in lipid levels likely relate to the decrease in estrogen. Estrogen affects VLDL synthesis, insulin sensitivity, LDL-receptors, and PCSK9.[36,37] Estrogen-replacement therapy leads to increases in HDL-c and decreases in LDL-c; however, progestins tend to decrease HDL-c.[38,39] In patients with an underlying predisposition to hypertriglyceridemia (because of genetics or other risk factors, such as diabetes, obesity, or insulin resistance) estrogen therapy can cause significant increases in TG levels and increase risk for pancreatitis. However, although this is not uncommonly seen in specific individuals, population-based studies have not found a significant increase of pancreatitis with estrogen therapy.[40]

Considerations for clinical management

Several decades ago the standard of care was to recommend hormone-replacement therapy (estrogen, with or without progestins for uterine protection) with the expectation this would decrease CVD risk in postmenopausal women. However, several large randomized controlled trials of estrogen ($\pm$ progestins) found increased CVD events, thought to be caused by increased thrombosis, especially when introduced late after onset of menopause (>60 years, or >10 years since last menstrual period).[41,42] Thus, most guidelines recommend caution for initiation of estrogen, especially in older women.

When menopause occurs early, regardless of whether it is spontaneous or surgically induced, CVD risk is increased: a younger age at menopause seems to be an independent risk factor for CVD.[43–46] The estimate is that the risk of ASCVD is 1.5-fold higher in women with menopause less than 40 years, and 1.3-fold higher in women with menopause occurring at age 40 to 44 years, compared with women who entered menopause at age 50 to 51 years.[46] Several recent guidelines now recognize early menopause as a cardiovascular risk factor. Statin therapy in postmenopausal women has been shown to lower CVD risk, for women using or not using hormone-replacement therapy.[47,48] As further evidence, a meta-analysis of estrogen therapy in younger women reported a significant reduction in CVD.[49] Thus, the Endocrine Society recommends use of statin therapy in postmenopausal women with dyslipidemia, or those on hormone therapy with other risk factors for CVD, and encourages consideration of CVD risk in patients who enter menopause early.

Thus, for the case vignette presented, there are several factors to consider. Her hypothyroidism is undertreated, her glucocorticoid dose is supraphysiologic, she has obesity, and she has early menopause. Although the 10-year risk calculator estimates her risk as fairly low (2.8%) none of these factors are included in that calculator. Collectively, this patient has several endocrine comorbidities that each confer increased CVD risk, and initiation of statin therapy would be expected to help reduce her risk. However, if the provider does not consider each of these comorbidities, the therapeutic opportunity may be missed.

OTHER LIPID-INFLUENCING ENDOCRINE DIAGNOSES

Beyond the topics raised by the case vignette, the Endocrine Society addressed several other endocrine diagnoses that affect lipid levels and CVD risk. These are summarized next.

Changes in Lipids with Polycystic Ovary Syndrome

Polycystic ovary syndrome (PCOS) is characterized by insulin resistance and often a similar lipid profile to that seen in metabolic syndrome: increased TG, low HDL-c, and normal or increased LDL-c.[50,51] In addition, increased levels of Lp(a) may be seen, particularly in nonobese women with PCOS.[52–54] The dyslipidemia exists throughout the reproductive years, tends to be worse in anovulatory women,[53,55] and may be further exacerbated after the onset of menopause. Thus, although the dyslipidemia may be mild, it may be of long duration. Despite the dyslipidemia, it is not clear if there is increased ASCVD risk in PCOS per se, or if the risk is explained by the obesity and metabolic syndrome components.[56]

Considerations for clinical management

Unlike the impact on dyslipidemia in obesity and metabolic syndrome, weight loss achieved via lifestyle therapy (diet and exercise) in PCOS seems to have minimal effects on the dyslipidemia, although improvements in body composition, insulin resistance, and ovulation are seen.[57,58] Other common therapies used in PCOS include metformin and oral contraceptives. Metformin monotherapy seems to have minimal effects on the dyslipidemia in PCOS, although metformin in combination with other medications, such as statins, thiazolidinediones, oral contraceptives, or inositol, can induce improvements.[59–61] However, treatment with oral contraceptives confers the risk of further elevations in TG in susceptible women, although beneficial effects of estrogen on LDL-c and HDL-c are seen.[62]

There have been several trials determining the effect of lipid-lowering medications (mainly statins) in PCOS; collectively, statins are efficacious at lipid-lowering in women with PCOS,[63–67] but cardiovascular outcomes and reproductive outcomes remain unclear.

The Endocrine Society recommends obtaining a lipid panel in all women with PCOS, but using lipid-lowering therapies only as indicated for lipid lowering, and not for the treatment of hyperandrogenism or infertility.

Changes in Lipids with Male Hypogonadism and Testosterone Therapy

Men with hypogonadism tend to have elevations in LDL-c and TG with lower levels of HDL-c[68]; however, repletion of testosterone tends to have minimal effects on lipid levels.[69,70] Thus, use of testosterone therapy is not recommended as a treatment of dyslipidemia. Furthermore, illicit use of testosterone or other androgens is not uncommon, and elevated (supraphysiologic) androgen levels can dramatically suppress HDL-c, increase ApoB and decrease Lp(a).[71,72]

Considerations for clinical management

Although hypogonadism is associated with increased CVD risk,[73] there are multiple factors involved, including insulin resistance, obesity, increased prevalence of metabolic syndrome, and increased free fatty acids, in addition to the dyslipidemia. However, it remains controversial if testosterone therapy alters CVD risk, with some benefit perhaps seen in appropriate dosing of certain subpopulations, but no global benefit.[74]

The Endocrine Society recommends using testosterone therapy for hypogonadism symptoms, but not as a treatment of dyslipidemia or CVD risk. Moreover, in patients with very low HDL-c but without high TG, androgen abuse should be considered as a cause of the dyslipidemia.

Changes in Lipids with Gender-Affirming Hormone Therapy

The use of gender-affirming hormone therapy is increasing, but there is still a paucity of long-term outcome data to guide CVD recommendations. Numerous small studies and a meta-analysis reported an increase in TG and LDL-c and a drop in HDL-c with use of testosterone therapy for transmen.[75–77] In transwomen treated with estrogen therapy most studies have reported an increase in TG with use of oral estrogens, but not with use of transdermal estrogens.[77] Although an increase in HDL-c may be expected, this has not always been confirmed.

Considerations for clinical management

There are minimal data to guide use of lipid-lowering therapy in the transgender population. The Endocrine Society recommends evaluation of CVD risk using the same guidelines as in cisgender adults.

Changes in Lipids with Growth Hormone Deficiency or Growth Hormone Excess

In the setting of growth hormone deficiency, elevations in TC and LDL-c are commonly seen, whereas TG and HDL-c changes are variable.[78–80] Conversely, in growth hormone excess, such as seen in acromegaly, increased TG is commonly observed with variable effects on cholesterol and LDL-c levels.[81,82] Growth hormone inhibits hepatic lipase and lipoprotein lipase activity[81,83] and can increase hepatic LDL-R expression and decrease PCSK9 expression.[84,85]

Considerations for clinical management

Hypopituitarism, of which growth hormone deficiency is the most common hormone abnormality, is associated with increased premature mortality, including increased risk of CVD.[86–88] Growth hormone deficiency itself may affect the myocardial and endothelial tissue, cardiac performance, and coronary calcification, although the direct mechanisms linking growth hormone deficiency and CVD are not fully understood. Although long-term growth hormone therapy improves the dyslipidemia in growth hormone deficiency[89–91] it is not clear that growth hormone therapy can decrease mortality.[92]

SUMMARY

Numerous endocrine disorders affect lipid levels, and thus may confer risk for CVD. Because the current CVD risk calculators that are widely used to guide lipid-lowering therapy decisions do not consider endocrine comorbidities, CVD risk may be underestimated, and thus lipid-lowering therapy may be underused in these populations. Consideration of the additional impact of endocrine diseases when assessing individuals for dyslipidemia, CVD risk, and lipid lowering therapy is urged.

CLINICS CARE POINTS

- Many endocrine diseases affect lipid levels and thus may confer CVD risk.
- CVD risk calculators do not currently assess the impact of endocrine comorbidities.
- Clinicians should consider impact of endocrine comorbidities on CVD risk when making treatment decisions regarding lipid-lowering medications.

ACKNOWLEDGMENTS

This work was supported in part by funding from the National Institutes of Health R01 HL147381 and the Department of Veterans Affairs BX004275.

DISCLOSURE

Dr L.R. Tannock has no conflicts to disclose.

REFERENCES

1. Grundy SM, Stone NJ, Bailey AL, et al. 2018 AHA/ACC/AACVPR/AAPA/ABC/ACPM/ADA/AGS/APhA/ASPC/NLA/PCNA Guideline on the management of blood cholesterol: a report of the American College of Cardiology/American Heart Association task force on clinical practice guidelines. Circulation 2019;139(25):e1082–143.

2. Newman CB, Blaha MJ, Boord JB, et al. Lipid management in patients with endocrine disorders: an endocrine society clinical practice guideline. J Clin Endocrinol Metab 2020;105(12):dgaa674.
3. Choi JW, Choi HS. The regulatory effects of thyroid hormone on the activity of 3-hydroxy-3-methylglutaryl coenzyme A reductase. Endocr Res 2000;26(1):1–21.
4. Duntas LH, Brenta G. The effect of thyroid disorders on lipid levels and metabolism. Med Clin North Am 2012;96(2):269–81.
5. Kuusi T, Taskinen MR, Nikkila EA. Lipoproteins, lipolytic enzymes, and hormonal status in hypothyroid women at different levels of substitution. J Clin Endocrinol Metab 1988;66(1):51–6.
6. Lithell H, Boberg J, Hellsing K, et al. Serum lipoprotein and apolipoprotein concentrations and tissue lipoprotein-lipase activity in overt and subclinical hypothyroidism: the effect of substitution therapy. Eur J Clin Invest 1981;11(1):3–10.
7. Lopez D, Abisambra Socarras JF, Bedi M, et al. Activation of the hepatic LDL receptor promoter by thyroid hormone. Biochim Biophys Acta 2007;1771(9):1216–25.
8. Kotwal A, Cortes T, Genere N, et al. Treatment of thyroid dysfunction and serum lipids: a systematic review and meta-analysis. J Clin Endocrinol Metab 2020;105(12):dgaa672.
9. Tanis BC, Westendorp GJ, Smelt HM. Effect of thyroid substitution on hypercholesterolaemia in patients with subclinical hypothyroidism: a reanalysis of intervention studies. Clin Endocrinol (Oxf) 1996;44(6):643–9.
10. Mya MM, Aronow WS. Subclinical hypothyroidism is associated with coronary artery disease in older persons. J Gerontol A Biol Sci Med Sci 2002;57(10):M658–9.
11. Razvi S, Jabbar A, Pingitore A, et al. Thyroid hormones and cardiovascular function and diseases. J Am Coll Cardiol 2018;71(16):1781–96.
12. Ferrau F, Korbonits M. Metabolic comorbidities in Cushing's syndrome. Eur J Endocrinol 2015;173(4):M133–57.
13. Giordano R, Picu A, Marinazzo E, et al. Metabolic and cardiovascular outcomes in patients with Cushing's syndrome of different aetiologies during active disease and 1 year after remission. Clin Endocrinol (Oxf) 2011;75(3):354–60.
14. Choi HK, Seeger JD. Glucocorticoid use and serum lipid levels in US adults: the Third National Health and Nutrition Examination Survey. Arthritis Rheum 2005;53(4):528–35.
15. Filipsson H, Monson JP, Koltowska-Haggstrom M, et al. The impact of glucocorticoid replacement regimens on metabolic outcome and comorbidity in hypopituitary patients. J Clin Endocrinol Metab 2006;91(10):3954–61.
16. Fardet L, Petersen I, Nazareth I. Risk of cardiovascular events in people prescribed glucocorticoids with iatrogenic Cushing's syndrome: cohort study. BMJ 2012;345:e4928.
17. Souverein PC, Berard A, Van Staa TP, et al. Use of oral glucocorticoids and risk of cardiovascular and cerebrovascular disease in a population based case-control study. Heart 2004;90(8):859–65.
18. Varas-Lorenzo C, Rodriguez LA, Maguire A, et al. Use of oral corticosteroids and the risk of acute myocardial infarction. Atherosclerosis 2007;192(2):376–83.
19. Wei L, MacDonald TM, Walker BR. Taking glucocorticoids by prescription is associated with subsequent cardiovascular disease. Ann Intern Med 2004;141(10):764–70.
20. Franssen R, Monajemi H, Stroes ES, et al. Obesity and dyslipidemia. Med Clin North Am 2011;95(5):893–902.

21. Klop B, Elte JW, Cabezas MC. Dyslipidemia in obesity: mechanisms and potential targets. Nutrients 2013;5(4):1218–40.
22. Paredes S, Fonseca L, Ribeiro L, et al. Novel and traditional lipid profiles in metabolic syndrome reveal a high atherogenicity. Sci Rep 2019;9(1):11792.
23. Couillard C, Bergeron N, Prud'homme D, et al. Postprandial triglyceride response in visceral obesity in men. Diabetes 1998;47(6):953–60.
24. Nieves DJ, Cnop M, Retzlaff B, et al. The atherogenic lipoprotein profile associated with obesity and insulin resistance is largely attributable to intra-abdominal fat. Diabetes 2003;52(1):172–9.
25. Taskinen MR, Adiels M, Westerbacka J, et al. Dual metabolic defects are required to produce hypertriglyceridemia in obese subjects. Arterioscler Thromb Vasc Biol 2011;31(9):2144–50.
26. Ohlson LO, Larsson B, Svardsudd K, et al. The influence of body fat distribution on the incidence of diabetes mellitus. 13.5 years of follow-up of the participants in the study of men born in 1913. Diabetes 1985;34(10):1055–8.
27. Ortega FB, Lavie CJ, Blair SN. Obesity and cardiovascular disease. Circ Res 2016;118(11):1752–70.
28. Yusuf S, Hawken S, Ounpuu S, et al. Obesity and the risk of myocardial infarction in 27,000 participants from 52 countries: a case-control study. Lancet 2005; 366(9497):1640–9.
29. Jensen MD, Ryan DH, Apovian CM, et al. 2013 AHA/ACC/TOS guideline for the management of overweight and obesity in adults: a report of the American College of Cardiology/American Heart Association Task Force on Practice Guidelines and The Obesity Society. Circulation 2014;129(25 Suppl 2):S102–38.
30. Zomer E, Gurusamy K, Leach R, et al. Interventions that cause weight loss and the impact on cardiovascular risk factors: a systematic review and meta-analysis. Obes Rev 2016;17(10):1001–11.
31. Hasan B, Nayfeh T, Alzuabi M, et al. Weight loss and serum lipids in overweight and obese adults: a systematic review and meta-analysis. J Clin Endocrinol Metab 2020;105(12):dgaa673.
32. Dattilo AM, Kris-Etherton PM. Effects of weight reduction on blood lipids and lipoproteins: a meta-analysis. Am J Clin Nutr 1992;56(2):320–8.
33. Wadden TA, Anderson DA, Foster GD. Two-year changes in lipids and lipoproteins associated with the maintenance of a 5% to 10% reduction in initial weight: some findings and some questions. Obes Res 1999;7(2):170–8.
34. Won KB, Hur SH, Nam CW, et al. Evaluation of the impact of statin therapy on the obesity paradox in patients with acute myocardial infarction: a propensity score matching analysis from the Korea acute myocardial infarction registry. *Medicine (Baltimore)* 2017;96(35):e7180.
35. Nicholls SJ, Tuzcu EM, Sipahi I, et al. Effects of obesity on lipid-lowering, anti-inflammatory, and antiatherosclerotic benefits of atorvastatin or pravastatin in patients with coronary artery disease (from the REVERSAL Study). Am J Cardiol 2006;97(11):1553–7.
36. Palmisano BT, Zhu L, Stafford JM. Role of estrogens in the regulation of liver lipid metabolism. Adv Exp Med Biol 2017;1043:227–56.
37. Ghosh M, Galman C, Rudling M, et al. Influence of physiological changes in endogenous estrogen on circulating PCSK9 and LDL cholesterol. J Lipid Res 2015;56(2):463–9.
38. Effects of estrogen or estrogen/progestin regimens on heart disease risk factors in postmenopausal women. The Postmenopausal Estrogen/Progestin

Interventions (PEPI) Trial. The Writing Group for the PEPI Trial. JAMA 1995;273(3): 199–208.

39. Godsland IF. Effects of postmenopausal hormone replacement therapy on lipid, lipoprotein, and apolipoprotein (a) concentrations: analysis of studies published from 1974-2000. Fertil Steril 2001;75(5):898–915.
40. Tetsche MS, Jacobsen J, Norgaard M, et al. Postmenopausal hormone replacement therapy and risk of acute pancreatitis: a population-based case-control study. Am J Gastroenterol 2007;102(2):275–8.
41. Hulley S, Grady D, Bush T, et al. Randomized trial of estrogen plus progestin for secondary prevention of coronary heart disease in postmenopausal women. Heart and Estrogen/progestin Replacement Study (HERS) Research Group. JAMA 1998;280(7):605–13.
42. Manson JE, Hsia J, Johnson KC, et al. Estrogen plus progestin and the risk of coronary heart disease. N Engl J Med 2003;349(6):523–34.
43. Lubiszewska B, Kruk M, Broda G, et al. The impact of early menopause on risk of coronary artery disease (PREmature Coronary Artery Disease In Women–PRECADIW case-control study). Eur J Prev Cardiol 2012;19(1):95–101.
44. Muka T, Oliver-Williams C, Kunutsor S, et al. Association of age at onset of menopause and time since onset of menopause with cardiovascular outcomes, intermediate vascular traits, and all-cause mortality: a systematic review and meta-analysis. JAMA Cardiol 2016;1(7):767–76.
45. Wellons M, Ouyang P, Schreiner PJ, et al. Early menopause predicts future coronary heart disease and stroke: the Multi-Ethnic Study of Atherosclerosis. Menopause 2012;19(10):1081–7.
46. Zhu D, Chung HF, Dobson AJ, et al. Age at natural menopause and risk of incident cardiovascular disease: a pooled analysis of individual patient data. Lancet Public Health 2019;4(11):e553–64.
47. Herrington DM, Vittinghoff E, Lin F, et al. Statin therapy, cardiovascular events, and total mortality in the Heart and Estrogen/Progestin Replacement Study (HERS). Circulation 2002;105(25):2962–7.
48. Berglind IA, Andersen M, Citarella A, et al. Hormone therapy and risk of cardiovascular outcomes and mortality in women treated with statins. Menopause 2015; 22(4):369–76.
49. Salpeter SR, Walsh JM, Greyber E, et al. Brief report: coronary heart disease events associated with hormone therapy in younger and older women. A meta-analysis. J Gen Intern Med 2006;21(4):363–6.
50. Legro RS, Kunselman AR, Dunaif A. Prevalence and predictors of dyslipidemia in women with polycystic ovary syndrome. Am J Med 2001;111(8):607–13.
51. Berneis K, Rizzo M, Lazzarini V, et al. Atherogenic lipoprotein phenotype and low-density lipoproteins size and subclasses in women with polycystic ovary syndrome. J Clin Endocrinol Metab 2007;92(1):186–9.
52. Berneis K, Rizzo M, Hersberger M, et al. Atherogenic forms of dyslipidaemia in women with polycystic ovary syndrome. Int J Clin Pract 2009;63(1):56–62.
53. Rizzo M, Berneis K, Hersberger M, et al. Milder forms of atherogenic dyslipidemia in ovulatory versus anovulatory polycystic ovary syndrome phenotype. Hum Reprod 2009;24(9):2286–92.
54. Enkhmaa B, Anuurad E, Zhang W, et al. Lipoprotein(a) and apolipoprotein(a) in polycystic ovary syndrome. Clin Endocrinol (Oxf) 2016;84(2):229–35.
55. Kim JJ, Chae SJ, Choi YM, et al. Atherogenic changes in low-density lipoprotein particle profiles were not observed in non-obese women with polycystic ovary syndrome. Hum Reprod 2013;28(5):1354–60.

56. Fauser BC, Tarlatzis BC, Rebar RW, et al. Consensus on women's health aspects of polycystic ovary syndrome (PCOS): the Amsterdam ESHRE/ASRM-Sponsored 3rd PCOS Consensus Workshop Group. Fertil Steril 2012;97(1):28–38.e25.

57. Moran LJ, Hutchison SK, Norman RJ, et al. Lifestyle changes in women with polycystic ovary syndrome. Cochrane Database Syst Rev 2011;(7):CD007506.

58. Haqq L, McFarlane J, Dieberg G, et al. The effect of lifestyle intervention on body composition, glycemic control, and cardiorespiratory fitness in polycystic ovarian syndrome: a systematic review and meta-analysis. Int J Sport Nutr Exerc Metab 2015;25(6):533–40.

59. Wang A, Mo T, Li Q, et al. The effectiveness of metformin, oral contraceptives, and lifestyle modification in improving the metabolism of overweight women with polycystic ovary syndrome: a network meta-analysis. Endocrine 2019; 64(2):220–32.

60. Zhao H, Xing C, Zhang J, et al. Comparative efficacy of oral insulin sensitizers metformin, thiazolidinediones, inositol, and berberine in improving endocrine and metabolic profiles in women with PCOS: a network meta-analysis. Reprod Health 2021;18(1):171.

61. Liu Y, Shao Y, Xie J, et al. The efficacy and safety of metformin combined with simvastatin in the treatment of polycystic ovary syndrome: a meta-analysis and systematic review. Medicine (Baltimore) 2021;100(31):e26622.

62. Herink M, Ito MK. Medication induced changes in lipid and lipoproteins. In: Feingold KR, Anawalt B, Boyce A, et al, editors. Endotext. 2000.

63. Banaszewska B, Pawelczyk L, Spaczynski RZ, et al. Effects of simvastatin and oral contraceptive agent on polycystic ovary syndrome: prospective, randomized, crossover trial. J Clin Endocrinol Metab 2007;92(2):456–61.

64. Puurunen J, Piltonen T, Puukka K, et al. Statin therapy worsens insulin sensitivity in women with polycystic ovary syndrome (PCOS): a prospective, randomized, double-blind, placebo-controlled study. J Clin Endocrinol Metab 2013;98(12): 4798–807.

65. Raja-Khan N, Kunselman AR, Hogeman CS, et al. Effects of atorvastatin on vascular function, inflammation, and androgens in women with polycystic ovary syndrome: a double-blind, randomized, placebo-controlled trial. Fertil Steril 2011;95(5):1849–52.

66. Raval AD, Hunter T, Stuckey B, et al. Statins for women with polycystic ovary syndrome not actively trying to conceive. Cochrane Database Syst Rev 2011;(10):CD008565.

67. Sathyapalan T, Kilpatrick ES, Coady AM, et al. The effect of atorvastatin in patients with polycystic ovary syndrome: a randomized double-blind placebo-controlled study. J Clin Endocrinol Metab 2009;94(1):103–8.

68. Feingold KR, Brinton EA, Grunfeld C. The effect of endocrine disorders on lipids and lipoproteins. In: Feingold KR, Anawalt B, Boyce A, et al, editors. Endotext. 2000.

69. Huo S, Scialli AR, McGarvey S, et al. Treatment of men for "low testosterone": a systematic review. PLoS One 2016;11(9):e0162480.

70. Pizzocaro A, Vena W, Condorelli R, et al. Testosterone treatment in male patients with Klinefelter syndrome: a systematic review and meta-analysis. J Endocrinol Invest 2020;43(12):1675–87.

71. Kuipers H, Wijnen JA, Hartgens F, et al. Influence of anabolic steroids on body composition, blood pressure, lipid profile and liver functions in body builders. Int J Sports Med 1991;12(4):413–8.

72. Hartgens F, Rietjens G, Keizer HA, et al. Effects of androgenic-anabolic steroids on apolipoproteins and lipoprotein (a). Br J Sports Med 2004;38(3):253–9.
73. Corona G, Rastrelli G, Di Pasquale G, et al. Endogenous testosterone levels and cardiovascular risk: meta-analysis of observational studies. J Sex Med 2018; 15(9):1260–71.
74. Corona G, Rastrelli G, Di Pasquale G, et al. Testosterone and cardiovascular risk: meta-analysis of interventional studies. J Sex Med 2018;15(6):820–38.
75. Velho I, Fighera TM, Ziegelmann PK, et al. Effects of testosterone therapy on BMI, blood pressure, and laboratory profile of transgender men: a systematic review. Andrology 2017;5(5):881–8.
76. Irwig MS. Testosterone therapy for transgender men. Lancet Diabetes Endocrinol 2017;5(4):301–11.
77. Maraka S, Singh Ospina N, Rodriguez-Gutierrez R, et al. Sex steroids and cardiovascular outcomes in transgender individuals: a systematic review and meta-analysis. J Clin Endocrinol Metab 2017;102(11):3914–23.
78. Abdu TA, Neary R, Elhadd TA, et al. Coronary risk in growth hormone deficient hypopituitary adults: increased predicted risk is due largely to lipid profile abnormalities. Clin Endocrinol (Oxf) 2001;55(2):209–16.
79. Beshyah SA, Johnston DG. Cardiovascular disease and risk factors in adults with hypopituitarism. Clin Endocrinol (Oxf) 1999;50(1):1–15.
80. de Boer H, Blok GJ, Van der Veen EA. Clinical aspects of growth hormone deficiency in adults. Endocr Rev 1995;16(1):63–86.
81. Takeda R, Tatami R, Ueda K, et al. The incidence and pathogenesis of hyperlipidaemia in 16 consecutive acromegalic patients. Acta Endocrinol (Copenh) 1982; 100(3):358–62.
82. Beentjes JA, van Tol A, Sluiter WJ, et al. Low plasma lecithin:cholesterol acyltransferase and lipid transfer protein activities in growth hormone deficient and acromegalic men: role in altered high density lipoproteins. Atherosclerosis 2000;153(2):491–8.
83. Tan KC, Shiu SW, Janus ED, et al. LDL subfractions in acromegaly: relation to growth hormone and insulin-like growth factor-I. Atherosclerosis 1997;129(1): 59–65.
84. Rudling M, Parini P, Angelin B. Effects of growth hormone on hepatic cholesterol metabolism. Lessons from studies in rats and humans. Growth Horm IGF Res 1999;9(Suppl A):1–7.
85. Persson L, Cao G, Stahle L, et al. Circulating proprotein convertase subtilisin kexin type 9 has a diurnal rhythm synchronous with cholesterol synthesis and is reduced by fasting in humans. Arterioscler Thromb Vasc Biol 2010;30(12): 2666–72.
86. Nielsen EH, Lindholm J, Laurberg P. Excess mortality in women with pituitary disease: a meta-analysis. Clin Endocrinol (Oxf) 2007;67(5):693–7.
87. Pappachan JM, Raskauskiene D, Kutty VR, et al. Excess mortality associated with hypopituitarism in adults: a meta-analysis of observational studies. J Clin Endocrinol Metab 2015;100(4):1405–11.
88. Rosen T, Bengtsson BA. Premature mortality due to cardiovascular disease in hypopituitarism. Lancet 1990;336(8710):285–8.
89. Deepak D, Daousi C, Javadpour M, et al. The influence of growth hormone replacement on peripheral inflammatory and cardiovascular risk markers in adults with severe growth hormone deficiency. Growth Horm IGF Res 2010; 20(3):220–5.

90. Maison P, Griffin S, Nicoue-Beglah M, et al. Impact of growth hormone (GH) treatment on cardiovascular risk factors in GH-deficient adults: a metaanalysis of blinded, randomized, placebo-controlled trials. J Clin Endocrinol Metab 2004; 89(5):2192–9.

91. Newman CB, Carmichael JD, Kleinberg DL. Effects of low dose versus high dose human growth hormone on body composition and lipids in adults with GH deficiency: a meta-analysis of placebo-controlled randomized trials. Pituitary 2015; 18(3):297–305.

92. van Bunderen CC, van Nieuwpoort IC, Arwert LI, et al. Does growth hormone replacement therapy reduce mortality in adults with growth hormone deficiency? Data from the Dutch National Registry of Growth Hormone Treatment in adults. J Clin Endocrinol Metab 2011;96(10):3151–9.

Dyslipidemia in Diabetes
When and How to Treat?

Ronald B. Goldberg, MD

KEYWORDS

- Diabetes • Dyslipidemia • Management • Pharmacotherapy

KEY POINTS

- Atherosclerotic cardiovascular disease (ASCVD) risk increases with duration and severity of both type 1 and type 2 diabetes beginning in young adults with the disease and increasing with age and the presence of risk factors and risk enhancers.
- Statin therapy reduces ASCVD in both type 1 and type 2 diabetes in proportion to the level of individual risk and should be initiated in all patients older than 40 years of age and in higher-risk younger adults, with individualization in adults greater than 75 years based on safety concerns.
- High-intensity statin treatment is favored for high-risk primary prevention and is recommended in patients with ASCVD, often requiring the alternate or additional use of nonstatin low-density lipoprotein cholesterol (LDL-C)–lowering agents.
- Although fibrates and high-dose omega 3 fatty acid preparations should be used to treat severe hypertriglyceridemia, there is little evidence that they reduce ASCVD risk, other than icosapent ethyl in those with established ASCVD.

Atherosclerotic cardiovascular disease (ASCVD) remains the major cause of morbidity and mortality in diabetes, and diabetes increases ASCVD risk two-fold compared with those without diabetes.[1] Dyslipidemia is a risk factor for ASCVD in diabetes and a therapeutic target for risk reduction. Despite a decrease in the absolute rate of ASCVD in the past 2 decades, which may be attributable in part to the success of cardioprevention management strategies,[2] uncertainties remain on when and how to treat diabetic dyslipidemia. There are several reasons for this, including gaps in the understanding of the nature and atherogenicity of dyslipidemia in diabetes, greater recognition of the heterogeneity of cardiovascular risk in the population with diabetes together with insufficient information in lower-risk younger as well as aging individuals, and recognition of the limitations in benefits of some available lipid-lowering agents. This review provides an up-to-date assessment of the nature of dyslipidemia in diabetes, evaluation of ASCVD risk, evidence for clinical benefit from lipid lowering, and current approaches to pharmacologic management.

Division of Endocrinology, Diabetes and Metabolism, Diabetes Research Institute, University of Miami Miller School of Medicine, 1450 Northwest 10th Avenue, Miami, FL 33136, USA
E-mail address: rgoldber@med.miami.edu

Endocrinol Metab Clin N Am 51 (2022) 603–624
https://doi.org/10.1016/j.ecl.2022.02.011
0889-8529/22/© 2022 Elsevier Inc. All rights reserved.

endo.theclinics.com

THE NATURE OF DYSLIPIDEMIA IN DIABETES

Dyslipidemia may be defined as an abnormality in lipid levels, usually referring to an elevation in low-density lipoprotein cholesterol (LDL-C), triglyceride levels, and/or a reduction in high-density lipoprotein cholesterol levels (HDL-C). Although it is known that people with diabetes do not have generally higher LDL-C levels than the general population matched for age and sex but are more likely to exhibit increased numbers of atherogenic particles,[3,4] the use of the term has been broadened to refer to an atherogenic lipoprotein phenotype and is used in this way herein. Furthermore, it is not always appreciated that the lipoprotein phenotype in most patients with type 1 diabetes is not characterized by elevated triglyceride and low HDL-C as it often is in type 2 diabetes[3] (**Table 1**). Recent studies of the prevalence of hypertriglyceridemia (>150 mg/dL) are based on large databases of patients with diabetes, most of whom have type 2 diabetes, and in the modern era most are taking statin medications, which lower triglyceride levels slightly. They indicate that the prevalence varies from 40% to 60%[5,6] and is associated with the level of glycemic control.[7] The hypertriglyceridemia is usually mild to moderate (151–499 mg/dL) but occasionally may be severe (>500 mg/dL).

PATHOPHYSIOLOGY OF DYSLIPIDEMIA IN DIABETES
Type 2 Diabetes

The primary driving force for dyslipidemia in people with type 2 diabetes is insulin resistance[3] aggravated by hyperglycemia.[7] Insulin resistance increases lipolysis in adipose tissue and hepatic and intestinal triglyceride-rich lipoprotein (TRL) production. This is coupled with impaired clearance of TRL particles by reduced activity of lipoprotein lipase or altered regulation of its cofactors, such as apolipoprotein C-III, as well as impaired hepatic clearance of the remnant particles produced by lipase-mediated

Table 1
Plasma lipids in cohorts with type 1 and type 2 diabetes in the prestatin era (mean [±SD])

	Type 1 Diabetes[a] DCCT/ EDIC		Type 2 Diabetes[b] UKPDS			
	Intensive Treatment (N = 698)	Conventional Treatment (N = 723)	Men		Women	
			At Diagnosis	Mean Change After 3 mo Diet	At Diagnosis	Mean Change After 3 mo Diet
Total cholesterol, mg/dL	180 ± 31	184 ± 38	213 ± 39	−11	224 ± 46	−4
Triglyceride, mg/dL	84 ± 53	88 ± 51	158 (96–270)[c]	−36	160 (99–260)[c]	−20
LDL-C, mg/dL	112 ± 27	115 ± 32	139 ± 39	−10	151 ± 43	−4
HDL-C, mg/dL	51 ± 13	52 ± 13	39 ± 9	+1	42 ± 10	+1
HbA$_{1c}$	7.4 ± 1.1	9.1 ± 1.5	8.9 ± 2.2	−2.0	9.1 ± 2.1	−1.8

[a] From Ref.[30] Data at the end of the DCCT trial, mean follow-up 6.5 y.
[b] From Manley SE, Stratton IM, Cull CA, et al; United Kingdom Prospective Diabetes Study Group. Effects of 3 months' diet after diagnosis of Type 2 diabetes on plasma lipids and lipoproteins (UKPDS 45). UK Prospective Diabetes Study Group. Diabet Med 2000;17:518-23.
[c] ±1 SD interval.

hydrolysis. The result is an increase in very-low- and intermediate-density lipoproteins, all of which are known to be atherogenic. The resultant hypertriglyceridemia leads to the formation of small, dense LDL and HDL particles as a result of an enhanced exchange of triglyceride in the accumulating TRL for cholesteryl ester in LDL and HDL through the action of cholesteryl ester transfer protein. Small dense LDL is thought to be more proinflammatory than larger LDL particles, and there is evidence that HDL from individuals with type 2 diabetes is dysfunctional, both contributing to the atherogenicity of this phenotype.[3] In addition, small HDL particles have an accelerated catabolism, which together with the lipid compositional changes in HDL leads to reduced HDL-C levels.

Because insulin resistance typically precedes the clinical presentation of diabetes, and dyslipidemia is prevalent in the prediabetic phase of type 2 diabetes,[8] these lipoprotein abnormalities are likely to have been present for many years preceding the diagnosis of diabetes. Other factors, such as relative insulin deficiency, obesity, demographic factors, and other secondary causes of hypertriglyceridemia, may influence and aggravate the severity of the dyslipidemia.[9] Recent genetic studies also indicate that the severity of hypertriglyceridemia may be influenced by rare monogenic and more common polygenic variants affecting clearance of TRL[10] and may account for the small but important fraction of dyslipidemic patients with type 2 diabetes developing the multifactorial chylomicronemia syndrome with its attendant risk of acute pancreatitis.[11]

Type 1 Diabetes

In contrast to type 2 diabetes, the primary factor leading to abnormalities in circulating lipoproteins in type 1 diabetes is insulin deficiency together with modest effects of hyperglycemia, and except for patients in poor control who may have hypertriglyceridemia or elevated LDL-C, for most patients, triglyceride and LDL-C levels are either normal or mildly reduced, whereas HDL-C levels are usually normal or increased (4; see **Table 1**). These effects are thought to be related to peripheral hyperinsulinemia and hyperadiponectinemia, leading to enhanced lipoprotein lipase activity and increased LDL receptor-mediated clearance. Despite the relatively normal-appearing lipid profile in most individuals with type 1 diabetes, several lipoprotein compositional abnormalities have been identified, some related to hyperglycemia and others not, that increase their atherogenicity. These include smaller, cholesteryl ester–enriched very-low-density lipoprotein, smaller, more highly oxidized LDL particles and oxidized LDL-immunoglobulin complexes, dysfunctional HDL, and increased apolipoprotein C-III, which inhibits lipoprotein lipase activity and hepatic remnant clearance.[5] In addition, as intensive insulin administration has allowed for more flexibility with food intake, overweight may develop in up to 25% of individuals, accompanied by insulin resistance, hypertriglyceridemia, and reduced HDL-C,[12] adding to ASCVD risk.[13]

ASSESSMENT OF ATHEROSCLEROTIC CARDIOVASCULAR DISEASE RISK

In 2001, the National Cholesterol Education Panel guidelines recommended that adults with diabetes and without CVD be considered to have a coronary heart disease (CHD) risk equivalent, assigning a 10-year ASCVD risk of at least 20%.[14] It subsequently became evident that although this may be true in older people with long-standing, complicated diabetes,[15] there is significant heterogeneity of risk for ASCVD in the population with diabetes,[16,17] which influences pharmacotherapeutic decision making. Among key determinants of risk are demographic factors, such as age, sex, race/ethnicity, and socioeconomic status, duration and type of diabetes, family history of ASCVD, and the number and severity of major risk factors as well as other risk enhancers, some of which are specific to diabetes and others that are not (**Table 2**).[9]

Demographic Factors

The absolute risk for ASCVD in diabetes increases with age in both type 1 and type 2 diabetes,[18,19] although the relative risk is highest in young adults and then decreases with age. It is now recognized that the incidence of diabetes diagnosed before 40 years is increasing especially among those with type 2 diabetes, and that it is a more severe, rapidly progressive form of the disease with a greater relative risk for ASCVD than age-matched individuals with type 1 diabetes or older-onset individuals.[20–22] Women with diabetes appear to lose their gender protection from CHD and stroke and have a greater relative risk compared with men but this decreases as they age and is similar in elderly men and women.[23] Most minority groups have lower rates of ASCVD compared with whites except for South Asians,[24] and lower socioeconomic status is associated with higher cardiovascular mortality in type 2 diabetes.[25]

Onset and Duration of Diabetes

ASCVD risk is related to duration of diabetes independent of aging.[26] Onset of diabetes is usually obvious in type 1 diabetes, but the onset of type 2 diabetes is more

Table 2
Risk enhancers for atherosclerotic cardiovascular disease in diabetes

Risk Enhancers in Primary Prevention	
Specific to Diabetes	**General**
Degree of hyperglycemia[32]	Family history of premature ASCVD
Long duration (≥10 y for type 2 diabetes mellitus[3,14] or ≥20 y for type 1 diabetes mellitus[72]	LDL-C levels ≥160 mg/dL
Albuminuria ≥30 µg of albumin/mg creatinine[43]	Metabolic syndrome
eGFR <60 mL/min/1.73 m²[43]	Chronic kidney disease
Retinopathy[41]	History of preeclampsia or premature menopause in women
Neuropathy[42]	Chronic inflammatory disorders
	High-risk ethnicity such as South Asian ancestry
	Triglyceride levels persistently >175 mg/dL
	If measured:
	Apolipoprotein B levels with elevations >130 mg/dL (may be useful if hypertriglyceridemia >200 mg/dL to rule out genetic disorders such as type III or clarify ASCVD risk)
	High-sensitivity C-reactive protein ≥2 mg/L
	Lp(a) levels with elevations >125 nmol/L (50 mg/dL). Elevated Lp(a) levels especially useful in those with a family history of ASCVD
	Reduced ankle brachial index

Modified from Goldberg RB, Stone NJ, Grundy SM. The 2018 AHA/ACC/AACVPR/AAPA/ABC/ACPM/ADA/AGS/APhA/ASPC/NLA/PCNA Guidelines on the Management of Blood Cholesterol in Diabetes. Diabetes Care. 2020 Aug;43(8):1673-1678.

insidious, and diabetes may be present for years before clinical diagnosis. In addition, up to 1 in 3 adults have prediabetes, many of whom will develop type 2 diabetes and who already have modestly increased ASCVD risk,[27] thus offering an opportunity for early intervention. Also uncertain is how much ASCVD risk is increased in newly diagnosed diabetes in the elderly.

Risk Factors

Major risk factors

Hypercholesterolemia, cigarette smoking, and hypertension, all considered major risk factors because of evidence that their effects can be ameliorated by effective management, are strongly related to the development of ASCVD in diabetes as in the general population, although compared with nondiabetic subjects matched for these 3 risk factors, the incidence of CHD mortality remains two-fold increased in diabetes, indicating the importance of other determinants of risk.[28]

Hyperglycemia, insulin resistance, and obesity

Much of the underlying substrate for increased ASCVD risk is related to hyperglycemia, insulin resistance, and obesity, and the accompanying proinflammatory and procoagulant states. The degree of hyperglycemia is related to CVD risk in populations without known diabetes,[29] although the associations are attenuated after adjustment for other risk factors, and this is true for obesity as well. Evidence for the importance of hyperglycemia in people with known diabetes comes largely from clinical trials studying the benefits of glucose-lowering medications. Although intensive treatment of hyperglycemia with insulin clearly reduced ASCVD after some years in type 1 diabetes,[30] assessment of the effects of hyperglycemia in type 2 diabetes has been confounded by off-target effects of the glucose-lowering agent being tested as well by concomitant management of dyslipidemia and hypertension in modern clinical trials. A recent survey of a large database with diabetes examining the relative importance of a large number of risk factors for ASCVD found that the glycohemoglobin level was the most powerful.[31] There is also evidence that insulin resistance is associated with ASCVD,[32] although this evidence in people with diabetes is often based on imperfect surrogate measures of insulin resistance. Obesity has also been shown to associate with ASCVD in diabetes,[33] but weight loss intervention over 7 years did not reduce ASCVD outcomes.[34]

Dyslipidemia: an atherogenic tetrad

The HDL-C level is inversely and strongly related to ASCVD and is included together with age, sex, total cholesterol, blood pressure, and smoking in the risk factor algorithms used to quantify ASCVD risk in diabetes.[35] Lack of benefit for ASCVD in clinical trials that raised HDL-C pharmacologically has led to the notion that the basis for the strong inverse association between HDL-C and ASCVD in the general population may be related to HDL dysfunctionality, which is not sufficiently captured by the HDL-C value in high-risk states. In support of this concept, very high HDL-C was shown paradoxically to be a direct ASCVD risk factor in type 1 diabetes[36] in whom HDL-C levels are often elevated.[37] Although elevated triglyceride levels are associated with risk for ASCVD in diabetes, triglyceride lowering with pharmacologic agents has not been shown per se to be associated with a reduction of ASCVD events. More likely hypertriglyceridemia is a marker for other metabolic abnormalities, such as dysfunctional HDL, atherogenic small dense LDL, and remnant lipoprotein particles, making up an atherogenic tetrad.[38] Methods that quantify lipoprotein subfractions have demonstrated that selected subfractions are strongly correlated with insulin resistance[39] and are currently in clinical use, although it remains for them to be shown to be independent predictors of ASCVD in diabetes.

Other risk enhancers

The concept of risk enhancers was recently incorporated into risk assessment[24] to include factors that are not typically included in risk factor algorithms yet are sufficiently associated with ASCVD event rates to warrant consideration in risk assessment (see **Table 2**). Of relevance to individuals with diabetes, these include hypertriglyceridemia, elevated apolipoprotein B as a marker of increased numbers of atherogenic particles, and chronic kidney disease, which is common in diabetes owing to the development of diabetic nephropathy, manifesting as albuminuria or as reduced glomerular filtration rate. Elevated lipoprotein(a) (Lp(a)) has been associated with an increased risk of ASCVD in type 2 diabetes as in the population without diabetes.[40] Subclinical tests of coronary artery disease, such as the coronary calcium (CAC) score measured by computed tomography, are strongly related to future occurrence of ASCVD in diabetes, and its clinical utility is under evaluation in diabetes risk assessment. Last, the presence of microangiopathy is associated with increased ASCVD risk possibly because of common pathways for vascular damage[41–44] and should be considered in risk assessment.

Risk Factor Algorithms

Although risk factor algorithms are central to assessment of ASCVD in the general population,[24] they have less utility in people with diabetes. Referred to as the pooled cohorts equations (PCE), the algorithm is based on data from 4 large prospective cohort studies of risk factors for ASCVD and was a significant advance on the previously used Framingham Risk Algorithm because it included a large number of people with diabetes. However, it does not have data on individuals less than 40 or greater than 75 years of age, nor does it differentiate between the types or severity of diabetes, and in the 40- to 75-year age range, there is little controversy about the benefit of statin therapy in diabetes. Nevertheless, the 2018 American College of Cardiology/American Heart Association (ACC/AHA) Guidelines on the Management of Blood Cholesterol in Diabetes recommends its use in refining risk assessment,[35] as discussed later.

EVIDENCE FROM RANDOMIZED CLINICAL TRIALS FOR ATHEROSCLEROTIC CARDIOVASCULAR DISEASE REDUCTION USING STATINS

Although LDL-C is typically within the normal range in diabetes, when it became evident that the clinical benefit from statin therapy was strongly related to global risk for ASCVD, treatment with statins has become the mainstay of lipid-lowering therapy in diabetes for the prevention of ASCVD. Although LDL-C is the primary measure of efficacy used in clinical trials, non-HDL-C and apolipoprotein B are alternative measures of efficacy and may better reflect ASCVD risk than LDL-C in people with diabetes.[1]

Secondary Prevention

Meta-analyses of 26 randomized controlled clinical trials (RCTs) comparing statins versus placebo or higher versus lower doses of statins and which included participants aged 40 to 75 years with both type 1 and type 2 diabetes and with and without ASCVD showed that the benefit of statin therapy was related to the extent of reduction of LDL-C, and this applied even to individuals with LDL-C in the normal range.[45] Based on this, it is recommended that individuals with established ASCVD should receive high-intensity statin therapy aimed at achieving at least 50% LDL-C lowering[35,45,46] (**Fig. 1**). Because it is recognized that absolute risk reduction with statins is related to the individual's baseline ASCVD risk level, in those with very high risk, the recommended goal for LDL-C is a level less than 70 mg/dL[35] (**Box 1**). Some recommend an LDL-C goal of less than 55 mg/dL for very-high-risk patients based on subgroup analyses of an RCT.[47] Most patients with diabetes and ASCVD fall into this category, and many will require nonstatin LDL-C–lowering agents in addition to statins to achieve this goal, as discussed later.

Primary Prevention in Those Aged 40 to 75 Years

Moderate-intensity statin therapy (30%–35% low-density lipoprotein cholesterol reduction)

Specific evidence for benefit from moderate intensity statin therapy for primary prevention in diabetes comes from 4 RCTs, which tested moderate-intensity statin therapy (30%–35% LDL-C lowering) in cohorts aged 40 to 75 years with diabetes. A meta-analysis of these studies, which included people with type 1 (n = 1466) and type 2 (n = 17,220) diabetes, found a 25% reduction in events, similar to what has been shown in cohorts without diabetes, although the absolute reduction in events was greater in those with diabetes, and the benefit was similar for type 1 and type 2 diabetes.[48]

Although there have been no RCTs in cohorts with type 1 diabetes only, a large registry study (n = 24,230) in people with type 1 diabetes without a history of ASCVD found a 40% reduction in ASCVD death among those receiving lipid-lowering therapy compared with those who did not.[49] The ACC/AHA guidelines recommend moderate-

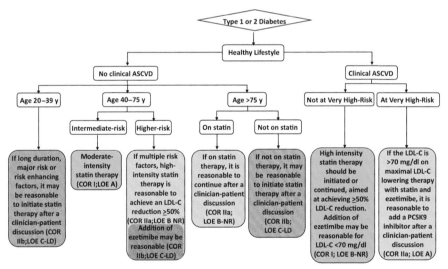

Fig. 1. AHA/ACC MultiSociety 2018 guidelines for cholesterol management in people with diabetes. COR, class of recommendation, encompassing the estimated magnitude and certainty of benefit in proportion to risk; COR I, strong (*green*); COR IIa, moderate (*yellow*); COR IIb, weak (*orange*); LOE, level of evidence; LOE A, high-quality: multiple high-quality RCTs/meta-analyses; LOE B-NR, moderate quality: one or more well-designed nonrandomized studies; LOE B-R, moderate quality: at least 1 RCT/meta-analysis; LOE C-LD, limited data. (*Modified from* Goldberg RB, Stone NJ, Grundy SM. The 2018 AHA/ACC/AACVPR/AAPA/ABC/ACPM/ADA/AGS/APhA/ASPC/NLA/PCNA Guidelines on the Management of Blood Cholesterol in Diabetes. Diabetes Care. 2020 Aug;43(8):1673-1678.)

Box 1
Definition of very high atherosclerotic cardiovascular disease risk status

History of multiple major ASCVD events
   Or

One major ASCVD event plus multiple high-risk conditions:
- Age greater than 65 years
- Heterozygous familial hypercholesterolemia
- Prior percutaneous coronary intervention/coronary artery bypass grafting
- Diabetes
- Hypertension
- Chronic kidney disease
- Current smoking
- History of heart failure
- LDL-C greater than 100 mg/dL on maximal statin plus ezetimibe

Modified from Goldberg RB, Stone NJ, Grundy SM. The 2018 AHA/ACC/AACVPR/AAPA/ABC/
ACPM/ADA/AGS/APhA/ASPC/NLA/PCNA Guidelines on the Management of Blood Cholesterol
in Diabetes. Diabetes Care. 2020 Aug;43(8):1673-1678.

---

intensity statin treatment for primary prevention in those 40 to 75 years of age,[35] a position supported by the American Diabetes Association.[50]

REFINEMENT OF RISK AND INCREASING INTENSITY OF STATIN THERAPY IN ADULTS AGED 40 TO 75 YEARS

Because of the heterogeneity of ASCVD risk in this population, further risk assessment is recommended using the PCE algorithm to refine risk estimates and therapeutic decision making, particularly for the purpose of identifying people at higher risk who are more likely to benefit from high-intensity statin therapy (see **Fig. 1**). This 3-tiered ASCVD risk score categorizes individuals into borderline (5% to 7.4%), intermediate (7.5% to 19.9%), and high (>20%) 10-year risk for ASCVD. Given the increased morbidity and mortality following a first cardiovascular event in diabetes,[1] the presence of a high residual risk following moderate-intensity statin therapy,[48] evidence in men greater than 50 years and women greater than 60 years for benefit from high-intensity statin therapy in primary prevention,[51] and the increased trajectory of risk over time in diabetes, it is reasonable to intensify statin therapy with age, presence of risk factors or risk enhancers, or a high-risk PCE score in people with diabetes.[35] Recently, the utility of CAC scoring as a subclinical marker of atherosclerosis offers a new opportunity to improve risk assessment in people with diabetes. In the Multiethnic Study of Atherosclerosis (mean age 62 years), 53% of those with diabetes were CAC positive and had a 10-year ASCVD event rate of greater than 15%,[52] supporting the use of high-intensity statin therapy. By contrast, in a younger cohort with type 1 diabetes from the Epidemiology of Diabetes Interventions and Complications study (mean age 43 years), 70% were CAC negative, 19% had CAC scores of 1 to 99 Agatston units with a 10-year ASCVD event rate of 2.8%, and only those who had a CAC score greater than 100 Agatston units ($\sim$10% of the cohort) had a 10-year event rate of 13.9% or greater.[53]

Indications for Nonstatin Agents that Lower Low-Density Lipoprotein Cholesterol

Statins are the primary agents recommended to lower LDL-C and reduce ASCVD risk. However, intolerance of statins, although its nature and prevalence continue to be debated,[54] is estimated to occur in from 1% to greater than 10% of individuals in

RCTs and may limit their use. Furthermore, in those with significant hypercholesterole-mia or even in those with established ASCVD who have average LDL-C levels, maximal intensity statin therapy may not achieve adequate LDL-C lowering particu-larly if full doses of rosuvastatin or atorvastatin, the 2 most potent statins, are not fully tolerable. Although statins increase the risk of diabetes development[55] and progres-sion[56] probably by increasing insulin resistance, the benefits owing to ASCVD risk reduction are thought to outweigh adverse effects in individuals with intermediate or greater levels of ASCVD risk.[57] In cases of statin intolerance, the maximum tolerable statin dose should remain the first choice because of the wealth of evidence for benefit, followed by the addition or replacement by nonstatin LDL-C–lowering agents. Preference in the choice of a nonstatin agent should be based on evidence for benefit and needed efficacy, although there are sufficient data to indicate that the benefit resulting from LDL-C lowering is related to the degree of lowering rather than to the particular agent used.[58] These agents, which like statins all up-regulate the LDL-receptor and enhance LDL clearance, include ezetimibe, proprotein convertase sub-tilisin/kexin 9 inhibitors (evolocumab and alirocumab, PCSKi), bile sequestrants, and bempedoic acid. Although niacin in large doses lowers LDL-C, there is no longer an indication for its use for this purpose. In situations where statins cannot be tolerated at any dose, then the choice for non-statin-lowering therapy is between a PCSK9i, which may lower LDL-C 45% to 60%, or a combination of at least 2 of the other agents, because they are less efficacious than statins or PCSK9i's.

Ezetimibe

Ezetimibe lowers LDL-C 15% to 25% by inhibiting the intestinal cholesterol trans-porter NPCL1, and addition of ezetimibe to moderate-intensity statin therapy can achieve the same percent LDL-C lowering as that achieved with high-intensity statin therapy and is well tolerated.[59] Evidence for benefit of ezetimibe on ASCVD events in diabetes comes from the subgroup analysis of participants with diabetes in a single RCT (IMPROVE-IT) comparing the addition of ezetimibe to 40 mg simvastatin versus statin plus placebo in patients with an acute coronary syndrome whose admission me-dian LDL-C was 89 mg/dL. Ezetimibe plus simvastatin safely reduced the LDL-C to 49 mg/dL and the rate of major CVD events by 5.5% compared with simvastatin plus placebo.[60] Thus, if maximally tolerable statin therapy does not achieve the required LDL-C lowering, ezetimibe, which is well tolerated and cost-effective, is rec-ommended for add-on therapy in both primary and secondary prevention[35] (see **Fig. 1**).

Proprotein convertase subtilisin/kexin type 9 serine protease inhibitors (PCSK9i)

The PCSK9i's evolocumab and alirocumab are monoclonal antibodies directed at PCSK9, a serum protease that regulates LDL-receptor degradation, thereby enhancing LDL clearance. These agents, which are indicated for treatment of primary hypercholesterolemia as well as established ASCVD, are administered parenterally 2 or 4 weekly and lower LDL-C 40% to 60% and Lp(a) by 20% to 30%. The ACC/AHA guidelines recommend that PCSK9i's may be considered for very-high-risk individuals with ASCVD in whom treatment with statins plus ezetimibe does not achieve an LDL-C less than 70 mg/dL[35] (see **Fig. 1**). The basis for this recommendation comes from an-alyses of 2 similar RCTs, one with evolocumab (FOURIER) and one with alirocumab (ODYSSEY), both of which randomized patients with ASCVD and an LDL-C greater than 70 mg/dL on statin therapy to PCSK9i or placebo and performed prespecified an-alyses in the subgroups with diabetes.[61,62] Evolocumab safely reduced LDL-C by 59% and ASCVD risk by 17% in those with diabetes at baseline over 2.2 years of follow-up and with no evidence of worsening hyperglycemia.[61] A similar result was obtained among those with diabetes treated with alirocumab. Alirocumab reduced ASCVD events by 16% over 2.8 years of follow-up, and in both trials the absolute benefit was greater in those who had diabetes versus those who did not. The guidelines[35] draw attention to evidence that most patients with ASCVD will reach an LDL-C goal of less than 70 mg/dL using statin with or without ezetimibe treatment,[63] that the RCTs with PCSK9i's lasted less than 3 years and thus did not exclude longer-term side effects, and unlike ezetimibe, PCSK9i's are not available in generic form so that their cost-effectiveness is relatively low.[64]

Bile Sequestrants

By inhibiting bile acid absorption, bile sequestrants upregulate hepatic LDL-receptors, thus lowering LDL-C. The 2 original bile sequestrants cholestyramine and colestipol have been succeeded by colesevelam, a bile sequestrant available in tablet or dissolvable powder form, which is more tolerable, although it may cause flatulence and constipation. Colesevelam reduces LDL-C by 15% to 25% and is the only LDL-C-lowering agent shown to modestly lower HbA_{1c}.[65] However, it has a tendency to raise triglyceride levels through its bile sequestrant action and is contraindicated in individuals with triglyceride levels greater than 350 mg/dL. It should therefore be used with caution in those with type 2 diabetes who have concomitant hypertriglyceridemia.

Bempedoic Acid

This is a synthetic dicarboxylic acid prodrug that is enzymatically activated in the liver to inhibit ATP citrate lyase, an enzyme upstream from HMGCoA reductase in the cholesterol synthetic pathway.[66] Like statins, which are HMGCoA reductase inhibitors, bempedoic acid inhibits cholesterol synthesis, upregulating LDL receptors and leading to a 15% to 25% reduction in LDL-C, with no differences reported between those with or without diabetes. It is also available in a fixed dose combination with ezetimibe that lowered LDL-C up to 36% in patients on maximally tolerated statin therapy.[67] Recently introduced, the available safety and efficacy data are from relatively short RCTs, although a long-term, ASCVD outcome-based RCT should be completed in about a year. In a meta-analysis of available data, bempedoic acid use was associated with a 25% reduction of ASCVD events as well as a 45% reduction in rates of new-onset or worsening diabetes.[68] Bempedoic acid is well tolerated, like statins lowers C-reactive protein possibly reflecting an anti-inflammatory effect, and has not been reported to cause myalgia, including in statin-intolerant patients. In some studies, it raised uric acid levels and has been reported to precipitate gout. Currently, it is indicated only as an add-on to maximally tolerated statin therapy, and because of expense, it is likely to be a third- or fourth-line LDL-C-lowering agent.

INDICATIONS FOR STATINS AND OTHER LOW-DENSITY LIPOPROTEIN CHOLESTEROL–LOWERING AGENTS IN THOSE LESS THAN 40 OR GREATER THAN 75 YEARS OF AGE

When to Begin Pharmacotherapy Before Age 40 Years

Aside from the fact that diabetes onset of patients less than 40 years of age carries with it a longer lifetime exposure to the disease compared with those with later onset, earlier-onset type 2 diabetes is a more rapidly progressive disease than it is in older adults[20–22] and is associated with a greater risk of ASCVD compared with similarly aged individuals with type 1 diabetes.[69] Furthermore, younger-onset type 2 diabetes is associated with a greater relative ASCVD risk than older-onset diabetes even when adjusted for duration of diabetes,[70] likely related to the higher prevalence of hypertension, hyperlipidemia, and metabolic syndrome and earlier development of microangiopathic complications.[22]

There are no ASCVD event-based RCTs with statins in cohorts with diabetes less than 40 years of age. Thus, recommendations for such treatment depend upon the few, long-term observational studies of risk of development of ASCVD, as well as evidence for safety and efficacy in young, high-risk adults.[71] It has been found that although rates of ASCVD are low in those less than 30 years of age, they increase with time,[26,27,72–74] and ASCVD risk may reach intermediate levels by 30 to 39 years of age in a sizable subgroup of individuals, especially those with longer duration of diabetes, namely 10 years' duration of type 2 diabetes[26,27] or 20 years' duration of type 1 diabetes.[72] In addition, about half of those with diabetes aged 40 to 49 years have intermediate levels of ASCVD risk.[73]

The use of chest computed tomography to detect subclinical coronary atherosclerosis has revealed that ~50% of individuals with type 2 diabetes aged 30 to 39 years (median diabetes duration 11 years) has coronary plaque and is 25% more likely to have CAC than nondiabetic controls after adjustment for known risk factors.[75] In a larger study of black and white participants aged 18 to 30 years (average age 25 years), the hazard ratio for CAC was 1.15 and 1.07 times higher for each 5-year-longer duration of diabetes and prediabetes, respectively.[76] In type 1 diabetes, CAC was present in 11% of a small group with average age of 20 years[77] and in 29% of a larger cohort, with average age of 40 years, whereby CAC presence was related to duration of diabetes and cardiovascular risk factors, and was significantly associated with an increased risk of CVD events.[53] Finally, a recent large registry study identifying individuals with first myocardial infarction (MI) before age 55 years (average age 45 years) demonstrated that 20% had diabetes of whom 91% had type 2 diabetes and 35% of these were insulin-treated, suggesting they had relatively severe diabetes.[78] The group with diabetes had double the long-term cardiovascular mortality in follow-up than those without diabetes and was relatively greater than that reported in older cohorts with MI, emphasizing the importance of preventing CVD in young adults with diabetes.

Therefore, a significant proportion of this population, particularly those greater than 30 years of age having prolonged diabetes (at least 10 years of type 2 diabetes or 20 years of type 1 diabetes), 1 or more major risk factors, microvascular disease or other risk enhancing factors (see **Table 2**) should be considered for initiation of statin treatment.[35] The National Lipid Association's Update on Coronary Calcium Scoring to Guide Preventive Strategies for ASCVD Risk Reduction recently extended these recommendations by stating that in adults 30 to 39 years of age with long-standing diabetes and risk factors or microangiopathy, CAC scoring may be reasonable to aid in ASCVD risk stratification and statin treatment shared decision making.[79] It was recommended that in those less than 40 years of age with a CAC score of greater than 100 Agatston units, it may be reasonable to choose high-intensity statin therapy.

Low-Density Lipoprotein Cholesterol Lowering Pharmacotherapy in Those Greater than 75 Years of Age

As in those less than 40 years of age, there are no RCTs with statins in people with diabetes greater than 75 years, and guidelines are based on observational data and extrapolation from studies in nondiabetic cohorts. ASCVD risk increases incrementally with age in diabetes.[18,19,26] In 1 long-term cohort study of type 2 diabetes without ASCVD, incident rates of MI averaged 25.6 per 1000 person-years in those greater than 75 years of age,[19] whereas another in a type 1 diabetes cohort found the 10-year fatal CVD risk in those greater than 75 years of age was 70% in men and 40% in women.[18] A meta-analysis of 2 recent statin trials in older nondiabetic subjects without CVD demonstrated similar benefits in ASCVD reduction among those greater than 70 of age versus less than 70 years of age.[80] In addition, a recent large retrospective study found that statin therapy in new users without preexisting ASCVD was associated with reduced ASCVD events in people with type 2 diabetes aged 75 to 84 years but not in those greater than 85 years of age, nor in those without diabetes.[81] These studies do support the continuation of moderate- or high-intensity statin therapy for primary prevention in those greater than 75 years of age with diabetes, who comprise a sizable 20% of the population in this age category especially in those with ASCVD.

The question of whether to initiate statin therapy in this group is more uncertain. CAC scoring may be used to assist with decision making.[79] Among subjects in the 75- to 84-year-old age group in the Multiethnic Study of Atherosclerosis in which 15% of the cohort had diabetes, as in all age groups, the severity of CAC was strongly associated with ASCVD events over an 8.5-year follow-up period.[52] It may therefore be reasonable to have a clinician-patient discussion in which the potential benefits and risks of initiating statin therapy in this age group are reviewed.[35] The clinician should note that the benefit may be offset by limited lifespan or increased susceptibility to adverse events in patients in this age group. This becomes even more relevant in those in whom the diagnosis of diabetes is recent.

EVALUATION AND MANAGEMENT OF HYPERTRIGLYCERIDEMIA
Clinical Impact of Hypertriglyceridemia

Hypertriglyceridemia and atherosclerotic cardiovascular disease risk
Triglyceride levels have been linked to development of ASCVD events independently of other cardiovascular risk factors, such as low HDL-C and body mass index in some,[82,83] but not in all[84] studies. There are fewer studies in cohorts with diabetes, and these are smaller in size, but again show a disparity in the findings.[85,86] The nonfasting triglyceride level appears to be more strongly associated with ASCVD, which may reflect the importance of postprandial remnant lipoproteins in atherogenesis.[87]

Hypertriglyceridemia also remains a residual risk factor for ASCVD in statin-treated individuals[88] and was found to be present in 40% of a representative sample of the US population with diabetes treated with statins.[6]

As mentioned above, the basis for the relationship between hypertriglyceridemia and ASCVD has been linked to insulin resistance, remnants of TRLs, small LDL particles, and dysfunctional HDL. Recent genetic developments have in addition incriminated 2 apoproteins carried on TRLs. A Mendelian randomization study using a rare genetic loss-of-function variant in *APOA5*, the gene for apo A-V, which is carried on TRL and is an important activator of lipoprotein lipase-mediated hydrolysis and a powerful determinant of triglyceride levels, suggested a direct causal relationship between triglyceride levels and coronary disease.[89] Apo C-III is also carried on TRL and is increased in hypertriglyceridemia. Loss-of-function variants of *APOC3*, some rare and some more common, are associated with low triglyceride levels and a significantly reduced risk of ASCVD, also suggesting a causal relationship.[90] On the other hand, clear-cut benefit from pharmacologic triglyceride lowering is lacking as discussed later. Thus, hypertriglyceridemia is linked to ASCVD development through multiple atherogenic pathways, providing the basis for significant heterogeneity in this relationship. Development of clinically useful biomarkers of these pathways may help to improve predictability of ASCVD risk in this population as well as provide potential specific targets for therapy.

Hypertriglyceridemia and the multifactorial chylomicronemia syndrome
Typically, type 2 diabetes, and occasionally chronically poorly controlled type 1 diabetes, is one of the common secondary factors that can cause chylomicronemia

(triglycerides >1000 mg/dL) in patients with polygenic hypertriglyceridemia and may lead to pancreatitis,[11] often a disastrous complication for patients with diabetes. Triglyceride levels may vary widely in these patients depending on the efficacy of their dietary and pharmacologic management and the presence of aggravating factors. Thus, until genetic testing for polygenic variants with high risk for the chylomicronemia syndrome is widely available,[91] it is probably prudent to regard all patients with hypertriglyceridemia as potentially at risk for this complication. This is especially true for those with triglyceride levels greater than 500 mg/dL in less-than-optimal glycemic control.

Hypertriglyceridemia and fatty liver

A recent survey estimated that approximately 47% of people with diabetes has nonalcoholic fatty liver disease (NAFLD) and a further 26% has nonalcoholic steatohepatitis (NASH).[92] In addition, in a cohort with diabetes, those with NAFLD had higher triglyceride levels than those who did not.[93] Given the impact of NAFLD and NASH on development of cirrhosis, hepatocellular carcinoma, and need for liver transplantation, hypertriglyceridemia should be regarded as a possible risk marker for NAFLD and NASH in type 2 diabetes.

Management of Hypertriglyceridemia

Triglyceride-lowering drugs to be considered for triglyceride lowering are fibrates and the omega 3 fatty acids (O3FA). Niacin is no longer recommended for add-on treatment to statin therapy because of its lack of benefit as well as side effects.[94] Rarely, it may be considered in patients who have severe hypertriglyceridemia despite combined fibrate and O3FA treatment. There are several other promising agents in development.[95] Among these are an anti-apo C-III antisense oligonucleotide and inhibitors of angiopoietin-like protein type 3, a circulating inhibitor of lipoprotein lipase activity, using either a monoclonal antibody or an antisense oligonucleotide.

Fibrates

Fibrates, which are peroxisome proliferator-receptor alpha (PPARα) agonists, are the first choice together with dietary management for treating severe hypertriglyceridemia and should be considered for use in patients with triglyceride levels greater than 500 to 1000 mg/dL to reduce the risk of development of chylomicronemia. Fibrates lower triglyceride levels 30% to 50% as well as lower apo C-III and are generally well tolerated. The benefits of long-term fibrate therapy are less clear. Older primary and secondary prevention RCTs using clofibrate and gemfibrozil in monotherapy demonstrated a significant reduction in ASCVD events.[96] However, clofibrate was withdrawn because of adverse effects and because there is a small but significant incidence of rhabdomyolysis when gemfibrozil is used together with statins, fenofibrate is preferred. Long-term RCTs using fenofibrate in cohorts with diabetes either used as monotherapy (Fenofibrate Intervention and Event Lowering in Diabetes – FIELD)[97] or added to statin therapy (Action to Control Cardiovascular Risk in Diabetes – ACCORD)[98] showed no significant overall benefit for ASCVD events. Interestingly in both of these RCTs, secondary analyses showed beneficial effects on retinopathy progression independent of effects on lipids.[99,100] The FIELD trial was conducted as the benefits of statin therapy were being recognized, and there was a significant "drop-in" use of statins in the study, so that may have affected the result. In addition, the presence of hypertriglyceridemia, which is the primary indication for fibrates, was not an inclusion criterion in either of these studies.

However, a prespecified subanalysis in ACCORD noted a benefit for fibrate therapy in men and the subgroup of participants with triglyceride levels greater than 204 mg/

dL and HDL-C levels less than 34 mg/dL,[101] a finding that was supported by a systematic review of fibrate RCTs.[102] Most guidelines[35,50] but not all[103] do not recommend fibrates as add-on therapy in statin-treated patients with diabetes for ASCVD prevention.

The development of a selective PPARα modulator, pemafibrate, which is more potent than fenofibrate and has fewer hepatic and renal side effects and greater anti-atherosclerosis benefit in experimental atherosclerosis, is currently being tested in a long-term RCT in cohorts of statin-treated hypertriglyceridemic patients with diabetes with as well as without ASCVD.[104]

Omega 3 fatty acids

Omega 3 fatty acids (O3FA) at a dose of 4 g daily lowers triglyceride levels by 20% to 40% principally by inhibiting hepatic triglyceride production and also by lowering apo C-III and is a useful adjunct to fibrate therapy in patients with severe hypertriglyceridemia.[105,106] Earlier long-term RCTs studying the effects of O3FA on ASCVD used low doses of omega 3 preparations that were mixtures of the 2 principal O3FA, docosahexaenoic acid (DHA) and eicosapentaenoic acid (EPA), and a recent RCT also using an O3FA formulation with both EPA and DHA at a dose of 4 g daily demonstrated no benefit.[106] However, the Reduction of Cardiovascular Events with Icosapent Ethyl–Intervention Trial (REDUCE-IT), which used a purified, synthetic EPA in statin-treated individuals with ASCVD (71%) or without ASCVD but with diabetes and 1 additional risk factor (29%) demonstrated a 25% reduction in the primary ASCVD outcome and a 20% reduction in cardiovascular death.[107] In subanalyses, there was significant benefit in those both with and without diabetes, but not in the primary prevention subgroup with diabetes. There was a small increase in bleeding and atrial fibrillation. These beneficial effects, which confirm an earlier lower-dose RCT of EPA in an open-label statin-treated cohort in Japan,[108] appear to have been independent of the triglyceride-lowering effect of the agent, suggest that the EPA in REDUCE-IT has other antiatherogenic effects,[109] and the use of icosapent ethyl ester has been recommended by the ADA in patients with ASCVD as an add-on to statin therapy.[50]

SUMMARY

The mainstay of lipid-lowering pharmacotherapy for the prevention of ASCVD in both type 1 and type 2 diabetes is directed at lowering the number of atherogenic particles, as reflected by lowering of LDL-C, using statin therapy. Where statins are insufficient or intolerable, adding or substituting other LDL-C-lowering agents is reasonable. Most people with diabetes over the age of 40 years without ASCVD have at least an intermediate-level ($\geq 7.5\%$) 10-year risk of ASCVD, which has been shown to benefit from 30% to 35% LDL-C lowering with statin therapy, and an LDL-C target of less than 100 mg/dL (non-HDL-C <130 mg/dL) is reasonable if they have hypercholesterolemia. Many individuals greater than 40 years will have high levels of risk and will receive greater benefit from high-intensity statin therapy, to which ezetimibe may be added to achieve 50% to 60% LDL-C lowering.

Younger adults are likely to have an intermediate ASCVD risk level or will develop it rapidly if they have relatively long-duration diabetes, risk factors, or risk enhancers and should be considered for moderate-intensity statin therapy. In people greater than 75 years of age in whom evidence for benefit is less robust and adverse effects are more common, the decision to continue or initiate pharmacotherapeutic LDL-C lowering should be individualized. CAC scoring may be helpful in assisting with decision making in primary prevention. Those with established ASCVD have a very high short to medium risk for recurrence and should receive high-intensity statin therapy that often will require add-on ezetimibe and/or PCSK9i treatment to reach the recommended LDL-C goal of less than 70 mg/dL (non-HDL-C <100 mg/dL) or even lower levels.

Patients with type 2 diabetes are at risk for severe hypertriglyceridemia (>500 mg/dL) and the chylomicronemia syndrome and should be evaluated for aggravating factors. They require dietary management and treatment with fenofibrate if they do not respond, to which high-dose O3FA can be added if necessary. In general, hypertriglyceridemia (>150–200 mg/dL) enhances ASCVD risk, and these patients should be considered for initiation or intensification of statin therapy. Clinical trials testing ther addition of fibrates or mixed DHA + EPA O3FA preparations to statin therapy have not shown any benefit, although both fibrates and O3FA lower the triglyceride level. Icosapent ethyl ester should be added to statin therapy in hypertriglyceridemic individuals with ASCVD because it has added benefit.

CLINICS CARE POINTS

- Atherosclerotic cardiovascular disease risk increases with age, duration, and severity of both type 1 and type 2 diabetes.
- Statin therapy reduces atherosclerotic cardiovascular disease events in both types of diabetes in proportion to the level of individual atherosclerotic cardiovascular disease risk.
- At least 50% low-density lipoprotein cholesterol–lowering pharmacotherapy is favored in high-risk primary prevention and is recommended in secondary prevention.
- Fibrates and high-dose omega 3 fatty acid preparations reduce elevated triglyceride, but there is little evidence that they reduce atherosclerotic cardiovascular disease risk, other than icosapentanyl ethyl ester in those with atherosclerotic cardiovascular disease.

DISCLOSURE

The author has no disclosures.

REFERENCES

1. Barrett-Connor E, Wingard D, Wong N, et al. Heart disease and diabetes. In: Cowie CC, Casagrande SS, Menke A, et al, editors. Diabetes in America. 3rd edition. Bethesda (MD): National Institute of Diabetes and Digestive and Kidney Diseases (US); 2018. CHAPTER 18.
2. Gregg EW, Cheng YJ, Saydah S, et al. Trends in death rates among U.S. adults with and without diabetes between 1997 and 2006: findings from the National Health Interview Survey. Diabetes Care 2012;35:1252–7.
3. Vergès B. Pathophysiology of diabetic dyslipidaemia: where are we? Diabetologia 2015;58:886–99.
4. Vergès B. Lipid disorders in type 1 diabetes. Diabetes Metab 2009;35:353–60.
5. Rana JS, Liu JY, Moffet HH, et al. Metabolic dyslipidemia and risk of coronary heart disease in 28,318 adults with diabetes mellitus and low-density lipoprotein cholesterol <100 mg/dl. Am J Cardiol 2015;116:1700–4.
6. Fan W, Philip S, Granowitz C, et al. Residual hypertriglyceridemia and estimated atherosclerotic cardiovascular disease risk by statin use in U.S. adults with diabetes: National Health and Nutrition Examination Survey 2007-2014. Diabetes Care 2019;42:2307–14.
7. Zheng D, Dou J, Liu G, et al. Association between triglyceride level and glycemic control among insulin-treated patients with type 2 diabetes. J Clin Endocrinol Metab 2019;104:1211–20.

8. Goldberg RB, Temprosa M, Haffner S, et al. Diabetes Prevention Program Research Group. Effect of progression from impaired glucose tolerance to diabetes on cardiovascular risk factors and its amelioration by lifestyle and metformin intervention: the Diabetes Prevention Program randomized trial by the Diabetes Prevention Program Research Group. Diabetes Care 2009;32:726–32.
9. Goldberg RB. Clinical approach to assessment and amelioration of atherosclerotic vascular disease in diabetes. Front Cardiovasc Med 2020;7:582826.
10. Dron JS, Hegele RA. Genetics of hypertriglyceridemia. Front Endocrinol (Lausanne) 2020;11:455.
11. Goldberg RB, Chait A. A comprehensive update on the chylomicronemia syndrome. Front Endocrinol (Lausanne) 2020;11:593931.
12. Purnell JQ, Braffett BH, Zinman B, et al. DCCT/EDIC Research Group. Impact of excessive weight gain on cardiovascular outcomes in type 1 diabetes: results from the diabetes control and complications trial/epidemiology of diabetes interventions and complications (DCCT/EDIC) Study. Diabetes Care 2017;40:1756–62.
13. Orchard TJ, Olson JC, Erbey JR, et al. Insulin resistance-related factors, but not glycemia, predict coronary artery disease in type 1 diabetes: 10-year follow-up data from the Pittsburgh Epidemiology of Diabetes Complications Study. Diabetes Care 2003;26:1374–9.
14. Expert Panel on Detection, Evaluation, and Treatment of High Blood Cholesterol in Adults Executive summary of the third report of the national cholesterol education program (NCEP) expert panel on detection, evaluation, and treatment of high blood cholesterol in adults (Adult Treatment Panel III). JAMA 2001;285:2486–97.
15. Haffner SM, Lehto S, Ronnemaa T, et al. Mortality from coronary heart disease in subjects with type 2 diabetes and in nondiabetic subjects with and without prior myocardial infarction. N Engl J Med 1998;339:229–34.
16. Gore MO, McGuire DK, Lingvay I, et al. Predicting cardiovascular risk in type 2 diabetes: the heterogeneity challenges. Curr Cardiol Rep 2015;17:607.
17. Sarwar N, Gao P, Seshasai SR, et al. Emerging risk factors collaboration: diabetes mellitus, fasting blood glucose concentration, and risk of vascular disease: a collaborative meta-analysis of 102 prospective studies. Lancet 2010;375:2215–22.
18. Soedamah-Muthu SS, Mulnier HE, Fuller JH, et al. High risk of cardiovascular disease in patients with type 1 diabetes in the U.K.: a cohort study using the general practice research database. Diabetes Care 2006;29:798–804.
19. Mulnier HE, Seaman HE, Raleigh VS, et al. Risk of myocardial infarction in men and women with type 2 diabetes in the UK: a cohort study using the General Practice Research Database. Diabetologia 2008;51:1639–45.
20. Lascar N, Brown J, Pattison H, et al. Type 2 diabetes in adolescents and young adults. Lancet Diabetes Endocrinol 2018;6:69–80.
21. Huo X, Gao L, Guo L, et al. Risk of non-fatal cardiovascular diseases in early-onset versus late-onset type 2 diabetes in China: a cross-sectional study. Lancet Diabetes Endocrinol 2016;4:115–24.
22. Dabelea D, Stafford JM, Mayer-Davis EJ, et al. Association of type 1 diabetes vs type 2 diabetes diagnosed during childhood and adolescence with complications during teenage years and young adulthood. JAMA 2017;317:825–35.
23. Kalyani RR, Lazo M, Ouyang P, et al. Sex differences in diabetes and risk of incident coronary artery disease in healthy young and middle-aged adults. Diabetes Care 2014;37:830–8.

24. Arnett DK, Blumenthal RS, Albert MA, et al. 2019 ACC/AHA Guideline on the primary prevention of cardiovascular disease: a report of the American College of Cardiology/American Heart Association Task Force on Clinical Practice Guidelines. J Am Coll Cardiol 2019;74:e177–232.

25. Connolly VM, Kesson CM. Socioeconomic status and clustering of cardiovascular disease risk factors in diabetic patients. Diabetes Care 1996;19:419–22.

26. Rana JS, Liu JY, Moffet H, et al. Diabetes and prior coronary heart disease are not necessarily risk equivalent for future coronary heart disease events. J Gen Intern Med 2016;31:387–93.

27. Huang Y, Cai X, Mai W, et al. Association between prediabetes and risk of cardiovascular disease and all cause mortality: systematic review and meta-analysis. BMJ 2016;355:i5953.

28. Stamler J, Vaccaro O, Neaton JD, et al. Diabetes, other risk factors, and 12-yr cardiovascular mortality for men screened in the Multiple Risk Factor Intervention Trial. Diabetes Care 1993;16:434–44.

29. Emerging Risk Factors Collaboration, Di Angelantonio E, Gao P, Khan H, et al. Glycated hemoglobin measurement and prediction of cardiovascular disease. JAMA 2014;311:1225–33.

30. Nathan DM, Cleary PA, Backlund JY, et al. Diabetes control and complications trial/epidemiology of diabetes interventions and complications (DCCT/EDIC) Study Research Group. Intensive diabetes treatment and cardiovascular disease in patients with type 1 diabetes. N Engl J Med 2005;353:2643–53.

31. Rawshani A, Rawshani A, Franzén S, et al. Risk factors, mortality, and cardiovascular outcomes in patients with type 2 diabetes. N Engl J Med 2018;379:633–44.

32. Rewers M, Zaccaro D, D'Agostino R, et al. Insulin Resistance Atherosclerosis Study Investigators: Insulin sensitivity, insulinemia, and coronary artery disease: the Insulin Resistance Atherosclerosis Study. Diabetes Care 2004;27:781–7.

33. Fox CS, Pencina MJ, Wilson PW, et al. Lifetime risk of cardiovascular disease among individuals with and without diabetes stratified by obesity status in the Framingham Heart Study. Diabetes Care 2008;31:1582–4.

34. The Look AHEAD Research Group, Wing RR, Bolin P, Brancati FL, et al. Cardiovascular effects of intensive lifestyle intervention in type 2 diabetes. N Engl J Med 2013;369:145–54.

35. Goldberg RB, Stone NJ, Grundy SM. The 2018 AHA/ACC/AACVPR/AAPA/ABC/ACPM/ADA/AGS/APhA/ASPC/NLA/PCNA Guidelines on the Management of Blood Cholesterol in Diabetes. Diabetes Care 2020;43:1673–8.

36. Costacou T, Evans RW, Orchard TJ. High-density lipoprotein cholesterol in diabetes: is higher always better? J Clin Lipidol 2011;5:387–94.

37. Alessa T, Szeto A, Chacra W, et al. High HDL-C prevalence is common in type 1 diabetes and increases with age but is lower in Hispanic individuals. J Diabetes Complications 2015;29:105–7.

38. Chait A, Ginsberg HN, Vaisar T. Remnants of the triglyceride-rich lipoproteins, diabetes, and cardiovascular disease. Diabetes 2020;69:508–16.

39. Shalaurova I, Connelly MA, Garvey WT, et al. Lipoprotein insulin resistance index: a lipoprotein particle-derived measure of insulin resistance. Metab Syndr Relat Disord 2014;12:422–9.

40. Ward NC, Vickneswaran S, Watts GF. Lipoprotein (a) and diabetes mellitus: causes and consequences. Curr Opin Endocrinol Diabetes Obes 2021;28:181–7.

41. Guo VY, Cao B, Wu X, et al. Prospective association between diabetic retinopathy and cardiovascular disease—a systematic review and meta-analysis of cohort studies. J Stroke Cerebrovasc Dis 2016;25:1688–95.

42. Brownrigg JR, de Lusignan S, McGovern A, et al. Peripheral neuropathy and the risk of cardiovascular events in type 2 diabetes mellitus. Heart 2014;100: 1837–43.

43. Svensson MK, Cederholm J, Eliasson B, et al. Albuminuria and renal function as predictors of cardiovascular events and mortality in a general population of patients with type 2 diabetes: a nationwide observational study from the Swedish National Diabetes Register. Diab Vasc Dis Res 2013;10:520–9.

44. Goldberg RB. Cytokine and cytokine-like inflammation markers, endothelial dysfunction, and imbalanced coagulation in development of diabetes and its complications. J Clin Endocrinol Metab 2009;94:3171–82.

45. Cholesterol Treatment Trialists' (CTT) Collaboration, Baigent C, Blackwell L, Emberson J, et al. Efficacy and safety of more intensive lowering of LDL cholesterol: a meta-analysis of data from 170,000 participants in 26 randomised trials. Lancet 2010;376:1670–81.

46. Grundy SM, Stone NJ, Bailey AL, et al. AHA/ACC/AACVPR/AAPA/ABC/ACPM/ ADA/AGS/APhA/ASPC/NLA/PCNA Guideline on the Management of Blood Cholesterol: Executive Summary: a report of the American College of Cardiology/American Heart Association Task Force on Clinical Practice Guidelines. Circulation 2019;139(25):e1046–81.

47. Jellinger PS, Handelsman Y, Rosenblit PD, et al. American Association of Clinical Endocrinologists and American College of Endocrinology Guidelines for management of dyslipidemia and prevention of cardiovascular disease. Endocr Pract 2017;23(Suppl 2):1–87.

48. de Vries FM, Denig P, Pouwels KB, et al. Primary prevention of major cardiovascular and cerebrovascular events with statins in diabetic patients: a meta-analysis. Drugs 2012;72:2365–73.

49. Hero C, Rawshani A, Svensson AM, et al. Association between use of lipid-lowering therapy and cardiovascular diseases and death in individuals with type 1 diabetes. Diabetes Care 2016;39:996–1003.

50. American Diabetes Association. 10. Cardiovascular disease and risk management: standards of medical care in diabetes-2021. Diabetes Care 2021; 44(Suppl 1):S125–50.

51. Ridker PM, Danielson E, Fonseca FA, et al. Rosuvastatin to prevent vascular events in men and women with elevated C-reactive protein. N Engl J Med 2008;359:2195–207.

52. Malik S, Budoff MJ, Katz R, et al. Impact of subclinical atherosclerosis on cardiovascular disease events in individuals with metabolic syndrome and diabetes: the multi-ethnic study of atherosclerosis. Diabetes Care 2011;34:2285–90.

53. Budoff M, Backlund JC, Bluemke DA, et al. DCCT/EDIC Research Group. The association of coronary artery calcification with subsequent incidence of cardiovascular disease in type 1 diabetes: the DCCT/EDIC Trials. JACC Cardiovasc Imaging 2019;12:1341–9.

54. Toth PP. That myalgia of yours is not from statin intolerance. J Am Coll Cardiol 2021;78(12):1223–6.

55. Sattar N, Preiss D, Murray HM, et al. Statins and risk of incident diabetes: a collaborative meta-analysis of randomised statin trials. Lancet 2010;375: 735–42.

56. Mansi IA, Chansard M, Lingvay I, et al. Association of statin therapy initiation with diabetes progression: a retrospective matched-cohort study. JAMA Intern Med 2021;181(12):1562–74.
57. Soran H, France M, Adam S, et al. Quantitative evaluation of statin effectiveness versus intolerance and strategies for management of intolerance. Atherosclerosis 2020;306:33–40.
58. Silverman MG, Ference BA, Im K, et al. Association between lowering LDL-C and cardiovascular risk reduction among different therapeutic interventions: a systematic review and meta-analysis. JAMA 2016;316:1289–97.
59. Cannon CP, Blazing MA, Giugliano RP, et al. Ezetimibe added to statin therapy after acute coronary syndromes. N Engl J Med 2015;372:2387–97.
60. Giugliano RP, Cannon CP, Blazing MA, et al. IMPROVE-IT (Improved Reduction of Outcomes: Vytorin Efficacy International Trial) Investigators. Benefit of adding ezetimibe to statin therapy on cardiovascular outcomes and safety in patients with versus without diabetes mellitus: results from IMPROVE-IT. Circulation 2018;137:1571–82.
61. Sabatine MS, Leiter LA, Wiviott SD, et al. Cardiovascular safety and efficacy of the PCSK9 inhibitor evolocumab in patients with and without diabetes and the effect of evolocumab on glycaemia and risk of new-onset diabetes: a prespecified analysis of the FOURIER randomised controlled trial. Lancet Diabetes Endocrinol 2017;5:941–50.
62. Leiter LA, Zamorano JL, Bujas-Bobanovic M, et al. Lipid-lowering efficacy and safety of alirocumab in patients with or without diabetes: a sub-analysis of ODYSSEY COMBO II. Diabetes Obes Metab 2017;19:989–96.
63. Cannon CP, Khan I, Klimchak AC, et al. Simulation of lipid-lowering therapy intensification in a population with atherosclerotic cardiovascular disease. JAMA Cardiol 2017;2:959–66.
64. Virani SS, Akeroyd JM, Nambi V, et al. Estimation of eligibility for proprotein convertase Subtilisin/Kexin type 9 inhibitors and associated costs based on the FOURIER trial (Further Cardiovascular Outcomes Research With PCSK9 Inhibition in Subjects With Elevated Risk): insights from the Department of Veterans Affairs. Circulation 2017;135:2572–4.
65. Goldberg RB, Fonseca VA, Truitt KE, et al. Efficacy and safety of colesevelam in patients with type 2 diabetes mellitus and inadequate glycemic control receiving insulin-based therapy. Arch Intern Med 2008;168:1531–40.
66. Smith W, Cheng-Lai A, Nawarskas J. Bempedoic acid: a new avenue for the treatment of dyslipidemia. Cardiol Rev 2021;29:274–80.
67. Ballantyne CM, Laufs U, Ray KK, et al. Bempedoic acid plus ezetimibe fixed-dose combination in patients with hypercholesterolemia and high CVD risk treated with maximally tolerated statin therapy. Eur J Prev Cardiol 2020;27:593–603.
68. Wang X, Zhang Y, Tan H, et al. Efficacy and safety of bempedoic acid for prevention of cardiovascular events and diabetes: a systematic review and meta-analysis. Cardiovasc Diabetol 2020;19:128.
69. Constantino MI, Molyneaux L, Limacher-Gisler F, et al. Long-term complications and mortality in young-onset diabetes: type 2 diabetes is more hazardous and lethal than type 1 diabetes. Diabetes Care 2013;36:3863–9.
70. Echouffo-Tcheugui JB, Niiranen TJ, McCabe EL, et al. An early-onset subgroup of type 2 diabetes: a multigenerational, prospective analysis in the Framingham Heart Study. Diabetes Care 2020;43:3086–93.

71. Braamskamp MJAM, Kastelein JJP, Kusters DM, et al. Statin initiation during childhood in patients with familial hypercholesterolemia: consequences for cardiovascular risk. J Am Coll Cardiol 2016;67:455–6.

72. Pambianco G, Costacou T, Ellis D, et al. The 30-year natural history of type 1 diabetes complications: the Pittsburgh Epidemiology of Diabetes Complications Study Experience. Diabetes 2006;55:1463–9.

73. Diabetes Control and Complications Trial/Epidemiology of Diabetes Interventions and Complications (DCCT/EDIC) Research Group. Risk factors for cardiovascular disease in type 1 diabetes. Diabetes 2016;65:1370–9.

74. Wong ND, Glovaci D, Wong K, et al. Global cardiovascular disease risk assessment in United States adults with diabetes. Diab Vasc Dis Res 2012;9:146–52.

75. Nezarat N, Budoff MJ, Luo Y, et al. Presence, characteristics, and volumes of coronary plaque determined by computed tomography angiography in young type 2 diabetes mellitus. Am J Cardiol 2017;119:1566–71.

76. Reis JP, Allen NB, Bancks MP, et al. Duration of diabetes and prediabetes during adulthood and subclinical atherosclerosis and cardiac dysfunction in middle age: the CARDIA Study. Diabetes Care 2018;41:731–8.

77. Starkman HS, Cable G, Hala V, et al. Delineation of prevalence and risk factors for early coronary artery disease by electron beam computed tomography in young adults with type 1 diabetes. Diabetes Care 2003;26:433–6.

78. Divakaran S, Singh A, Biery D, et al. Diabetes is associated with worse long-term outcomes in young adults after myocardial infarction: the Partners YOUNG-MI Registry. Diabetes Care 2020;43:1843–50.

79. Orringer CE, Blaha MJ, Blankstein R, et al. The National Lipid Association scientific statement on coronary artery calcium scoring to guide preventive strategies for ASCVD risk reduction. J Clin Lipidol 2021;15:33–60.

80. Ridker PM, Lonn E, Paynter NP, et al. Primary prevention with statin therapy in the elderly: new meta-analyses from the contemporary JUPITER and HOPE-3 randomized trials. Circulation 2017;135:1979–81.

81. Ramos R, Comas-Cufí M, Martí-Lluch R, et al. Statins for primary prevention of cardiovascular events and mortality in old and very old adults with and without type 2 diabetes: retrospective cohort study. BMJ 2018;362:1–4.

82. Hokanson JE, Austin MA. Plasma triglyceride level is a risk factor for cardiovascular disease independent of high-density lipoprotein cholesterol level: a meta-analysis of population-based prospective studies. J Cardiovasc Risk 1996;3:213–9.

83. Sarwar N, Danesh J, Eiriksdottir G, et al. Triglycerides and the risk of coronary heart disease: 10,158 incident cases among 262,525 participants in 29 Western prospective studies. Circulation 2007;115:450–8.

84. Emerging Risk Factors Collaboration, Danesh J, Erqou S, Walker M, et al. Eur J Epidemiol 2007;22:839–69.

85. Turner RC, Millns H, Neil HA, et al. Risk factors for coronary artery disease in non-insulin dependent diabetes mellitus: United Kingdom Prospective Diabetes Study (UKPDS: 23). BMJ 1998;316:823–8.

86. Fontbonne A, Eschwege E, Cambien F, et al. Hypertriglyceridaemia as a risk factor of coronary heart disease mortality in subjects with impaired glucose tolerance or diabetes. Results from the 11-year follow-up of the Paris Prospective Study. Diabetologia 1989;32:300–4.

87. Nordestgaard BG, Benn M, Schnohr P, et al. Nonfasting triglycerides and risk of myocardial infarction, ischemic heart disease, and death in men and women. JAMA 2007;298:299–308.

88. Nichols GA, Philip S, Reynolds K, et al. Increased residual cardiovascular risk in patients with diabetes and high versus normal triglycerides despite statin-controlled LDL cholesterol. Diabetes Obes Metab 2019;21:366–71.

89. Triglyceride Coronary Disease Genetics Consortium and Emerging Risk Factors Collaboration, Sarwar N, Sandhu MS, Ricketts SL, et al. Triglyceride-mediated pathways and coronary disease: collaborative analysis of 101 studies. Lancet 2010;375:1634–9.

90. TG and HDL Working Group of the Exome Sequencing Project, National Heart, Lung, and Blood Institute, Crosby J, Peloso GM, Auer PL, et al. Loss-of-function mutations in APOC3, triglycerides, and coronary disease. N Engl J Med 2014; 371:22–31.

91. Paquette M, Amyot J, Fantino M, et al. Rare variants in triglycerides-related genes increase pancreatitis risk in multifactorial chylomicronemia syndrome. J Clin Endocrinol Metab 2021;106:e3473–82.

92. Cusi K. Time to include nonalcoholic steatohepatitis in the management of patients with type 2 diabetes. Diabetes Care 2020;43:275–9.

93. Bril F, Barb D, Portillo-Sanchez P, et al. Metabolic and histological implications of intrahepatic triglyceride content in nonalcoholic fatty liver disease. Hepatology 2017;65:1132–44.

94. The AIM-HIGH Investigators, Boden WE, Probstfield JL, et al. Niacin in patients with low HDL cholesterol levels receiving intensive statin therapy. N Engl J Med 2011;365:2255–67.

95. Akoumianakis I, Zvintzou E, Kypreos K, et al. ANGPTL3 and apolipoprotein C-III as novel lipid-lowering targets. Curr Atheroscler Rep 2021;23:20.

96. Khoury N, Goldberg AC. The use of fibric acid derivatives in cardiovascular prevention. Curr Treat Options Cardiovasc Med 2011;13:335–42.

97. Keech RJ, Simes P, Barter J, et al. Effects of long-term fenofibrate therapy on cardiovascular events in 9795 people with type 2 diabetes mellitus. Lancet 2005;365:1849–61.

98. Friedewald WT, Buse JB, Bigger JT, et al. Effects of combination lipid therapy in type 2 diabetes mellitus. N Engl J Med 2010;362:1563–73.

99. Keech AC, Mitchell P, Summanen PA, et al. Effect of fenofibrate on the need for laser treatment for diabetic retinopathy (FIELD study): a randomised controlled trial. Lancet 2007;370:1687–97.

100. Chew EY, Davis MD, Danis RP, et al. The effects of medical management on the progression of diabetic retinopathy in persons with type 2 diabetes: the Action to Control Cardiovascular Risk in Diabetes (ACCORD) Eye Study. Ophthalmology 2014;121:2443–51.

101. Pisano E, Gatsonis C, Boineau R, et al. Effects of combination lipid therapy in type 2 diabetes mellitus. N Engl J Med 2010;362:1563–74.

102. Bruckert E, Labreuche J, Deplanque D, et al. Fibrates effect on cardiovascular risk is greater in patients with high triglyceride levels or atherogenic dyslipidemia profile: a systematic review and meta-analysis. J Cardiovasc Pharmacol 2011;57:267–72.

103. Chapman MJ, Ginsberg HN, Amarenco P, et al. European Atherosclerosis Society Consensus Panel. Triglyceride-rich lipoproteins and high-density lipoprotein cholesterol in patients at high risk of cardiovascular disease: evidence and guidance for management. Eur Heart J 2011;32:1345–61.

104. Pradhan AD, Paynter NP, Everett BM, et al. Rationale and design of the pemafibrate to reduce cardiovascular outcomes by reducing triglycerides in patients with diabetes (PROMINENT) study. Am Heart J 2018;206:80–93.

105. Roth EM, Bays HE, Forker AD, et al. Prescription omega-3 fatty acid as an adjunct to fenofibrate therapy in hypertriglyceridemic subjects. J Cardiovasc Pharmacol 2009;54:196–203.

106. Kapoor K, Alfaddagh A, Stone NJ, et al. Update on the omega-3 fatty acid trial landscape: a narrative review with implications for primary prevention. J Clin Lipidol 2021;S1933–2874.

107. Bhatt DL, Steg PG, Miller M, et al. REDUCE-IT Investigators. Cardiovascular risk reduction with icosapent ethyl for hypertriglyceridemia. N Engl J Med 2019; 380(1):11–22.

108. Yokoyama M, Origasa H, Matsuzaki M, et al. Japan EPA Lipid Intervention Study (JELIS) Investigators. Effects of eicosapentaenoic acid on major coronary events in hypercholesterolaemic patients (JELIS): a randomised open-label, blinded endpoint analysis. Lancet 2007;369:1090–8.

109. Budoff MJ, Bhatt DL, Kinninger A, et al. Effect of icosapent ethyl on progression of coronary atherosclerosis in patients with elevated triglycerides on statin therapy: final results of the EVAPORATE trial. Eur Heart J 2020;41:3925–32.

Big Fish or No Fish; Eicosapentaenoic Acid and Cardiovascular Disease

Ira J. Goldberg, MD[a],*, Jana Gjini, MS[a], Edward A. Fisher, MD, PhD[b]

KEYWORDS

• Triglyceride • Chylomicron • VLDL • Atherosclerosis • Cholesterol

KEY POINTS

- Omega 3 fatty acids, both docosahexaenoic acid (DHA) and eicosapentaenoic acid (EPA), reduce circulating triglyceride levels. The reductions seem to be due to reduced production of both very low-density lipoprotein (VLDL) and chylomicrons.
- Omega 3 fatty acids can be used to prevent recurrent episodes of hypertriglyceridemia-induced pancreatitis. Recent data show that triglyceride reduction will decrease events.
- There is controversy on the interpretation of the data on the role of EPA to prevent cardiovascular events. The use of different controls, mineral versus corn oil, might have affected the trial outcome.

The epidemiology of cardiovascular disease (CVD) especially that due to atherosclerosis (AS) forms the basis for our approaches to reducing circulating low-density lipoprotein (LDL)-cholesterol (LDL-C) levels and to recommending "heart healthy" eating patterns. This has led to recommendations to replace saturated fats with more mono- and poly-unsaturated fats. Included in these recommendations is a switch from animal-to fish-derived protein. In addition, the use of the highly unsaturated fatty acids in fish, especially oily fish, as a supplement or pharmaceutical was shown to reduce circulating triglyceride levels.[1]

Human intravascular ultrasound studies show that lesions stabilize or regress in up to ~2/3 of patients on high-dose statin therapy and with LDL-C levels that averages ~70 mg/dL.[2] Whose lesions fail to stabilize or regress when LDL-C is reduced? In one meta-analysis, one marker in humans for defective regression is hypertriglyceridemia.[3] In addition, a number of recent genetic studies have implicated hypertriglyceridemia with more CVD events.[4] Thus far studies to confirm that triglyceride reduction

[a] Division of Endocrinology, Diabetes and Metabolism, New York University Grossman School of Medicine, 435 First Avenue, SB 617, New York, NY 10016, USA; [b] Division of Cardiology and Center for the Prevention of Cardiovascular Disease, New York University Grossman School of Medicine, 435 First Avenue, SB 704, New York, NY 10016, USA
* Corresponding author. 435 East 30th Street, SB 617, New York, NY 10016.
E-mail address: Ira.Goldberg@nyulangone.org

Endocrinol Metab Clin N Am 51 (2022) 625–633
https://doi.org/10.1016/j.ecl.2022.02.012
0889-8529/22/© 2022 Elsevier Inc. All rights reserved.

reduces CVD have not reached the level required for generalized clinical recommendations.[5–7] However, it is generally accepted that the reduction of severe hypertriglyceridemia will reduce risk of pancreatitis.

Docosahexaenoic acid (DHA) and eicosapentaenoic acid (EPA) are long-chain fatty acids with 6 or 5, respectively, double bonds, including one between the 3rd and 4th carbon from the omega (the nonacidic) end of the molecule. They differ by 2 carbons; 20 carbon EPA can be converted to 22 carbon DHA via the addition of a carboxyl-terminal end acetyl group. Although some DHA and EPA in humans can be synthesized by the elongation of shorter omega 3 fatty acids (linolenic acid, C18, found in plants), the origin of most of these fatty acids is in oceanic algae, which are eaten by the fish that become rich in DHA and EPA. DHA is a major component of human brain phospholipids, suggesting an important role in neurologic function. This review will, however, focus on the possible roles of omega 3 fatty acids as a therapy to reduce hypertriglyceridemia and the less than conclusive data that some of these fatty acids reduce CVD. We will review human studies that show the benefits and potential side effects of this therapy (**Fig. 1**)

POPULATIONS EATING MORE FISH HAVE REDUCED CARDIOVASCULAR DISEASE

In the last quarter of the 20th century, population epidemiologists were intrigued by the relatively low incidence of atherosclerotic cardiovascular disease (ASCVD) in first peoples of the north of Canada (Eskimos).[8] These people consume a high-fat diet, but the fat predominantly came from fish and oceanic mammals. A number of other population diet analyses support the hypothesis that fish intake reduces CVD (reviewed in[9]). Although it has become commonplace for physicians and other health providers to recommend a Mediterranean diet, which is characterized by more fresh vegetables and use of olive oil, the industrialized country with the greatest longevity and lowest rates of ASCVD is Japan. Why is this? A major source of protein in Japan is fish, rather than animal protein. Furthermore, circulating levels of omega 3 fatty acids are much greater in Japanese than Americans.[10] Levels of LDL-C as well as average body weight index (BMI) are also lower in the Japanese population, so the importance of omega 3 fatty acids alone cannot be dissected. Measurements of EPA and DHA in populations suggest that high blood levels of these fatty acids associate with less

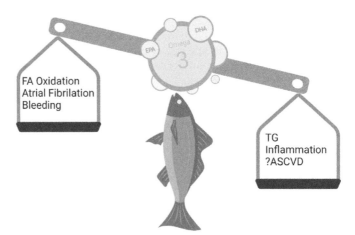

Fig. 1. Benefits and Downsides of Omega 3 Fatty Acids. (Created with BioRender.com.)

CVD and, surprisingly (see later in discussion) less atrial fibrillation.[11] In a large meta-analysis, Harris and colleagues reported a strong negative correlation between blood omega fatty acid levels and CVD.[12] Together, these correlative data make the case that changes in diet associated with the ingestion of more fish is beneficial and this recommendation has crept into many dietary recommendations for CVD reduction.

OMEGA 3 FATTY ACIDS REDUCE CIRCULATING TRIGLYCERIDE LEVELS

Although many postulated benefits of omega 3 fatty acids have been touted (see later in discussion) their single confirmed medical use is to lower circulating levels of triglycerides. The current American Heart Association[13] and Endocrine Society 6 Guidelines recommend the use of greater than 3 g of EPA/DHA as a monotherapy or adjunct to other drugs as a treatment of hypertriglyceridemia.[13] This therapy will reduce triglyceride levels greater than 30% in most cases.

Omega 3 fatty acids reduce hepatic and intestinal triglyceride secretion. Both de novo synthesis of fatty acids from carbohydrate and assembly of triglycerides are reduced, while fatty acid oxidation is increased.[14] Large number of double bonds also allows for greater oxidation, which may lead to more intracellular degradation of apolipoprotein (apo) B, the major structural protein of very low-density lipoprotein (VLDL) and LDL.[15] This would be consistent with human studies showing VLDL-apoB production decreased in subjects consuming diets enriched in omega 3 fatty acids.[16,17]

The reduction in circulating triglyceride levels seems to be similar using 4 g of either EPA or a mixture of DHA/EPA. As with other triglyceride-reducing therapies, such as fibrates, reduced VLDL is sometimes accompanied by increases in circulating LDL-C levels.[18–20] In part, this might indicate greater VLDL to LDL conversion via lipoprotein lipase. More likely, the reduction in triglyceride-rich lipoproteins reduces lipid transfer via cholesteryl ester transfer protein, which during hypertriglyceridemia increases LDL triglyceride content and production of smaller, relatively cholesterol-poor LDL. Icosapent ethyl (IPE) capsules, a clinically prescribed EPA, do not seem to increase LDL-C.[21]

EXPERIMENTAL DATA ON OMEGA 3 FATTY ACID PROVIDE MECHANISTIC INSIGHTS INTO POSSIBLE BENEFICIAL ACTIONS OF THESE COMPOUNDS

How and if EPA reduces CVD is largely unexplained. Some possibilities include beneficial effects on circulating lipoproteins, altered coagulation, or production of specialized proresolving lipid mediators (SPMs). SPMs decrease in the aorta during high-fat diets, and treatment with the SPMs Resolvin D2 and Maresin1 reduced AS, vascular inflammation, and necrotic cores.[22] Two receptors, GPR120 and ChemR23, are thought to mediate anti-inflammatory effects of EPA.[23,24]

Omega 3 fatty acids in experimental studies associate with changes in cardiac electrical conduction, perhaps via altering ion channels.[25,26] Initially such effects were proposed to reduce cardiac arrhythmias and sudden death,[27] but, as noted later in discussion, data from human clinical trials have not supported this.

Another possible beneficial action of omega 3 fatty acids is its effects on coagulation, specifically on platelet function. Omega 3 fatty acids reduce platelet activation and adhesion, thromboxane A2 (TXA2) synthesis, and plasminogen activator inhibitor-1 plasma concentrations.[28,29] Such an effect is supported by a trend to increased GI hemorrhage in some clinical trials.[30]

There are some biological differences between DHA and EPA. For example, both are incorporated into membrane phospholipids and affect membrane characteristics, such as fluidity and flexibility. This, in turn, modulates the activities of transmembrane proteins, with consequences on ion transport, enzyme activities, and cell signaling.[31][32] Nevertheless, DHA (vs EPA) seems to have a predominant role in vision and the developing brain because of its selective incorporation into retinal cell membranes and postsynaptic neuronal cell membranes.[33]

Another distinction between DHA and EPA relates to the aforementioned SPM class of molecules. Both the enzymatic steps as well as the products differ for each n-3 fatty acid. For example, the synthesis of the E-series (derived from EPA) resolvins involves 5-lipoxygenase, but some of the D-series resolvins additionally require the action of 15-lipoxygenase. Also, SPMs derived from DHA do not only include resolvins, but also other inflammation-resolving molecules called maresins and protectins.[34] While there are many overlapping effects of the different species of SPMs on inflammation, there are also a number of distinct differences among them (summarized in[34]). Thus, while it is plausible that a tissue-selective aspect of EPA or DHA metabolism (such as the degree of incorporation into membranes) or a difference in the effects of E-resolvins, D-resolvins, maresins, and protectins is the basis for the discrepant clinical results reported, rigorous evidence is lacking to make any firm conclusions.

ACUTE BENEFITS OF OMEGA 3 FATTY ACIDS

Supplementation with DHA ethyl esters or DHA triglycerides required 1 to 3 months to substantially increase DHA concentrations in plasma and red blood cells in humans.[35] Similarly, incorporation of EPA and DHA into the membrane phospholipids in immune cells with fish oil consumption requires 30 days in healthy human subjects.[36] In rats, maximum incorporation of omega 3 fatty acids in cardiac phospholipids was achieved after 8 weeks of oral ingestion.[37] Thus, oral intake or ingestion of omega 3 fatty acid supplements requires a prolonged period, over days to weeks, to achieve substantial cellular enrichment through which they may yield protective effects on CVD.

Aside from studies using omega 3 fatty acids as an oral dietary supplement, these lipids have been used in acute infusion studies.[38] Omega 3 fatty acids seem to have acute anti-inflammatory effects in stroke[39] and ischemic heart models[40] when these lipids are given as intravenous infusions. Some clinicians recommend that patients with severe respiratory compromise who receive parenteral nutrition are administered lipid emulsions that contain a greater concentration of omega 3 fatty acids, although the data for this are less than definitive.[41] Whether the benefits of this approach derive from anti-inflammatory or anti-thrombotic effects, or changes in lung lipids, for example, surfactants, is unclear.

ONE DOUBLE-BLIND TRIAL IN HUMANS SHOWS A SIGNIFICANT REDUCTION IN CARDIOVASCULAR DISEASE EVENTS WITH AN ORAL ESTER OF EICOSAPENTAENOIC ACID

These data excited a field littered with positive fish oil-related trials that were mowed down by larger negative outcomes. In 1999 the Gruppo Italiano per lo Studio della Sopravvivenza nell'Insufficienza Cardiaca-Heart Failure (GISSI) reported that 1 g of a mixed DHA/EPA supplement reduced vascular CVD events.[42] Attempts to reproduce these benefits failed.[43–45] In contrast, 1.8 g/d of EPA in statin-treated patients in Japan led to a 19% reduction in CVD events (the JELIS trial[46]).

When the Reduction of Cardiovascular Events with Icosapent Ethyl–Intervention Trial (REDUCE-IT 30) first appeared it was hailed at first as a real test of the role of omega 3 fatty acid supplements in CVD. The patient population was chosen to be high risk (>57% with diabetes) and hypertriglyceridemic (triglycerides>150 mg/dL), although some subjects had levels as low as 135 mg/dL. In addition, the therapy, 4 g per day of IPE, is the therapeutic dose used to treat hypertriglyceridemia. The subjects in REDUCE-IT were taking statins to reduce circulating LDL-C levels and had an average level at a baseline of 74 mg/dL. The benefits of IPE, which were a reduction of events from 22% to 17.2%, occurred in subjects with all levels of triglyceride and did not seem to correlate with the degree of triglyceride reduction, nor were the benefits reduced when only US subjects were separately analyzed.[47]

The striking benefits of IPE found in REDUCE-IT led the FDA to specifically include IPE as an added CVD preventive therapy. REDUCE-IT also generated considerable controversy. The control group in REDUCE-IT received 4 g of mineral oil, a nonabsorbable oil obtained from petroleum that is sometimes used as a laxative. Unlike in studies using corn oil as the control, the mineral oil group had an increase in both LDL-C and CRP during the trial. A separate IPE study assessing vascular lesions using serial multi-detector computed tomography, Effect of Vascepa on Improving Coronary Atherosclerosis in People With High Triglycerides Taking Statin Therapy (EVAPO-RATE) showed an overall 17% reduction in plaque with IPE, but a doubling of (109%) volume after 18 months in the mineral oil group.[48] Although all subjects were on statin, the LDL-C levels were between 40 and 115 mg/dL and did not increase in the mineral oil group. A companion study using a cellulose-based control claimed that this control led to a similar effect on vascular lesions as did the mineral oil.[49] The 2 studies are difficult to compare as baseline and changes in LDL-C and CRP were not included.

Shortly after the publication of REDUCE-IT, another larger CVD outcome trial, Long-Term Outcomes Study to Assess Statin Residual Risk with Epanova in High Cardiovascular Risk Patients with Hypertriglyceridemia (STRENGTH), using an EPA/DHA combination, failed to show a CVD benefit in subjects chosen for greater CVD risk (70% with diabetes), median triglyceride levels of 240 mg/dL, and LDL-C on statin 75 mg/dL.[50] Even the subgroup of subjects with the greatest increase in circulating EPA levels did not benefit including subjects achieving circulating EPA levels similar to those in REDUCE-IT.[51] A recent analysis performed by matching subjects in REDUCE-IT and STRENGTH with those in the Copenhagen Heart Study concluded that most of the difference in CVD events between the IPE and mineral oil groups in REDUCE-IT were attributable to the detrimental effects of the mineral oil.[52,53] Nonetheless, because both JELIS and REDUCE-IT, but no studies using DHA or DHA/EPA combinations, showed benefit, the available data suggest that EPA alone should be used when physicians are adding omega 3 fatty acids for CVD reduction.

One side effect of high dose omega 3 fatty acids was an increase in atrial fibrillation from 2.1% to 3.1% (IPE group vs placebo) in REDUCE-IT and from 1.3% to 2.2% in STRENGTH. This has led to some concern that the less than definitively beneficial therapy of omega 3 fatty acid could, overall, have negative effects on aspects of CVD other than coronary artery disease.

SUMMARY

Aside from the small changes in atrial fibrillation and possible bleeding risk, high doses of omega 3 fatty acids seem to be relatively harmless. They certainly lower triglyceride levels and provide an alternative or addition to fibrates for the prevention of pancreatitis in patients with triglyceride levels more than 500 mg/dL. Fibrates are generic and often easier to take on a regular basis and viewed by some clinicians as the first-line therapy, with the addition of prescription of over-the-counter omega 3 fatty acids at 4 g per day as the second approach. New molecular and immunologic methods to more effectively lower triglycerides for pancreatitis prevention are on the horizon and likely will enter general clinical practice soon.

The importance of both fasting and postprandial triglycerides as causative for CVD events remains uncertain. As described elsewhere in this issue, while genetic associations of triglyceride-regulating proteins and CVD risk implies causality, definitive clinical trials and even preclinical data demonstrating the atherogenicity of triglyceride-rich lipoproteins are missing. Definite data showing CVD benefit due to fibrate therapy are not available. The clinical trial data using omega 3 fatty acids or IPE reduction of triglycerides must also be viewed cautiously. Nonetheless, EPA seems to have some benefit, while DHA and DHA/EPA combinations have none. As we await further trials of omega fatty acids and other triglyceride-reducing medications physicians will be forced to choose between a therapy with little harm but uncertain benefits. until newer and less controversial therapies arrive.

CLINICS CARE POINTS

- Patients with hypertriglyceridemia more than 500 mg/dL should be treated with omega 3 fatty acids or/or in addition to fibrates to prevent pancreatitis.
- If patients have and are at increased risk of atrial fibrillation be aware that these omega 3 fatty acids could exacerbate this condition.

ACKNOWLEDGMENTS

Work on omega 3 fatty acids by Drs. Goldberg and Fisher is funded by PPG HL: 151328

DISCLOSURE

Dr I.J. Goldberg has received consulting fees from IONIS and Arrowhead Pharmaceuticals. Dr E.A. Fisher has received fees as an expert witness for Hikma Pharmaceuticals and Dr Reddy's Laboratories, both of which have EPA products.

REFERENCES

1. Kris-Etherton PM, Harris WS, Appel LJ. American heart association. nutrition C. Fish consumption, fish oil, omega-3 fatty acids, and cardiovascular disease. Circulation 2002;106(21):2747–57.
2. Nicholls SJ, Ballantyne CM, Barter PJ, et al. Effect of two intensive statin regimens on progression of coronary disease. N Engl J Med 2011;365(22):2078–87.
3. Bayturan O, Kapadia S, Nicholls SJ, et al. Clinical predictors of plaque progression despite very low levels of low-density lipoprotein cholesterol. J Am Coll Cardiol 2010;55(24):2736–42.
4. Dron JS, Hegele RA. Genetics of Triglycerides and the Risk of Atherosclerosis. Curr Atheroscler Rep 2017;19(7):31.
5. Miller M, Stone NJ, Ballantyne C, et al. Triglycerides and cardiovascular disease: a scientific statement from the American Heart Association. Circulation 2011;123: 2292–333.
6. Newman CB, Blaha MJ, Boord JB, et al. Lipid management in patients with endocrine disorders: an endocrine society clinical practice guideline. J Clin Endocrinol Metab 2020;105(12).

7. Ginsberg HN, Packard CJ, Chapman MJ, et al. Triglyceride-rich lipoproteins and their remnants: metabolic insights, role in atherosclerotic cardiovascular disease, and emerging therapeutic strategies-a consensus statement from the European Atherosclerosis Society. Eur Heart J 2021;42(47):4791–806.

8. Leaf A. Historical overview of n-3 fatty acids and coronary heart disease. Am J Clin Nutr 2008;87:1978S–80S.

9. Jayedi A, Shab-Bidar S. Fish consumption and the risk of chronic disease: an umbrella review of meta-analyses of prospective cohort studies. Adv Nutr 2020;11: 1123–33.

10. Sekikawa A, Curb JD, Ueshima H, et al. Marine-derived n-3 fatty acids and atherosclerosis in Japanese, Japanese-American, and white men: a cross-sectional study. J Am Coll Cardiol 2008;52(6):417–24.

11. Kapoor K, Alfaddagh A, Al Rifai M, et al. Association between Omega-3 fatty acid levels and risk for incident major bleeding events and atrial fibrillation: MESA. J Am Heart Assoc 2021;10:e021431.

12. Harris WS, Tintle NL, Imamura F, et al. Blood n-3 fatty acid levels and total and cause-specific mortality from 17 prospective studies. Nat Commun 2021;12(1): 2329.

13. Skulas-Ray AC, Wilson PWF, Harris WS, et al. Omega-3 fatty acids for the management of hypertriglyceridemia: a science advisory from the american heart association. Circulation 2019;140(12):e673–91.

14. Jump DB. Fatty acid regulation of hepatic lipid metabolism. Curr Opin Clin Nutr Metab Care 2011;14(2):115–20.

15. Pan M, Cederbaum AI, Zhang Y-L, et al. Lipid peroxidation and oxidant stress regulate hepatic apolipoprotein B degradation and VLDL production. J Clin Invest 2004;113:1277–87.

16. Nestel PJ, Connor WE, Reardon MF, et al. Suppression by diets rich in fish oil of very low density lipoprotein production in man. J Clin Invest 1984;74(1):82–9.

17. Ng TW, Ooi EM, Watts GF, et al. Atorvastatin plus omega-3 fatty acid ethyl ester decreases very-low-density lipoprotein triglyceride production in insulin resistant obese men. Diabetes Obes Metab 2014;16(6):519–26.

18. Roth EM, Bays HE, Forker AD, et al. Prescription omega-3 fatty acid as an adjunct to fenofibrate therapy in hypertriglyceridemic subjects. J Cardiovasc Pharmacol 2009;54(3):196–203.

19. Chan DC, Watts GF, Barrett PH, et al. Regulatory effects of HMG CoA reductase inhibitor and fish oils on apolipoprotein B-100 kinetics in insulin-resistant obese male subjects with dyslipidemia. Diabetes 2002;51(8):2377–86.

20. Bays HE, Tighe AP, Sadovsky R, et al. Prescription omega-3 fatty acids and their lipid effects: physiologic mechanisms of action and clinical implications. Expert Rev Cardiovasc Ther 2008;6(3):391–409.

21. Sharp RP, Gales BJ, Sirajuddin R. Comparing the impact of prescription Omega-3 fatty acid products on low-density lipoprotein cholesterol. Am J Cardiovasc Drugs 2018;18:83–92.

22. Viola JR, Lemnitzer P, Jansen Y, et al. Resolving lipid mediators maresin 1 and resolvin D2 prevent atheroprogression in mice. Circ Res 2016;119(9):1030–8.

23. Oh DY, Talukdar S, Bae EJ, et al. GPR120 is an omega-3 fatty acid receptor mediating potent anti-inflammatory and insulin-sensitizing effects. Cell 2010;142(5): 687–98.

24. Back M, Hansson GK. Omega-3 fatty acids, cardiovascular risk, and the resolution of inflammation. FASEB J 2019;33(2):1536–9.

25. Calo L, Martino A, Tota C. The anti-arrhythmic effects of n-3 PUFAs. Int J Cardiol 2013;170(2 Suppl 1):S21–7.

26. Geleijnse JM, Giltay EJ, Grobbee DE, et al. Blood pressure response to fish oil supplementation: metaregression analysis of randomized trials. J Hypertens 2002;20(8):1493–9.

27. Leaf A. Omega-3 fatty acids and prevention of arrhythmias. Curr Opin Lipidol 2007;18:31–4.

28. Lagarde M, Calzada C, Guichardant M, et al. In vitro and in vivo bimodal effects of docosahexaenoic acid supplements on redox status and platelet function. Prostaglandins Leukot Essent Fatty Acids 2018;138:60–3.

29. Phang M, Lincz LF, Garg ML. Eicosapentaenoic and docosahexaenoic acid supplementations reduce platelet aggregation and hemostatic markers differentially in men and women. J Nutr 2013;143(4):457–63.

30. Bhatt DL, Steg PG, Miller M, et al. Cardiovascular risk reduction with icosapent ethyl for hypertriglyceridemia. N Engl J Med 2019;380:11–22.

31. Jump DB, Tripathy S, Depner CM. Fatty acid-regulated transcription factors in the liver. Annu Rev Nutr 2013;33:249–69.

32. Stillwell W, Wassall SR. Docosahexaenoic acid: membrane properties of a unique fatty acid. Chem Phys Lipids 2003;126(1):1–27.

33. Jump DB. The biochemistry of n-3 polyunsaturated fatty acids. J Biol Chem 2002; 277(11):8755–8.

34. Basil MC, Levy BD. Specialized pro-resolving mediators: endogenous regulators of infection and inflammation. Nat Rev Immunol 2016;16(1):51–67.

35. Witte TR, Salazar AJ, Ballester OF, et al. RBC and WBC fatty acid composition following consumption of an omega 3 supplement: lessons for future clinical trials. Lipids Health Dis 2010;9:31.

36. Kew S, Mesa MD, Tricon S, et al. Effects of oils rich in eicosapentaenoic and docosahexaenoic acids on immune cell composition and function in healthy humans. Am J Clin Nutr 2004;79(4):674–81.

37. Ayalew-Pervanchon A, Rousseau D, Moreau D, et al. Long-term effect of dietary {alpha}-linolenic acid or decosahexaenoic acid on incorporation of decosahexaenoic acid in membranes and its influence on rat heart in vivo. Am J Physiol Heart Circ Physiol 2007;293(4):H2296–304.

38. Zirpoli H, Chang CL, Carpentier YA, et al. Novel approaches for Omega-3 fatty acid therapeutics: chronic versus acute administration to protect heart, brain, and spinal cord. Annu Rev Nutr 2020;40:161–87.

39. Williams JJ, Mayurasakorn K, Vannucci SJ, et al. N-3 fatty acid rich triglyceride emulsions are neuroprotective after cerebral hypoxic-ischemic injury in neonatal mice. PLoS One 2013;8(2):e56233.

40. Zirpoli H, Abdillahi M, Quadri N, et al. Acute administration of n-3 rich triglyceride emulsions provides cardioprotection in murine models after ischemia-reperfusion. PLoS One 2015;10(1):e0116274.

41. Vanek VW, Seidner DL, Allen P, et al. A.S.P.E.N. position paper: Clinical role for alternative intravenous fat emulsions. Nutr Clin Pract 2012;27(2):150–92.

42. Dietary supplementation with n-3 polyunsaturated fatty acids and vitamin E after myocardial infarction: results of the GISSI-Prevenzione trial. Gruppo Italiano per lo Studio della Sopravvivenza nell'Infarto miocardico. Lancet 1999;354(9177): 447–55.

43. Bosch J, Gerstein HC, Dagenais GR, et al. n-3 fatty acids and cardiovascular outcomes in patients with dysglycemia. N Engl J Med 2012;367:309–18.

44. Bowman L, Mafham M, Wallendszus K, et al. Effects of n-3 fatty acid supplements in diabetes mellitus. N Engl J Med 2018;379:1540–50.
45. Manson JE, Cook NR, Lee I-M, et al. Marine n-3 Fatty acids and prevention of cardiovascular disease and cancer. N Engl J Med 2019;380:23–32.
46. Yokoyama M, Origasa H. Effects of eicosapentaenoic acid on cardiovascular events in Japanese patients with hypercholesterolemia: rationale, design, and baseline characteristics of the Japan EPA lipid intervention study (JELIS). Am Heart J 2003;146:613–20.
47. Bhatt DL, Miller M, Brinton EA, et al. REDUCE-IT USA: results from the 3146 patients randomized in the United States. Circulation 2020;141:367–75.
48. Budoff MJ, Bhatt DL, Kinninger A, et al. Effect of icosapent ethyl on progression of coronary atherosclerosis in patients with elevated triglycerides on statin therapy: final results of the EVAPORATE trial. Eur Heart J 2020;41:3925–32.
49. Lakshmanan S, Shekar C, Kinninger A, et al. Comparison of mineral oil and non-mineral oil placebo on coronary plaque progression by coronary computed tomography angiography. Cardiovasc Res 2020;116(3):479–82.
50. Nicholls SJ, Lincoff AM, Garcia M, et al. Effect of high-dose Omega-3 Fatty acids vs corn oil on major adverse cardiovascular events in patients at high cardiovascular risk: the strength randomized clinical trial. JAMA 2020;324:2268–80.
51. Nissen SE, Lincoff AM, Wolski K, et al. Association between achieved omega-3 fatty acid levels and major adverse cardiovascular outcomes in patients with high cardiovascular risk: a secondary analysis of the STRENGTH trial. JAMA Cardiol 2021;6(8):1–8.
52. Doi T, Langsted A, Nordestgaard BG. A possible explanation for the contrasting results of REDUCE-IT vs. STRENGTH: cohort study mimicking trial designs. Eur Heart J 2021;42(47):4807–17.
53. Deckelbaum RJ, Calder PC. Editorial: Is it time to separate EPA from DHA when using omega-3 fatty acids to protect heart and brain? Curr Opin Clin Nutr Metab Care 2020;23(2):65–7.

New and Emerging Therapies for Dyslipidemia

Alberto Zambon, MD, PhD[a],*, Maurizio Averna, MD[b], Laura D'Erasmo, MD, PhD[c],
Marcello Arca, MD[c], Alberico Catapano, MD, PhD[d,e]

KEYWORDS

- Atherosclerotic cardiovascular disease (ASCVD) • Inclisiran • SiRNA
- Selective PPAR alpha modulators • SPPARM • Volanesorsen
- Angiopoietin-like protein 3 • ANGPTL3

KEY POINTS

- Genetic studies have informed on biological pathways modulating lipid and lipoprotein metabolism, which have been exploited to design new drugs
- Inhibition of PCSK9 expression by long-acting siRNA is effective in lowering LDL-C
- Bi-annual administration of long-acting siRNA will improve adherence and represents a novel therapeutic strategy in high and very high CV risk patients
- Selective PPARa modulator (SPPARM) pemafibrate might represent a new option for combination LLT to decrease the risk of macro and microvascular complications in diabetes.
- Targeting ANGPTL3 is showing highly effective in reducing LDL-C and total triglycerides
- Targeting ApoCIII reduces TGRL by an LPL-independent mechanism

INTRODUCTION

Atherosclerotic cardiovascular disease (ASCVD) continues to represent a growing global health challenge. Despite guideline-recommended treatment of ASCVD risk, including antihypertensive, high-intensity statin therapy, and antiaggregant agents, high-risk patients, especially those with established ASCVD and patients with type 2 diabetes, continue to experience cardiovascular events.[1]

Robust and growing evidence from epidemiologic and genetic studies, as well as randomized clinical trials, suggest that triglyceride (TG)-rich VLDL (very-low-density lipoprotein) and their remnants, lipoprotein (a) [Lp(a)], and inflammation are causally related to risk of ASCVD in individuals already treated with statin therapy (**Fig. 1**).

[a] University of Padova, Clinica Medica 1, Department of Medicine - DIMED, Via Giustiniani 2, Padova 35128, Italy; [b] Policlinico, Paolo Giaccone, Via del Vespro 149, Palermo 90127, Italy; [c] Department of Translational and Precision Medicine, University of Rome, Viale dell' Università 37, Sapienza 00161, Italy; [d] Department of Pharmacological and Biomolecular Sciences, Università degli Studi di Milano, Via G. Balzaretti 9, Milan 20133, Italy; [e] IRCCS MultiMedica, Via Milanese 300, Sesto San Giovanni (MI) 200099, Italy
* Corresponding author.
E-mail address: alberto.zambon@unipd.it

Endocrinol Metab Clin N Am 51 (2022) 635–653
https://doi.org/10.1016/j.ecl.2022.02.004
0889-8529/22/© 2022 Elsevier Inc. All rights reserved.

endo.theclinics.com

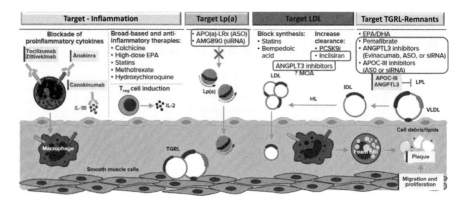

Fig. 1. Current and emerging therapeutic strategies to reduce cardiovascular risk. (*Adapted from* Hussain A, Ballantyne CM. New Approaches for the Prevention and Treatment of Cardiovascular Disease: Focus on Lipoproteins and Inflammation. Annu Rev Med. 2021 Jan 27;72:431-446.)

Recent years have brought significant developments in lipid and atherosclerosis research. Several lipid drugs owe their existence, in part, to human genetic evidence.[2] Although statins remain the mainstay of guideline-recommended lipid-lowering strategies, new and effective lipid-lowering therapies (LLT) are, or will be soon, available to lower risk of ASCVD events by further reducing atherogenic apoB-containing particles, such as LDL but also Lp(a), TG-rich VLDL, and their remnants (see **Fig. 1**).

These emerging therapeutic strategies will likely translate into a significant clinical benefit for individuals with severe dyslipidemias that are resistant to existing treatments, those who experience intolerable or harmful adverse effects from existing therapies, and most importantly for patients at significant residual ASCVD risk, despite apparently acceptable response to the current standard of care. Here, the authors briefly review the mechanisms, the effect on lipid parameters, and safety profiles of some of the most promising new lipid-lowering approaches that will be soon available in our daily clinical practice.

Inclisiran

The primary and secondary prevention of ASCVD is based on the achievement of the goals for the major risk factors recommended by the Guidelines.[3] LDL-cholesterol (LDL-C) is considered a causal factor of ASCVD, and the evidence collected suggests that the strategies aimed to reduce LDL-C are the most effective in reducing cardiovascular morbidity and mortality. Statins alone, and in combination with ezetimibe, have represented the conventional drug strategies to reduce ASCVD events, and recently the discovery of the role of PCSK9 as one of the main regulators of the LDL receptor degradation pathway[4,5] has prompted the development of novel approaches targeting this protein, which increase the number of LDL receptors and reduce plasma levels of LDL-C. The inhibition of PCSK9 by monoclonal antibodies is today a well-established strategy sustained by a large body of evidence based on efficacy, safety, and CVD outcomes trials (review). Evolocumab and alirocumab have received approval from regulatory authorities and are currently used in real-world clinical settings. The anti-PCSK9 monoclonal antibodies inhibit the circulating

PSK9 protein without interfering with the molecular mechanisms of PCSK9 gene expression, transcription, and translation.[6]

The pharmacologic development of inclisiran represents a new and promising approach to target PCSK9 at the RNA level in the liver. Inclisiran is a small interfering RNA (siRNA) molecule obtained by chemical synthesis and shares the mechanism of action with the siRNA family by interfering with the expression of the PCSK9 gene, as its complementary nucleotide sequences produce the degradation of PCSK9 messenger RNA (mRNA) once transcripted, preventing its translation.

The appealing features of inclisiran are the durability—it is a long-acting siRNA—and the liver specificity conferred by the conjugation to triantennary N-acetyl galactosamine carbohydrates that bind to asialoglycoprotein receptors highly abundant in hepatocytes.[7–9]

In 2020 and 2021, inclisiran was approved in Europe and the United States for reducing LDL-C in adults with primary hypercholesterolemia (heterozygous familial and nonfamilial) or mixed dyslipidemia, as an adjunct to diet, and in combination with a statin or a statin plus other LLT, who are unable to reach LDL-C goals. Inclisiran is also approved for adults on other LLT who cannot tolerate a statin or for whom a statin is contraindicated. The dose is 284 mg sc to be repeated at 3 months, 6 months, and subsequently every 6 months. Inclisiran, 284 mg, is equivalent to inclisiran sodium salt, 300 mg.

Phase I Trials

In 2014[9] a phase I trial demonstrated the safety and efficacy of ALN-PCS (inclisiran). Thirty-two healthy volunteers with plasma LDL-C levels of 3 mmol/L or higher were allocated in 6 single-dose cohorts with a ratio 3:1 to receive inclisiran intravenously or placebo. The incidence of adverse events (AEs) was not different in treatment and placebo groups, and the pharmacodynamic studies showed that the plasma increase of ALN-PCS was dose dependent. The plasma levels of PCSK9 and LDL-C were significantly reduced with the highest dose of ALN-PCS (0·4 mg/kg) by 70% and 40%, respectively. In 2017 the results of a phase I trial, aimed to assess safety and efficacy of single- and multiple-dose regimens of inclisiran administered subcutaneously, were published.[10] No serious AEs were registered and the more frequent AEs (≥5% of the inclisiran treated subjects) were cough, musculoskeletal pain, and nasopharyngitis. The highest reduction of PCSK9 plasma levels (74.5%), which was maintained at day 180, was seen in the group treated with a single 300 mg dose. In the multiple dose arm of the trial, plasma LDL-C and PCSK9 levels were reduced by about 60% and 80%, respectively. LDL-C levels remained reduced at day 180 with doses of 300 mg or higher.

The Orion/Victorion Program

The clinical development of inclisiran has been conducted by the Orion/Victorion program.[11] The Orion-1 and -2 (phase II trials) and Orion-8, -9, -10, and -11 (phase III trials)[12] have been completed. In these studies, the efficacy and safety of inclisiran have been tested in several categories of patients such as the following: (1) patients with ASCVD or ASCVD risk equivalents and elevated LDL-C (Orion-1 and Orion-11); (2) patients with familial homozygous hypercholesterolemia (HoFH) (ORION-2); (3) patients with familial heterozygous hypercholesterolemia (HeFH) (Orion-9); (4) patients with ASCVD and elevated LDL-C (Orion-10).

Inclisiran sodium has been used at single or multiple subcutaneous injections (Orion-1) or at a dose of 300 mg subcutaneously at day 1, day 90, and then every 6 months (Orion- 9, -10, and 11).

PATIENTS WITH ATHEROSCLEROTIC CARDIOVASCULAR DISEASE OR ATHEROSCLEROTIC CARDIOVASCULAR DISEASE RISK EQUIVALENT AND ELEVATED LEVEL OF LDL-C (ORION-1, -10, AND -11)

Inclisiran at a dose of 284 mg subcutaneously every 6 months for 18 months reduced LDL-C by about 50% at day 540 in about 1500 patients, with placebo-corrected reduction in PCSK9 plasma levels of about 80%.[13] The safety and tolerability were good.

PATIENTS WITH HOMOZYGOUS HYPERCHOLESTEROLEMIA (ORION-2) AND HETEROZYGOUS HYPERCHOLESTEROLEMIA (ORION-9)

Inclisiran has been studied in 2 "difficult-to-treat settings" HoFH and HeFH; in the Orion-2 pilot study, 4 patients with a genetic or clinical diagnosis of HoFH (untreated LDL-C >500 mg/d–13 mmol/L) completed the study. The background treatment was combination therapy for high-intensity statin plus ezetimibe. Inclisiran sodium was administered at a dose of 300 mg subcutaneously on day 1 and eventually repeated based on the reduction of PCSK9 levels. All 4 patients showed a durable reduction of PCSK9 plasma levels (up to 80%) and 3 out of 4 a durable reduction of LDL-C (up to 37%). The results of the Orion-9 trial that enrolled 481 HeFH subjects have shown that inclisiran significantly reduced LDL-C levels by about 48% and that the effect was sustained up to day 540 with an LDL-C reduction of about 44%. A dose of 300 mg, or a placebo, was administered subcutaneously on days 1, 90, 270, and 450. No differences of AEs or serious AEs in comparison with the placebo group were found.

The other Orion/Victorion trials are still in the recruiting phase.

Outcome Trials

The ORION-4 trial[14] is the large ongoing outcome trial that will evaluate the effect of inclisiran on MACE; at the end of the enrolment period, 15,000 subjects older than 55 years with ASCVD will be randomized to inclisiran sodium, 300 mg, subcutaneously every 180 days or placebo. The primary endpoint is the 5-year occurrence of coronary heart disease death, myocardial infarction, fatal or nonfatal ischemic stroke, and urgent coronary revascularization procedures. The other outcome trial—VICTORION-2 PREVENT—in 16,000 patients with established ACVD[15] has a composite primary endpoint of cardiovascular death, nonfatal myocardial infarction, and nonfatal ischemic stroke. In this trial, inclisiran sodium will be administered subcutaneously at the dose of 300 mg subcutaneously injected on day 1, day 90, and every 6 months until the end of the study.

Conclusions

Taken together, all these studies show that inclisiran, a long-acting siRNA belonging to the family of "sirans," is effective in lowering LDL-C in several populations of patients at high and very high risk of cardiovascular disease: patients with HoFH, HeFH, ASCVD, and ASCVD risk equivalent, including patients with diabetes. The appealing feature is the frequency of administration (twice/year) that will likely be associated with a much greater adherence than currently available lipid-lowering approaches (ie, statins and ezetimibe) allowing for a better time-averaged LDL-C reduction in the medium long term. In about 60% of patients a durable LDL-C reduction greater than 50% was obtained. A pooled analysis has shown that inclisiran is safe and well tolerated even in patients with chronic kidney disease and a creatinine clearance level of 15 to 29 mL/min, and the rate of AEs was not different from the placebo arm with the exception for minor and transient injection site reactions. In addition, no AEs have been reported for platelet counts or immunogenicity.[12] The ongoing trials will answer several relevant questions regarding the impact of inclisiran on therapeutic adherence and ASCVD clinical events, the safety and efficacy in special populations such as children and older people, the clinical use in postacute coronary syndromes, and, not less relevant, economic sustainability.

SELECTIVE PEROXISOME PROLIFERATOR–ACTIVATED RECEPTOR ALPHA MODULATORS

Growing evidence has established that triglyceride-rich lipoproteins (TRLs) and their remnants are also causal factors in ASCVD, and their contribution to atherothrombotic processes seems statistically independent of, and additional to, that of LDL.[16,17] A key investigational drug to address the residual vascular risk related to TRL remnants is a member of the nuclear peroxisome proliferator–activated receptors (PPARs) family, PPAR alpha (PPARα). PPARα, is mainly expressed in metabolically active tissues, such as the liver, kidney, heart, muscle, and macrophages, and has a key role in modulating the expression of genes involved in fatty acid oxidation, lipoprotein metabolism, and inflammation.[18,19] Guidelines recommend fibrates (PPARα agonists) and omega-3 fatty acids for the management of hypertriglyceridemia, usually as an add-on to primary statin treatment.[3] Clinicians are, however, well aware that current PPARα agonists, that is, fenofibrate, have proved disappointing in cardiovascular outcome studies either as monotherapy (FIELD)[20] or against a background of best evidence-based treatment including statin therapy,[21] with the possible exception of subgroups of patients with elevated baseline triglyceride levels (TG > 200 mg/dL–2.3 mmol/L). Pemafibrate is a selective PPARα modulator (SPPARM) that has been shown to reduce TG levels and elevate HDL-C levels. It is approved in Japan for use in dyslipidemia and is still undergoing phase III trials in the United States and Europe.

Preclinical Studies

Preclinical studies have revealed that enhanced potency, selectivity, and cofactor binding profile differentiate this novel SPPARMα agent, pemafibrate, from traditional nonselective PPARα agonists (**Fig. 2**). Compared with fenofibrate, pemafibrate resulted in greater TG lowering and elevation in HDL-C in animals with hypertriglyceridemia and more effective attenuation of postprandial hypertriglyceridemia, by suppressing the postprandial increase in chylomicrons and accumulation of chylomicron remnants.[22] Clinically relevant genes regulated by this SPPARMα agonist include those involved in regulation of lipoprotein metabolism, such as VLDLR and ABCA1. In addition, pemafibrate has been associated with an increased expression of genes involved in the regulation of the innate immune system (mannose-binding lectin 2), inflammation, and fibroblast growth factor (FGF),[23] a metabolic regulator with favorable effects on glucose- and lipid-mediated energy metabolism (FGF21), implying the potential for effects beyond lipid metabolism. Finally, this SPPARMα agonist may produce beneficial microvascular benefits, with evidence of reduction of diabetic nephropathy in diabetic db/db mice, attributed, at least partly, to inhibition of renal lipid content and oxidative stress.[24] Interestingly, the positive effect on microvascular complications supports data from FIELD[20] and ACCORD[21] where the use of fenofibrate in patients with type 2 diabetes was associated with a significant reduction in the progression of microvascular complications such as diabetic retinopathy and worsening of the albumin/creatinine ratio.

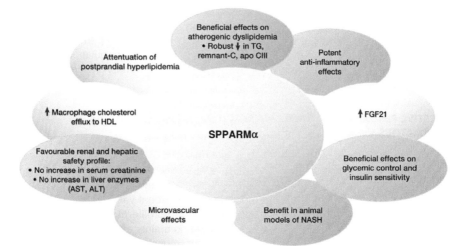

Fig. 2. Unique pharmacologic profile of pemafibrate (SPPARMα). (*From* Fruchart JC, Santos RD, Aguilar-Salinas C, Aikawa M, Al Rasadi K, Amarenco P, Barter PJ, Ceska R, Corsini A, Després JP, Duriez P, Eckel RH, Ezhov MV, Farnier M, Ginsberg HN, Hermans MP, Ishibashi S, Karpe F, Kodama T, Koenig W, Krempf M, Lim S, Lorenzatti AJ, McPherson R, Nuñez-Cortes JM, Nordestgaard BG, Ogawa H, Packard CJ, Plutzky J, Ponte-Negretti CI, Pradhan A, Ray KK, Reiner Ž, Ridker PM, Ruscica M, Sadikot S, Shimano H, Sritara P, Stock JK, Su TC, Susekov AV, Tartar A, Taskinen MR, Tenenbaum A, Tokgözoğlu LS, Tomlinson B, Tybjærg-Hansen A, Valensi P, Vrablík M, Wahli W, Watts GF, Yamashita S, Yokote K, Zambon A, Libby P. The selective peroxisome proliferator-activated receptor alpha modulator (SPPARMα) paradigm: conceptual framework and therapeutic potential : A consensus statement from the International Atherosclerosis Society (IAS) and the Residual Risk Reduction Initiative (R3i) Foundation. Cardiovasc Diabetol. 2019 Jun 4;18(1):71.)

Clinical Trial Evidence and Safety

A phase II dose-ranging trial in Japanese patients with elevated TG ($\geq$2.3 mmol/L) and low HDL-C (<1.3 mmol/L) showed that, after 12 weeks, this agent produced reductions from baseline in TG (up to 42.7%), VLDL-cholesterol (up to 48.4%), remnant-cholesterol (up to 50.1%), apoB-48 (up to 55.9%), and apolipoprotein C-III (apoC-III) (up to 34.6%), compared with both placebo and micronized fenofibrate 100 mg/d, with maximal effects at a dose of 0.2 to 0.4 mg daily.[25] Phase II/III trials in Japanese and European patients with elevated TG with or without type 2 diabetes mellitus (T2DM) confirmed the lipid-modifying activity of this SPPARMα agonist, in particular robust and sustained lowering of remnant cholesterol (by up to 80%) and TG and apoC-III (by ~50%). Treatment with pemafibrate, 0.2 to 0.4 mg/d, significantly reduced the postprandial area under the curve for TG, apoB-48, and remnant cholesterol for patients with and without T2DM.

Across published trials, this SPPARMα agonist was generally well tolerated both as monotherapy and in combination with statins, particularly with respect to renal and hepatic safety signals[26] with no difference as compared with the placebo groups. Importantly, and in contrast to studies with fenofibrate, which showed reversible increases in serum creatinine,[20,21] pemafibrate at any studied dose showed no increase in serum creatinine in studies up to 52 weeks in patients with or without preexisting renal dysfunction.[26]

Therefore, pemafibrate may offer a novel approach to target residual cardiovascular risk in high-risk patients with atherogenic dyslipidemia, especially those with T2DM, on a background of best evidence-based treatment including statin therapy.

The PROMINENT study (Pemafibrate to Reduce cardiovascular OutcoMes by reducing triglycerides IN diabetic patiENTs) will address this critical question.[27] PROMINENT has been designed with the goal of evaluating cardiovascular outcomes in more than 10,000 patients with elevated TG (baseline 200–500 mg/dL) and reduced HDL-C ($\leq$55 mg/dL). Thus, unlike the previous fibrate trials, PROMINENT will specifically target a hypertriglyceridemic population. Patients will be randomized to pemafibrate, 0.2 mg, BID versus placebo in addition to optimized statin therapy and followed-up for 4 years.[27] The primary endpoint is a composite of nonfatal myocardial infarction, nonfatal ischemic stroke, hospitalization for unstable angina requiring urgent coronary revascularization, and cardiovascular death. The trial should take 4 to 5 years to be completed. Within PROMINENT, a prospective nested substudy will investigate whether pemafibrate will significantly slow the progression of diabetic retinopathy in patients with nonproliferative diabetic retinopathy.[28] PROMINENT will determine whether therapeutic application of the SPPARMα concept translates to reduction in cardiovascular events in high-risk patients with T2DM already receiving evidence-based treatment. The results will provide additional information on the combination of LLT for elevated apoB-containing lipoproteins. A prior study, Reduction of Cardiovascular Events with Icosapent Ethyl-Intervention (REDUCE-IT), showed significant cardiovascular event reduction in patients with elevated TG taking statins when treated with 2 g twice daily of highly purified eicosapentaenoic acid ethyl ester.[29]

APOLIPOPROTEIN C-III TARGETING APPROACHES

Apolipoprotein C-III (apoC-III) has a key role in triglyceride-rich lipoprotein metabolism. ApoC-III is a 79 amino acid protein expressed mainly in the liver and intestine and found primarily on chylomicrons and VLDL. ApoC-III inhibits lipoprotein lipase (LPL) activity.

Robust data show that high levels of apoC-III lead to hypertriglyceridemia and, thereby, may influence the risk of cardiovascular disease. In humans, loss-of-function (LOF) mutations in apoC-III have been associated with low TG levels and reduced risk of atherosclerotic disease (**Fig. 3**).[30] Moreover, recent findings indicate that apoC-III might also modulate glucose homeostasis, monocyte adhesion, activation of inflammatory pathways, and modulation of the coagulation cascade.[31] These observations highlight the possibility of therapeutically targeting apoC-III in hypertriglyceridemia. Based on these findings, significant efforts have been undertaken to find a therapy specifically targeting apoC-III.[32]

Volanesorsen

Volanesorsen, a second-generation chimeric antisense inhibitor of Apo-CIII production, binds to apoC-III mRNA, triggering degradation by RNase H1.[31] ApoC-III inhibits LPL and hepatic uptake of TG-rich particles, which can lead to hypertriglyceridemia. Inhibition of apoC-III production thus allows for increased uptake of TG particles and reduces TG levels. It is administered as a subcutaneous once weekly injection with a follow-up dose after 3 months. It is eliminated by the kidneys after being metabolized by tissue endonucleases and exonucleases. The efficacy of volanesorsen was first published from a study of 3 patients with a rare syndrome of familial chylomicronemia syndrome (FCS). FCS is a rare autosomal recessive disease generally caused by mutations in the gene encoding LPL or genes encoding proteins involved in LPL function

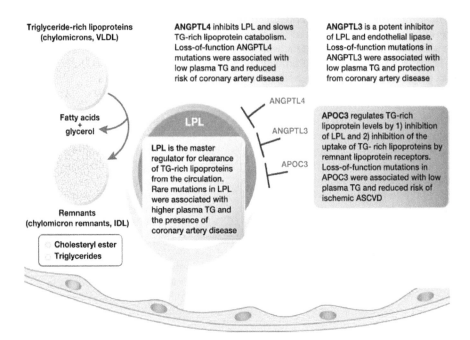

Triglyceride-rich lipoproteins (chylomicrons, VLDL)

ANGPTL4 inhibits LPL and slows TG-rich lipoprotein catabolism. Loss-of-function ANGPTL4 mutations were associated with low plasma TG and reduced risk of coronary artery disease

ANGPTL3 is a potent inhibitor of LPL and endothelial lipase. Loss-of-function mutations in ANGPTL3 were associated with low plasma TG and protection from coronary artery disease

Fatty acids + glycerol

LPL

ANGPTL4

ANGPTL3

APOC3

APOC3 regulates TG-rich lipoprotein levels by 1) inhibition of LPL and 2) inhibition of the uptake of TG- rich lipoproteins by remnant lipoprotein receptors. Loss-of-function mutations in APOC3 were associated with low plasma TG and reduced risk of ischemic ASCVD

LPL is the master regulator for clearance of TG-rich lipoproteins from the circulation. Rare mutations in LPL were associated with higher plasma TG and the presence of coronary artery disease

Remnants (chylomicron remnants, IDL)

Cholesteryl ester
Triglycerides

Fig 3. Novel approaches for the management of hypertriglyceridemia and key targets in the regulation of triglyceride-rich lipoprotein metabolism: apolipoprotein C-III (encoded by *APOC3*), angiopoietin-like proteins (ANGPTL) 3 and 4. (*From* Fruchart JC, Santos RD, Aguilar-Salinas C, Aikawa M, Al Rasadi K, Amarenco P, Barter PJ, Ceska R, Corsini A, Després JP, Duriez P, Eckel RH, Ezhov MV, Farnier M, Ginsberg HN, Hermans MP, Ishibashi S, Karpe F, Kodama T, Koenig W, Krempf M, Lim S, Lorenzatti AJ, McPherson R, Nuñez-Cortes JM, Nordestgaard BG, Ogawa H, Packard CJ, Plutzky J, Ponte-Negretti CI, Pradhan A, Ray KK, Reiner Ž, Ridker PM, Ruscica M, Sadikot S, Shimano H, Sritara P, Stock JK, Su TC, Susekov AV, Tartar A, Taskinen MR, Tenenbaum A, Tokgözoğlu LS, Tomlinson B, Tybjærg-Hansen A, Valensi P, Vrablík M, Wahli W, Watts GF, Yamashita S, Yokote K, Zambon A, Libby P. The selective peroxisome proliferator-activated receptor alpha modulator (SPPARMα) paradigm: conceptual framework and therapeutic potential : A consensus statement from the International Atherosclerosis Society (IAS) and the Residual Risk Reduction Initiative (R3i) Foundation. Cardiovasc Diabetol. 2019 Jun 4;18(1):71.)

(see Alan Chait's article, "Hypertriglyceridemia," in this issue); FCS is characterized by elevated levels of plasma chylomicrons, resulting in severe hypertriglyceridemia and increased risk of recurrent acute pancreatitis and other complications.[33] In this study, TG were found to decrease by 56% to 86% through LPL-independent pathways.[34] All patients achieved TG levels less than 500 mg/dL (<5.7 mmol/L) with treatment. TG levels in chylomicrons, apoB-48 levels, and non-HDL-C were also reduced.

Phase II Clinical Trials

Subsequent phase II studies showed similar TG reductions (40%–80%) compared with placebo when used as monotherapy or in combination with statins/fibrates.[35] In a phase II clinical trial of patients with hypertriglyceridemia (www.clinicaltrials. gov: NCT01529424), volanesorsen, 300 mg, given weekly reduced plasma apoC-III and TG levels by 79.6% and 70.9%, respectively.[36] In 80 patients from phase

II studies treated for 85 days or less, volanesorsen, 300 mg, was associated with greater than 80% reductions in apoC-III in various lipoprotein classes. In 15 adults with T2DM and hypertriglyceridemia treated for 15 weeks, volanesorsen reduced TG by 69%, with significant improvements in glycemia, glucose disposal, and insulin sensitivity.[37] In a study of 17 patients with hypertriglyceridemia, volanesorsen significantly reduced TG, apoC-II, and apoC-III and increased apoA-I and apoA-II.

Phase III Clinical Trials

Two phase III randomized, double-blind, placebo-controlled trials have been completed. APPROACH (www.clinicaltrials.gov:NCT02211209) evaluated 66 patients with FCS who had fasting TG greater than or equal to 8.4 mmol/L ($\geq$750 mg/dL).[38] Participants were randomized to 52 weeks of weekly subcutaneous volanesorsen, 300 mg, or matching placebo. At 3 months, TG decreased by 77% in 33 volanesorsen-treated patients but increased by 18% in 33 placebo-treated patients ($P < .0001$); the effect was sustained during 52 weeks. There were 3 placebo-treated patients with 4 acute pancreatitis events, whereas 1 volanesorsen-treated patient had 1 event 9 days after the end of therapy. The most common AE was injection-site reactions, most of which were mild to moderate (mean of 11.8% of all volanesorsen injections). However, declines in platelet counts led to 5 early terminations; 2 patients had platelet count less than 25 000/μL, which recovered after cessation of volanesorsen. The COMPASS study (clinicaltrials.gov: NCT02300233) randomized 113 patients with fasting TG greater than or equal to 500 mg/dL ($\geq$5.7 mmol/L; mean TG, 1261 $\pm$ 955 mg/dL or 14.3 $\pm$ 10.8 mmol/L) in a 2:1 ratio to receive either volanesorsen, 300 mg, or placebo subcutaneously once weekly for 26 weeks.[39] Patients treated with volanesorsen achieved a 71.8% reduction in TG from baseline after 3 months, compared with a 0.8% reduction in placebo-treated patients ($P < .0001$). Treatment effects were sustained after 26 weeks. Pancreatitis episodes were reduced on treatment, with 5 events in 3 patients occurring with placebo arm versus none with volanesorsen ($P = .036$). In contrast to APPROACH, there were no serious platelet events in the COMPASS study. However, injection-site reactions, nasopharyngitis, fatigue, arthralgias, myalgias, and thrombocytopenia are important AEs observed in trials.

Although the mechanism of the thrombocytopenia is unclear, development of a next-generation N-acetylgalactosamine (GalNac)-conjugated antisense oligonucleotide (ASO) targeting apoC-III may mitigate this risk. In a double-blind, placebo-controlled, dose-escalation phase I/IIa study in healthy volunteers with TG levels greater than or equal to 200 mg/dL, multiple doses of AKCEA-APO-CIII-LRx resulted in mean reductions of apoC-III of 83% and TGs of 65%, as well as significant reductions in total cholesterol, ApoB, non–HDL-C, and VLDL-C and increases in HDL-C. AKCEA-APO-CIIIL therapy was well tolerated with no flulike reactions, no platelet count reductions, and no liver or renal safety signals.[40] An ongoing multicenter, randomized, placebo-controlled, double-blind, phase II/III trial, BROADEN study (NCT02639286), has been planned to determine the benefit of volanesorsen in patients with familial partial lipodystrophy.[41] The primary objective of this study is to evaluate the efficacy and safety of volanesorsen therapy compared with placebo in reducing TG levels after 3 months of drug therapy. The study will last 52 weeks and involve 60 patients.

Because of the potential severity of side effects, caution is needed when evaluating the benefit/risk of medications under development for hypertriglyceridemia. Nevertheless, data strongly support the importance of apoC-III as a modulator of the lipolytic cascade and its inhibition as a major strategy for the development of new therapies for hypertriglyceridemia. It remains to be established if this approach may be useful also in controlling the residual cardiovascular risk associated with elevated TG and metabolic disorders.

On 28 February 2019, the Committee for Medicinal Products for Human Use of the European Medicines Agency recommended the conditional marketing authorization of volanesorsen for patients with genetically confirmed FCS and at high risk of pancreatitis, in whom the response to diet and TG reduction therapy is inadequate.[42] Volanesorsen has not been approved by the FDA because of safety concerns—low platelet counts and bleeding.

A phase I single and multiple dose-escalating study to evaluate the safety, tolerability, pharmacokinetics, and pharmacodynamic effects of ARO-APO CIII, a GalNAc–siRNA conjugate targeting Apo CIII, in adult healthy volunteers as well as in severely hypertriglyceridemic patients and patients with familial chylomicronemia syndrome is currently ongoing [ClinicalTrials.gov Identifier: NCT03783377].[43]

ANGIOPOIETIN-LIKE PROTEIN 3 TARGETING APPROACHES
The Role of Angiopoietin-like Protein 3 in Lipoprotein Metabolism

ANGPTL3 is a glycoprotein of 45 kDa protein that is only synthesized and secreted by the liver.[44,45] It belongs to a family of secretory proteins with structural homologies with angiopoietins, the key factors that regulate angiogenesis.[44] It is composed by an N-terminal coiled-coil domain, which is the functional portion of the protein, and a fibrinogen-like C-terminal domain.[44,45] Original studies conducted in mice have clearly established that ANGPTL3 is an important regulator of plasma TG levels due to its role as circulating inhibitor of LPL (see **Fig. 3**), the enzyme catalyzing the hydrolysis of TG contained in circulating VLDL and chylomicrons.[44,45] Furthermore, ANGPTL3 raises plasma HDL-C levels by inhibiting endothelial lipase.[44,45] Genome-wide association studies in humans have linked single nucleotide polymorphisms near to and within the *ANGPTL3* gene to TG variation in the population.[46] Later, homozygous LOF mutations in the ANGPTL3 gene were found to cause a lipid phenotype in humans, defined as familial combined hypolipidemia (FHBL2, OMIM #605019).[47,48] Noteworthy, this human model of ANGPTL3 deficiency has provided the unique opportunity to study ANGPTL3 function and the favorable consequences associated with its absence.[44] FHBL2 is characterized by a marked reduction of ApoA1- and ApoB-containing lipoprotein VLDL and LDL, an increase in LPL activity, and a markedly accelerated removal of TG-rich lipoproteins with an almost abolished postprandial lipemia.[48–52] The mechanism determining LDL-C reduction in ANGPLT3 deficiency is still unknown, even though it seems to be independent from the LDLR pathway. Indeed, Mendelian randomization studies have shown that subjects carrying LOF variants in *ANGPTL3* exhibit a reduced risk of atherosclerotic cardiovascular disease.[44] Altogether, these data have clearly established the rationale for developing pharmacologic strategies to inactivate ANGPTL3 and, thereby, to reduce plasma levels of atherogenic lipoproteins and cardiovascular risk.

Strategies to Pharmacologically Inactivate Angiopoietin-like Protein 3

To date, 2 different approaches have been used to inactivate ANGPTL3[53–55]: the administration of a human mAb against ANGPTL3 (REGN1500—evinacumab) or an ASO targeting Angptl3 (vupanorsen). The main difference between these treatments is that vupanorsen acts inside the nucleus of the hepatocyte, whereas evinacumab inhibits circulating ANGPTL3. Nevertheless, in animal models both therapies have been found to decrease TG, LDL-C, and HDL-C. Therefore, several clinical trials have been developed to evaluate the effectiveness and safety of these investigational drugs in humans.[53–55]

Evinacumab

Evinacumab is a fully humanized antibody that binds with high-affinity ANGPTL3. Phase I clinical trials have showed that the administration of evinacumab (75–250 mg subcutaneously or 5–20 mg/kg intravenously) to 83 healthy human volunteers with mild-to-moderate hypertriglyceridemia (150–450 mg/dL) or LDL-C greater than or equal to 100 mg/dL was associated with a dose-dependent, placebo-adjusted reduction of TG and LDL-C up to 76% and 23%, respectively.[53–55] Later, evinacumab was tested in a phase II, open-label, proof-of-concept study involving 9 patients with HoFH. HoFH is a rare autosomal dominant genetic disorder causing severe elevation of LDL-C and, consequently, accelerated atherosclerosis.[54,55] Results showed that the addition of evinacumab to background LLT determined in these patients a reduction in LDL-C, TG, and HDL-C levels by about 50%, 47%, and 36%, respectively.[53–55] Given these promising results, the Evinacumab Lipid Study in Patients with Homozygous Familial Hypercholesterolemia (ELIPSE HoFH trial), a phase III, double-blind, placebo-controlled trial, was conducted to assess the efficacy and safety of evinacumab in 65 patients with HoFH selected irrespectively of the molecular diagnosis and background LLT.[53–55] This trial found that monthly administration of evinacumab, in addition to background LLT, reduced LDL-C by 49%. More importantly, the reduction of LDL-C was independent from the residual LDLR activity with patients with HoFH carrying null/null *LDLR* variants exhibiting LDL-C reductions of about 70% compared with placebo.[53–55] The combined safety analysis of placebo-controlled studies showed that the most common adverse reactions (>3% of patients) after 24 weeks of therapy in patients in the evinacumab group versus placebo were nasopharyngitis (16% vs 13%), influenza-like illness (7% vs 6%), dizziness (6% vs 0%), rhinorrhea (5% vs 0%), nausea (5% vs 2%), extremity pain (4% vs 0% placebo), and asthenia (4% vs 0%).[53–55]

Therefore, evinacumab may offer a safe and effective option to significantly ameliorate atherogenic lipoprotein levels, thus possibly reducing cardiovascular events in patients with HoFH. Indeed, the Food and Drug Administration has approved evinacumab (Evkeeza) injection as an add-on treatment of patients with HoFH aged 12 years and older.[56]

Vupanorsen

Vupanorsen (IONIS-ANGPTL3-LRx or AKCEA-ANGPTL3-LRx) is a second-generation Gal-NAc-conjugated ASO targeting ANGPTL3 mRNA.[53,54] The Gal-NAc conjugation specifically directs the ASO to the liver (where ANGPTL3 is exclusively produced), allowing the use of a lower drug dosage, thus possibly preventing the most common adverse effect observed with ASO, namely thrombocytopenia.[57] Vupanorsen was first tested in a randomized, double-blind, placebo-controlled, phase I clinical trial designed to evaluate the safety, side-effect profile, pharmacokinetics, and pharmacodynamics of single ascending doses (N = 12) and multiple ascending doses (N = 32) of ANGPTL3-LRx in healthy adults aged 18 to 65 years.[53,54] Results of this trial indicated that inhibition of hepatic ANGPTL3 led to lowering of TG, LDL VLDL cholesterol, and apoC-III levels.[53,54] Later, a double-blind, placebo-controlled, dose-ranging, phase II study tested this drug in a broader spectrum of subjects (N = 105): (1) with elevated fasting plasma TG levels (>150 mg/dL), (2) type 2 diabetes with HbA1c greater than 6.5% and less than or equal to 10%, (3) hepatic steatosis.[53,54] Patients were treated for 6 months with placebo or vupanorsen at doses of 40 or 80 mg every

4 weeks (Q4W) or 20 mg every week (QW) given subcutaneously. Results of these trials showed that the maximal TG reduction of 53% from baseline was obtained with the 80 mg Q4W regimen and was associated with an LDL-C reduction of about 7%.[53,54] It must be noted that treatment with vupanorsen was not associated with any significant change in platelet count, and the injection site reactions were generally mild.[53,54]

Currently an ongoing phase II single-center, open-label trial is evaluating the efficacy of vupanorsen for triglyceride reduction in participants with familial chylomicronaemia syndrome (NCT03360747), and a phase II, double-blind, placebo-controlled, parallel group study is studying the efficacy, safety, tolerability, and pharmacokinetics of various doses and regimens of vupanorsen in participants with mixed dyslipidemia (NCT04516291).

It seems that there are differences in the LDL-lowering potency between evinacumab and vupanorsen. Further studies are needed to clarify if the strategy used to inhibit ANGPTL3 (mAb vs ASO) or the treatment protocol used (intravenous vs subcutaneous) might be the basis of the differences in lipid-lowering efficacy of these 2 approaches.

Future Perspectives

In the era of precision medicine, innovative therapeutic approaches targeting non-LDLR pathways as ANGPLT3 are currently in development; this includes RNA-based and gene-editing technologies.

siRNA Against ANGPTL3

ANGPTL3-targeted siRNA (ARO-ANG3) is an N-acetylgalactosamine-conjugated RNA silencing (siRNA) investigational therapy targeting ANGPTL3 mRNA.[58] ARO-ANG3 is administered subcutaneously and specifically directed at the liver, where it induces degradation of ANGPLT3 mRNA. Preliminary results of the phase I study in healthy volunteers have been presented at the European Atherosclerosis Society 2020 meeting.[59] The administration of ARO-ANG3 induced dose-dependent silencing of the ANGPTL3 gene, apparently avoiding off-target effects. This treatment was associated with a marked reduction of all lipoprotein fractions comparable to that observed in FHBL2. Indeed, maximal mean reductions in fasting lipid, lipoprotein, and apolipoprotein concentrations were −71% in TG, −50% in LDL-C, −42% in ApoB, −34% in non-HDL-C, and −47% in HDL-C.

In addition, initial results following repeated doses of ARO-ANG3 in 17 patients with HeFH and presenting LDL-C of 130 mg/dL despite intensive LLT, showed a reduction in LDL-C and TG of about 23% to 37% and 25% to 43%, respectively, at all doses.[60]

An ongoing phase II trial is currently recruiting patients with mixed dyslipidemia to assess the efficacy and safety of ARO-ANG3 in this population (NCT04832971).

CRISPR-Cas9 System for Gene Editing

A great interest is growing around CRISPR-based gene editing, which in recent years has emerged as a promising new strategy for treating patients with genetic disorders, including those with atherogenic dyslipidemia.[61,62] DNA strands at the target site are cleaved by an RNA-guided nuclease. When the standard DNA repair system of the cell attempts to repair the DNA, the engineered donor DNA provided by the CRISPR-Cas9 system is inserted into the target site.[55] As compared with ASO or antibody technologies that transiently reduce levels of the targeted protein, the CRISPR-Cas9 gene editing permanently repairs a mutated gene or inserts a missing gene in the edited cells, possibly inducing long-term therapeutic effects.[55,61,62]

Only preliminary studies on mouse models are available to date. Results have shown that both in-vivo adenoviral-mediated[63] and the nonviral lipid nanoparticle–mediated[64] editing of ANGPTL3 are associated with significantly reduced plasma levels of ANGPTL3, TG, and LDL-C.

Although these data are promising, further studies in humans are needed to establish the efficacy, safety, and durability of this method of inhibition of ANGPTL3.[62]

LIPOPROTEIN (A)-LOWERING APPROACHES: ANTISENSE OLIGONUCLEOTIDE AND SMALL INTERFERING RNA AGAINST APOLIPOPROTEIN (A)

Apolipoprotein B100 (apoB) containing lipoproteins are key players in atherogenesis and contribute causally to cardiovascular disease.[65] The apoB concentration in plasma is an excellent marker of cardiovascular risk.[66] Lp(a) is an apoB-containing lipoprotein bound to a hydrophilic, highly glycosylated protein called apolipoprotein (a) [apo(a)][67,68] (see Wann Jia Loh and Gerald F. Watts' article, "The Inherited Hypercholesterolemias," in this issue).

Epidemiologic, genome-wide association, and Mendelian randomization data[69–73] clearly demonstrate a causal role for Lp(a) in the development of ASCVD. To date, however, the definitive proof that specific interventions lowering Lp(a) reduce the risk of cardiovascular outcomes is missing. Still, some clinicians have a secondary goal of lowering Lp(a) in addition to lowering LDL-C and apoB in high-risk patients, in particular when recurrent ASCVD events occur despite aggressive LDL-C lowering.

Results from studies of dietary intervention show very modest effects on Lp(a) levels.[74] The most effective clinically available intervention for Lp(a) lowering is lipoprotein apheresis where the Lp(a) concentration is acutely lowered by approximately 50% to 85%, in association with comparable reductions in oxidized phospholipids. In addition to lowering Lp(a), lipoprotein apheresis with some systems also lowers LDL concentrations by 60% to 85%.[75,76] Limited clinical trial data suggest that Lp(a) lowering with lipoprotein apheresis may reduce the risk of ASCVD events,[77] but definitive studies are needed.

Currently available LDL-C lowering treatments have minor effects on Lp(a), with statins slightly increasing Lp(a) levels.[1,78] Data from trials of monoclonal antibodies directed against PCSK9 demonstrate dramatic LDL-C lowering by an average of 50% to 60% but a modest Lp(a)-lowering of 25% to 30%. The results of a recent analysis suggest that alirocumab-mediated Lp(a)-lowering independently contributed to major adverse cardiovascular event reduction.[79] Moreover, in patients with recent acute coronary syndrome on optimal statin therapy and LDL-C less than 70 mg/dL, alirocumab only lowered major adverse cardiovascular events in patients with mildly elevated (>13.7 mg/dL) Lp(a); there was no such interaction between Lp(a) levels and alirocumab benefit when LDL-C was greater than or equal to 70 mg/dL.[80] How to interpret these data remains difficult, given the multiple tests and the difficulties in knowing the contribution of Lp(a) cholesterol to the measurement of LDL cholesterol in subjects with high Lp(a) and low LDL. Niacin may dose-dependently lower Lp(a) up to 25% to 40%, but the cardiovascular benefit of this intervention is unknown, and the adverse side-effect profile of niacin in the setting of statins is a concern.[81,82]

Several experimental therapies targeting the apo(a) moiety of Lp(a) are under development.

Two mendelian randomization analyses aimed at estimating the extent of Lp(a) reduction required to observe a clinical benefit showed that large absolute reductions in Lp(a) levels (70–100 mg/dL) may be required to show a CHD risk reduction comparable to that observed with a 1 mmol/L ($\approx$39 mg/dL) LDL-C reduction.[83,84] Such large reduction cannot be achieved with conventional LLT but requires RNA therapeutics targeting selectively the hepatic synthesis of apo(a), which are currently under development. An ASO targeting apo(a) mRNA was shown to reduce Lp(a) by up to 80% at the highest dose (corresponding to ≈190 nmol/L, or 75 mg/dL) in patients with elevated Lp(a) levels,[85] with 98% of subjects treated with the ASO reaching on-treatment Lp(a) levels less than 125 nmol/L (<50 mg/dL). The ongoing phase 3 Lp(a) HORIZON outcomes trial will evaluate the effect of the ASO against apo(a) mRNA or placebo in patients after myocardial infarction with high levels of Lp(a).[86] The primary outcome is the time to the first occurrence of major ASCVD events in patients with Lp(a) greater than or equal to 70 mg/dL or greater than or equal to 90 mg/dL; the estimated completion date is June 2022.

Olpasiran is an siRNA designed to reduce the production of Lp(a) by targeting messenger RNA transcription. In a Phase I study (https://clinicaltrials.gov/ct2/show/record/NCT03626662), the safety, tolerability, pharmacokinetics (PK), and pharmacodynamics of olpasiran was evaluated. Adults with plasma concentrations at screening of Lp(a) greater than or equal to 70 to less than or equal to 199 nmol/L (cohorts 1 5) or greater than or equal to 200 nmol/L (cohorts 6 7) were randomized 3:1 to receive a single subcutaneous dose of olpasiran or placebo. The primary endpoints were treatment emergent AEs, safety laboratory analytes, vital signs, and electrocardiograms. Secondary endpoints included PK parameters and percent change from baseline in Lp(a). In olpasiran-allocated subjects, no safety concerns nor clinically relevant changes in liver or renal tests, platelets, or coagulation parameters were identified. In adults with elevated Lp(a) (median Lp(a) = 122 nmol/L [cohorts 1–5] and 253 nmol/L [cohorts 6 and 7]), a single dose of olpasiran significantly reduced Lp(a) with observed approximate median percent reductions of greater than 90% at doses of greater than or equal to 9 mg in a dose-dependent manner. The response persisted for 3 to 6 months at doses of greater than or equal to 9 mg. A phase II study is currently evaluating the efficacy, safety, and tolerability of an N-acetylgalactosamine–conjugated siRNA in 240 subjects with Lp(a) greater than 60 mg/dL (>150 nmol/L) (https://clinicaltrials.gov/ct2/show/record/NCT04270760).[87]

SUMMARY

In conclusion, despite national and international guideline recommendations to use statins as the first-line lipid therapy for ASCVD prevention, clinically relevant residual ASCVD risk, as observed in our daily clinical practice, emphasizes the need for additional therapies. Emerging agents offer options for further LDL-C reduction as well as alternative targets including TG and TG-rich lipoproteins, Lp(a), and inflammation. The clinical benefits in terms of ASCVD are being studied in ongoing clinical trials, including large outcomes studies. Combining many of these strategies will likely improve ASCVD outcomes, highlighting the role of health care professionals in selecting the correct patient population for each treatment modality to maximize benefits with the fewest medications and low sustainable costs.

CLINICS CARE POINTS

- In ASCVD and ASCVD risk equivalent patients Inclisiran is effective and safe in reducing LDL-C up to 50%
- In HeFH patients Inclisiran 300 mg s.c results in a durable reduction of LDL-C

- The efficacy of Inclisiran in reducing the cardiovascular outcomes will be highlighted by the results of the ORION-4 and VICTORION-2 Trials
- Pemafibrate, a selective PPARa modulator (SPPARM) is a "next generation" fibrate characterized by an enhanced potency as TG-lowering agent and greater safety profile compared to traditional non-selective PPARa agonists
- The presence of severe, resistant hypertriglyceridemia is suggestive of familial chylomicronemia syndrome
- The concomitant presence of low cholesterol and reduced HDL-C is suggestive of familial combined hypolipidemia (FHBL2)
- Evinacumab, a fully humanized mAb against ANGPTL3, may offer a safe and effective option to significantly decrease LDL-C and thus possibly reducing cardiovascular events in patients with HoFH independently of the residual LDL receptor activity
- Lp(a) is causal for CVD: the absolute weight of elevated plasma levels and the extent of Lp(a) reduction required to achieve a significant benefit are unknown
- Antisense oligonucleotide targeting apo(a) mRNA and small interfering RNA designed to reduce the production of Lp(a), represent the first specific and highly effective pharmacological approaches reducing plasma Lp(a) up to 80-85%.

REFERENCES

1. Hoogeveen RC, Ballantyne CM. Residual Cardiovascular Risk at Low LDL: Remnants, Lipoprotein(a), and Inflammation. Clin Chem 2021;67(1):143–53.
2. Kathiresan S. Developing medicines that mimic the natural successes of the human genome: lessons from NPC1L1, HMGCR, PCSK9, APOC3, and CETP. J Am Coll Cardiol 2015;65:1562–6.
3. Mach F, Baigent C, et al. 2019 ESC/EAS Guidelines for the management of dyslipidaemias: lipid modification to reduce cardiovascular risk. Eur Heart J 2020; 41(1):111–88.
4. Seidah NG, et al. The secretory proprotein convertase neural apoptosis-regulated convertase 1 (NARC-1): Liver regeneration and neuronal differentiation. Proc Natl Acad Sci USA 2003;100:928–33.
5. Cohen JC, et al. Sequence variations in PCSK9, low LDL, and protection against coronary heart disease. N Engl J Med 2006;354:1264–72.
6. Preis D, et al. Lipid-Modifying Agents,From Statins to PCSK9 Inhibitors. Am Coll Cardiol 2020;75:1945–55.
7. Nair JK, et al. Multivalent N-acetylgalactosamine-conjugated siRNA localizes in hepatocytes and elicits robust RNAi-mediated gene silencing. J Am Chem Soc 2014;136:16958–61.
8. Frank-Kamenetsky M, et al. Therapeutic RNAi targeting PCSK9 acutely lowers plasma cholesterol in rodents and LDL cholesterol in nonhuman primates. Proc Natl Acad Sci U.S.A 2008;105:11915–20.
9. Fitzgerald K, et al. Effect of an RNA interference drug on the synthesis of proprotein convertase subtilisin/kexin type9 (PCSK9) and the concentration of serum LDL cholesterol in healthy volunteers: A randomized, single-blind, placebo-controlled, phase 1 trial. Lancet 2014;383:60–8.
10. Fitzgerald K, et al. A Highly Durable RNAi Therapeutic Inhibitor of PCSK9. N Engl J Med 2017;376:41–51.
11. Henney NC, et al. RNA Silencing in the Management of Dyslipidemias. Curr Atheroscler Rep 2021;23:69.

12. Scott Wright R, et al. Pooled Patient-Level Analysis of Inclisiran Trials in Patients With Familial Hypercholesterolemia or Atherosclerosis. Am Coll Cardiol 2021;77: 1182–93.
13. Ray KK, Wright RS, Kallend D, et al. Two Phase 3 Trials of Inclisiran in Patients with Elevated LDL Cholesterol. NEJM 2020;382:1507–19.
14. NCT03705234 Available at: https://www.clinicaltrials.gov/ct2/show/NCT03705234. Accessed October 20, 2021.
15. NCT04929249 Available at: https://www.clinicaltrials.gov/ct2/show/NCT05030428. Accessed October 20, 2021.
16. Laufs U, Parhofer KG, Ginsberg HN, et al. Clinical review on triglycerides. Eur Heart J 2020;41:99–109.
17. Quispe R, Martin SS, Michos ED, et al. Remnant cholesterol predicts cardiovascular disease beyond LDL and ApoB: a primary prevention study. Eur Heart J 2021;42:4324–32.
18. Fruchart JC, Duriez P, Staels B. Peroxisome proliferator-activated receptor alpha activators regulate genes governing lipoprotein metabolism, vascular inflammation and atherosclerosis. Curr Opin Lipidol 1999;10:245–57.
19. Gervois P, Fruchart JC, Staels B. Drug Insight: mechanisms of action and therapeutic applications for agonists of peroxisome proliferator-activated receptors. Nat Clin Pract Endocrinol Metabol 2007;3:14556.
20. Keech A, Simes RJ, Barter P, et al. Effects of long-term fenofibrate therapy on cardiovascular events in 9795 people with type 2 diabetes mellitus (the FIELD study): randomized controlled trial. Lancet 2005;366(9500):1849–61.
21. ACCORD Study Group, Ginsberg HN, Elam MB, Lovato LC, et al. Effects of combination lipid therapy in type 2 diabetes mellitus. N Engl J Med 2010;362: 1563e74.
22. Sairyo M, Kobayashi T, Masuda D, et al. A novel selective PPAR Modulator (SPPARM), K-877 (pemafibrate), attenuates postprandial hypertriglyceridemia in mice. J Atheroscler Thromb 2018;25:142–52.
23. Raza-Iqbal S, Tanaka T, Anai M, et al. Transcriptome analysis of K-877 (a novel Selective PPARα Modulator (SPPARMα))-regulated genes in primary human hepatocytes and the mouse liver. J Atheroscler Thromb 2015;22:754–72.
24. Maki T, Maeda Y, Sonoda N, et al. Renoprotective effect of a novel selective PPARα modulator K-877 in db/db mice: a role of diacylglycerol-protein kinase C-NAD(P)H oxidase pathway. Metabolism 2017;71:33–45.
25. Ishibashi S, Yamashita S, Arai H, et al. Effects of K-877, a novel selective PPARα modulator (SPPARMα), in dyslipidaemic patients: a randomized, double blind, active- and placebo controlled,phase 2 trial. Atherosclerosis 2016;249:36–43.
26. Yokote K, Yamashita S, Arai H, et al. A pooled analysis of pemafibrate Phase II/III clinical trials indicated significant improvement in glycemic and liver function-related parameters. Atheroscler Suppl 2018;32:155.
27. Pradhan AD, Paynter NP, Everett BM, et al. Rationale and design of the pemafibrate to Reduce Cardiovascular Outcomes by Reducing Triglycerides in Patients with Diabetes (PROMINENT) study. Am Heart J 2018;206:80–93.
28. PROMINENT-Eye Ancillary Study (Protocol AD). ClinicalTrials.gov IdentifierNCT03345901. https://clinicaltrials.gov/ct2/show/NCT03345901. Accessed 7 Aug 2018.
29. Bhatt DL, Steg PG, Miller M, et al. Cardiovascular risk reduction with icosapent ethyl for hypertriglyceridemia. N Engl J Med 2019;380(1):11–22.
30. Crosby J, Peloso GM, Auer PL, et al. TG and HDL Working Group of the Exome Sequencing Project, National Heart, Lung, and Blood Institute. Loss-of-function

mutations in APOC3, triglycerides, and coronary disease. N Engl J Med 2014; 371(1):22–31.

31. Norata GD, Tsimikas S, Pirillo A, et al. Apolipoprotein C-III: from pathophysiology to pharmacology. Trends Pharmacol Sci 2015;36:675–87.

32. D'Erasmo L, Gallo A, Di Costanzo A, et al. Evaluation of efficacy and safety of antisense inhibition of apolipoprotein C-III with volanesorsen in patients with severe hypertriglyceridemia. Expert Opin Pharmacother 2020;21(14):1675–84.

33. Chait A, Brunzell JD. Chylomicronemia syndrome. Adv Intern Med 1992;37: 249–73.

34. Gaudet D, Brisson D, Tremblay K, et al. Targeting APOC3 in the familial chylomicronemia syndrome. N Engl J Med 2014;371(23):2200–6.

35. Yang X, Lee SR, Choi YS, et al. Reduction in lipoprotein-associated apoC-III levels following volanesorsen therapy: phase 2 randomized trial results. J Lipid Res 2016;57(4):706–13.

36. Gaudet D, Alexander VJ, Baker BF, et al. Antisense inhibition of apolipoprotein C-III in patients with hypertriglyceridemia. N Engl J Med 2015;373:438–47.

37. Digenio A, Dunbar RL, Alexander VJ, et al. Antisense-mediated lowering of plasma apolipoprotein C-III by volanesorsen improves dyslipidemia and insulin sensitivity in type 2 diabetes. Diabetes Care 2016;39(8):1408–15.

38. Gaudet D, Digenio A, Alexander VJ, et al. The APPROACH study: a randomized double-blind placebo-controlled, phase 3 study of volanesorsen administered subcutaneously to patients with FCS. Athero Suppl 2017;263:e10.

39. Gouni-Berthold I, Alexander V, Digenio A, et al. Apolipoprotein C-III Inhibition with volanesorsen in patients with hypertriglyceridemia (COMPASS): a randomized, double-blind, placebo-controlled trial. Athero Suppl 2017;28:e1–2.

40. Alexander VJ, Digenio A, Xia S, et al. Inhibition of apolipoprotein C-III with GalNac conjugated antisense drug potently lowes fasting serum apolipoprotein C-III and triglyceride levels in healthy volunteers with elevated triglycerides. J Am Coll Cardiol 2018;71:A1724.

41. The BROADEN study: a study of volanesorsen (Formerly ISIS-APOCIIIRx) in patients with familial partial lipodystrophy. Available at: https://clinicaltrials.gov/ct2/show/NCT02527343.

42. European Medicines Agency. 2018. Available at: https://www.ema.europa.eu/en/medicines/human/EPAR/waylivra. Accessed November 19, 2021.

43. Butler AA, Price GA, Graham JL, et al. Fructose-induced hypertriglyceridemia in rhesus macaques is attenuated with fish oil or ApoC3 RNA interference. J Lipid Res 2019;60:805–18.

44. Arca M, D'Erasmo L, Minicocci I. Familial combined hypolipidemia: angiopoietin-like protein-3 deficiency. Curr Opin Lipidol 2020;31(2):41–8.

45. Bini S, D'Erasmo L, Di Costanzo A, et al. The Interplay between Angiopoietin-Like Proteins and Adipose Tissue: Another Piece of the Relationship between Adiposopathy and Cardiometabolic Diseases? Int J Mol Sci 2021;22(2):742.

46. Kathiresan S, Melander O, Guiducci C, et al. Six new loci associated with blood low-density lipoprotein cholesterol, high-density lipoprotein cholesterol or triglycerides in humans. Nat Genet 2008;40(2):189–97. Erratum in: Nat Genet. 2008 Nov;40(11):1384.

47. Musunuru K, Pirruccello JP, Do R, et al. Exome sequencing, ANGPTL3 mutations, and familial combined hypolipidemia. N Engl J Med 2010;363(23):2220–7.

48. Minicocci I, Montali A, Robciuc MR, et al. Mutations in the ANGPTL3 gene and familial combined hypolipidemia: a clinical and biochemical characterization. J Clin Endocrinol Metab 2012;97(7):E1266–75.

49. Minicocci I, Santini S, Cantisani V, et al. Clinical characteristics, and plasma lipids in subjects with familial combined hypolipidemia: a pooled analysis. J Lipid Res 2013;54(12):3481–90.

50. Minicocci I, Tikka A, Poggiogalle E, et al. Effects of angiopoietin-like protein 3 deficiency on postprandial lipid and lipoprotein metabolism. J Lipid Res 2016; 57(6):1097–107.

51. Tikkanen E, Minicocci I, Hällfors J, et al. Metabolomic Signature of Angiopoietin-Like Protein 3 Deficiency in Fasting and Postprandial State. Arterioscler Thromb Vasc Biol 2019;39(4):665–74.

52. Ruhanen H, Haridas PAN, Minicocci I, et al. ANGPTL3 deficiency alters the lipid profile and metabolism of cultured hepatocytes and human lipoproteins. Biochim Biophys Acta Mol Cell Biol Lipids 2020;1865(7):158679.

53. Kersten S. ANGPTL3 as therapeutic target. Curr Opin Lipidol 2021;32(6):335–41.

54. D'Erasmo L, Bini S, Arca M. Rare Treatments for Rare Dyslipidemias: New Perspectives in the Treatment of Homozygous Familial Hypercholesterolemia (HoFH) and Familial Chylomicronemia Syndrome (FCS). Curr Atheroscler Rep 2021;23(11):65.

55. Cesaro A, Fimiani F, Gragnano F, et al. New Frontiers in the Treatment of Homozygous Familial Hypercholesterolemia. Heart Failure Clin 2022;18(1):177–88.

56. Available at: https://www.fda.gov/drugs/news-events-human-drugs/fda-approves-add-therapy-patients-genetic-form-severely-high-cholesterol-0. Accessed 17 November 2021.

57. Debacker AJ, Voutila J, Catley M, et al. Delivery of Oligonucleotides to the Liver with GalNAc: From Research to Registered Therapeutic Drug. Mol Ther 2020; 28(8):1759–71.

58. Ruotsalainen AK, Mäkinen P, Ylä-Herttuala S. Novel RNAi-Based Therapies for Atherosclerosis. Curr Atheroscler Rep 2021;23(8):45.

59. Available at: https://doi.org/10.1093/ehjci/ehaa946.3331. Accessed November 19, 2021.

60. Available at: https://doi.org/10.1161/circ.142.suppl_3.15751. Accessed November 19, 2021.

61. Sander JD, Joung JK. CRISPR-Cas systems for editing, regulating and targeting genomes. Nat Biotechnol 2014;32(4):347–55.

62. Behr M, Zhou J, Xu B, et al. In vivo delivery of CRISPR-Cas9 therapeutics: Progress and challenges. Acta Pharm Sin B 2021;11(8):2150–71.

63. Chadwick AC, Evitt NH, Lv W, et al. Reduced Blood Lipid Levels With In Vivo CRISPR-Cas9 Base Editing of ANGPTL3. Circulation 2018;137(9):975–7.

64. Qiu M, Glass Z, Chen J, et al. Lipid nanoparticle-mediated codelivery of Cas9 mRNA and single-guide RNA achieves liver-specific in vivo genome editing of Angptl3. Proc Natl Acad Sci U S A 2021;118(10). https://doi.org/10.1073/pnas.2020401118. e2020401118.

65. Sniderman AD, Thanassoulis G, Glavinovic T, et al. Apolipoprotein B Particles and Cardiovascular Disease: A Narrative Review. JAMA Cardiol 2019;4:1287–95.

66. Grundy SM, Stone NJ. Elevated apolipoprotein B as a risk-enhancing factor in 2018 cholesterol guidelines. J Clin Lipidol 2019;13:356–9.

67. Berg K. A New Serum Type System in Man–the Lp System. Acta Pathol Microbiol Scand 1963;59:369–82.

68. Kostner KM, Kostner GM. Lipoprotein (a): a historical appraisal. J Lipid Res 2017; 58:1–14.

69. Erqou S, Kaptoge S, Perry PL, et al. Lipoprotein(a) concentration and the risk of coronary heart disease, stroke, and nonvascular mortality. Jama 2009;302: 412–23.
70. Bennet A, Di Angelantonio E, Erqou S, et al. Lipoprotein(a) levels and risk of future coronary heart disease: large-scale prospective data. Arch Intern Med 2008;168:598–608.
71. Afshar M, Kamstrup PR, Williams K, et al. Estimating the Population Impact of Lp(a) Lowering on the Incidence of Myocardial Infarction and Aortic Stenosis-Brief Report. Arterioscler Thromb Vasc Biol 2016;36:2421–3.
72. Saleheen D, Haycock PC, Zhao W, et al. Apolipoprotein(a) isoform size, lipoprotein(a) concentration, and coronary artery disease: a mendelian randomisation analysis. Lancet Diabetes Endocrinol 2017;5:524–33.
73. Clarke R, Peden JF, Hopewell JC, et al. Genetic variants associated with Lp(a) lipoprotein level and coronary disease. N Engl J Med 2009;361:2518–28.
74. Enkhmaa B, Petersen KS, Kris-Etherton PM, et al. Diet and Lp(a): Does Dietary Change Modify Residual Cardiovascular Risk Conferred by Lp(a)? Nutrients 2020;12.
75. Waldmann E, Parhofer KG. Lipoprotein apheresis to treat elevated lipoprotein (a). J Lipid Res 2016;57:1751–7.
76. Pokrovsky SN, Afanasieva OI, Ezhov MV. Therapeutic Apheresis for Management of Lp(a) Hyperlipoproteinemia. Curr Atheroscler Rep 2020;22:68.
77. Roeseler E, Julius U, Heigl F, et al. Lipoprotein Apheresis for Lipoprotein(a)-Associated Cardiovascular Disease: Prospective 5 Years of Follow-Up and Apolipoprotein(a) Characterization. Arterioscler Thromb Vasc Biol 2016;36:2019–27.
78. Fras Z. Increased cardiovascular risk associated with hyperlipoproteinemia (a) and the challenges of current and future therapeutic possibilities. Anatol J Cardiol 2020;23:60–9.
79. Bittner VA, Szarek M, Aylward PE, et al. Effect of Alirocumab on Lipoprotein(a) and Cardiovascular Risk After Acute Coronary Syndrome. J Am Coll Cardiol 2020;75:133–44.
80. Schwartz GG, Szarek M, Bittner VA, et al. Lipoprotein(a) and Benefit of PCSK9 Inhibition in Patients With Nominally Controlled LDL Cholesterol. J Am Coll Cardiol 2021;78:421–33.
81. Landray MJ, Haynes R, Hopewell JC, et al. Effects of extended-release niacin with laropiprant in high-risk patients. N Engl J Med 2014;371:203–12.
82. Albers JJ, Slee A, O'Brien KD, et al. Relationship of apolipoproteins A-1 and B, and lipoprotein(a) to cardiovascular outcomes: the AIM-HIGH trial (Atherothrombosis Intervention in Metabolic Syndrome with Low HDL/High Triglyceride and Impact on Global Health Outcomes). J Am Coll Cardiol 2013;62:1575–9.
83. Burgess S, Ference BA, Staley JR, et al. Association of LPA variants with risk of coronary disease and the implications for lipoprotein(a)-lowering therapies: a Mendelian randomization analysis. JAMA Cardiol 2018;3:619–27.
84. Lamina C, Kronenberg F, Lp GC. Estimation of the Required Lipoprotein(a)-Lowering Therapeutic Effect Size for Reduction in Coronary Heart Disease Outcomes: A Mendelian Randomization Analysis. JAMA Cardiol 2019;4:575–9.
85. Tsimikas S, Karwatowska-Prokopczuk E, Gouni-Berthold I, et al. Lipoprotein(a) Reduction in Persons with Cardiovascular Disease. N Engl J Med 2020;382:244–55.
86. Tsimikas S, Moriarty PM, Stroes ES. Emerging RNA Therapeutics to Lower Blood Levels of Lp(a) 2021. J Am Coll Cardiol 2021;77:1576–89.
87. Available at: https://clinicaltrials.gov/ct2/show/record/NCT04270760. Accessed on November 21, 2021.

Safety of Statins and Nonstatins for Treatment of Dyslipidemia

Connie B. Newman, MD*

KEYWORDS

- Dyslipidemia • Safety • Statins • Nonstatins • Ezetimibe • PCSK9 inhibitors
- Bempedoic acid

KEY POINTS

- Myopathy and/or rhabdomyolysis (both with markedly increased CK), are rare, and reversible, adverse effects of statins, and are possibly related to an interacting drug.
- Statin intolerance with muscle or other symptoms (with a normal CK) is not pharmacologically related to the statin in the vast majority of patients, but rather to another etiology or the nocebo effect.
- Newly diagnosed diabetes due to statins occurs in about 0.2% of patients a year, usually those with risk factors such as obesity, high blood pressure, and impaired fasting glucose. The benefit exceeds the risk, and the statin should be continued and lifestyle changes intensified.
- Adverse effects for bempedoic acid include increased gout in patients with a history of gout.
- Omega-3-fatty acids have been associated with an increased risk of atrial fibrillation.

INTRODUCTION

Randomized controlled trials (RCTs) have demonstrated that lowering low-density lipoprotein cholesterol (LDL-C) with statins, alone and in combination with ezetimibe and/or proprotein convertase subtilisin/kexin type 9 (PCSK9) inhibitors, reduces atherosclerotic cardiovascular disease (ASCVD).[1–4] Reduction of very high triglycerides (TGs) with statins, fibrates, and other TG lowering drugs is anticipated to prevent pancreatitis. For an individual patient, potential benefits must be balanced by the risks associated with treatment. This article reviews the safety and tolerability of lipid-lowering medications (**Box 1**).

Division of Endocrinology, Diabetes and Metabolism, New York University Grossman School of Medicine, 435 East 30th street, Sixth floor, New York, NY 10016, USA
* Corresponding author.
E-mail address: connie.newman@nyulangone.org

Endocrinol Metab Clin N Am 51 (2022) 655–679
https://doi.org/10.1016/j.ecl.2022.01.004
0889-8529/22/© 2022 Elsevier Inc. All rights reserved.

endo.theclinics.com

Box 1
Safety terminology

- Adverse event: any medically undesirable event
- Adverse effect: an undesirable event caused by a medication
- Serious adverse event: an adverse event that may be life-threatening or cause disability, hospitalization, death, or is a congenital anomaly
- Well tolerated: refers to a medication with few adverse effects

---

Reliable information about adverse effects of a medication comes from RCTs that are double-blind and placebo-controlled.[5] Observational studies, which are not randomized, are subject to biases and cannot prove causality. Observational studies may be useful when adverse effects are so rare that they are not captured in RCTs. One example is statin-related myopathy and rhabdomyolysis, estimated incidence 0.1% and 0.01%, respectively, which were identified from case reports[5]

STATINS

The statin safety database is the largest of all lipid lowering medications.

Statins have been evaluated in numerous double-blind randomized placebo-controlled trials, with over 170,000 patients, followed for a median of 4.9 years.[6–8]

Skeletal Muscle

Myopathy and rhabdomyolysis

The hallmark adverse effect of statins is myopathy, defined here and in the original FDA-approved prescribing information as unexplained muscle pain or weakness accompanied by elevations in creatine kinase (CK) above 10-fold the upper limit of normal (ULN) (**Table 1**).[5] The most serious form of myopathy is rhabdomyolysis, characterized by markedly elevated CK, generally above 40-fold ULN, muscle necrosis, and often myoglobinuria, and/or renal impairment. Rhabdomyolysis is rare (<1 in 10,000) and potentially life-threatening because of renal injury.

CK levels are sex-specific, with higher levels in males,[9] and people of African ancestry. Nevertheless, most reference ranges are not specific to sex or race.

Statin myopathy and rhabdomyolysis occur with all statins, are generally dose-related (with the possible exception of atorvastatin[10,11]) and are rare. Myopathy can occur shortly after starting a statin or many years later, especially if it is caused by an interacting medication. Muscle symptoms are bilateral, often in the proximal muscles of the legs. Risk factors include older age, female sex, diabetes, hypothyroidism, and East Asian ancestry.[12] Interacting medications, which increase plasma levels of the statin, can precipitate myopathy/rhabdomyolysis. These include gemfibrozil and cyclosporine (for all statins) and macrolide antibiotics and antifungal azoles for those statins metabolized by cytochrome P450 3A 4 (CYP 3A4) (simvastatin, lovastatin, and to a lesser extent atorvastatin).[13,14] Many antiretroviral drugs inhibit cytochrome P450 enzymes, and are associated with increased risk of myopathy in patients taking statins.[15,16]

When evaluating a patient with muscle symptoms, it is important to consider the many etiologies. These include physical activity, trauma, hypothyroidism, polymyalgia

Table 1
Muscle adverse events caused by statin therapy

Term	CK Level	Frequency	Evidence
Myopathy[a] (muscle injury)	> 10× ULN[b]	<0.1% (<1 in 1000)	Case reports, RCTs
Rhabdomyolysis[a] (muscle injury and/or myoglobinuria)	40× ULN or >10,000 IU/L	<0.01% (<1 in 10,000)	Case reports
Autoimmune myopathy with muscle weakness (autoantibodies to HMG-CoA reductase)	> 10× ULN	<0.003% <3 in 100,000)	Case reports
Myalgia and normal CK	Normal	<1%[c]	RCTs with placebo

[a] May be associated with hypothyroidism, preexisting muscle disease, renal impairment, interacting drugs, and variant alleles that reduce organic anion transporter activity.
[b] The value for ULN is sex-specific; higher in men compared with women.
[c] This refers to the percent of patients with myalgia causally related own as the nocebo ef to the pharmacologic properties of the statin.
Data from Ref.[5]

rheumatica, inflammatory myopathies, seizure, illicit drug overdoses, thrombosis, embolism, severe infection, temperature extremes, and genetic muscle diseases.

Management of myopathy and rhabdomyolysis[17] is summarized in **Table 2**. For more detailed information, see Ref. 17.[17] Important steps include discontinuation of the statin, evaluation of creatinine to assess for rhabdomyolysis, and monitoring of CK. Should rhabdomyolysis be suspected, intensive intravenous hydration and monitoring of renal function and electrolytes, with correction as needed, are critical. Myopathy is usually reversible after statin discontinuation.

Table 2
Management of statin-induced myopathy and rhabdomyolysis

Myopathy CK > 10× ULN and Symptoms	Rhabdomyolysis CK > 40× ULN or Myoglobinuria
Discontinue statin immediately	Discontinue statin immediately
Follow-up with a repeat visit	Hospitalization may be needed, especially if the patient is very ill or weak
Rule out rhabdomyolysis (CK level, renal function)	Hydrate with intravenous normal saline
Assess interacting medications & other contributing factors	Check renal function, electrolytes, interacting medications
Monitor symptoms, examination, CK	Treat severe hyperkalemia
After resolution of myopathy, the decision to start a statin depends on multiple factors, including the cause of the myopathy, discontinuation of interacting medications, patient age, and patient preference	Hemodialysis may be needed for acute renal failure
	Monitor symptoms, examination, urine output, CK, creatinine, electrolytes, calcium

Data from Ref.[17]

Another very rare form of myopathy possibly related to statins is autoimmune myopathy, characterized by proximal muscle weakness, extreme CK elevations, and autoantibodies to HMG-CoA reductase.[18] It usually does not resolve after statin discontinuation.

Muscle symptoms with CK 5-10× ULN

Management of patients with muscle symptoms and CK 5-10× ULN depends on clinical judgment and risk factors for myopathy. In patients without extreme weakness or severe muscle pain, the statin may be continued and the CK repeated within 5 days. If the CK falls, the statin may be continued with monitoring of symptoms and repeat CK measurement.[5] If the CK rises, the statin should be discontinued and underlying etiologies evaluated.

Prevention of statin myopathy/rhabdomyolysis involves the assessment of all medications to avoid a serious drug interaction. It may be necessary to adjust the statin dose, or use a different statin during short-term treatment with an interacting medication. Special care is recommended for elderly patients, ensuring they remain hydrated, and understand their medications. Although it can be useful to measure CK before statin treatment, to screen for possible muscle disease, routine CK measurement during statin therapy is not helpful unless the patient has muscle symptoms.

Muscle symptoms with normal CK

Muscle symptoms without significant elevations in CK (CK < 3× ULN) are a common complaint, and may lead to statin discontinuation (statin intolerance). These symptoms are real to the patient, but generally not pharmacologically related to the statin.[19,20] The muscle symptoms may have another cause, or may be caused by expectation of harm, known as the nocebo effect (**Box 2**).[21,22] This explanation is supported by data from several double-blind RCTs. Analysis of pooled data from 12 large placebo-controlled trials found no difference in rates of myalgia in the statin and placebo groups (11.7% vs 11.4%, respectively, $P = .10$).[23]

Muscle and other symptoms believed by the patient to be caused by a statin, also occur when the patient is taking a placebo in double-blind trials. In ODYSSEY ALTERNATIVE[24] and GAUSS-3,[25] which enrolled patients with statin intolerance due to muscle symptoms, the vast majority of patients did not complain of muscle symptoms when blinded to study treatment. Subsequently, a double-blind proof of concept N-of-1 single patient crossover trial in 8 patients with statin-associated muscle symptoms found no difference in symptom scores between the placebo and statin treatment periods.[26] These data were confirmed in 2 larger double-blind N-of-1 trials in

---

Box 2
Nocebo effect

- Nocebo is a Latin word that means "I will harm."
- The nocebo effect refers to adverse symptoms that are caused by expectation of harm.
- Nocebo effects have been seen with many therapeutic interventions.
- Nocebo effect symptoms are the result of human neuropsychology, and are real to the patient.
- In double-blind studies, the nocebo effect increases adverse events equally in the active treatment arm and the placebo arm.

60 patients[27] and 200 patients[28] with a history of statin intolerance because of muscle or other symptoms. These 12-month trials allocated atorvastatin 20 mg or placebo for a period of 1 month[27] or 2 months[28] and found no difference in symptom scores in the placebo and atorvastatin 20 mg treatment periods. After the end of the trials, most patients had either successfully restarted statin therapy[27] or intended to do so. These N-of-1 trials and the RCTs discussed earlier provide strong evidence of a nocebo effect in patients with statin intolerance due to muscle symptoms.

The recommended approach to a patient with normal CK and statin intolerance is acknowledgment of the symptoms, reducing the statin dose, or switching to a different statin, after a discussion with the patient. Should muscle symptoms persist after a trial of at least 3 statins, a nonstatin lipid-lowering medication, such as ezetimibe, or a PCSK9 inhibitor, or a bile acid sequestrant, or a combination of these medications, should be considered to achieve the desired LDL-C reduction. The use of a lower dose of a long-acting statin such as rosuvastatin 2 or 3 times a week, with the aim of titration to once a day, may be helpful to improve tolerance, but data on cardiovascular disease (CVD) risk reduction are not available. Various methods to potentially prevent a statin-related nocebo effect have been suggested.[21] These include informing patients that myopathy/rhabdomyolysis is rare, occurring in fewer than 1 in 1000 patients, and that it can be detected by a simple blood test; explaining that the cardiovascular benefits of statins far outweigh the risk of serious muscle side effects, which are usually reversible; and explaining that muscle aches and pains are common symptoms in middle age and older people (**Box 3**).[21]

Diabetes Mellitus

After 20 years of marketed use, statins were found to cause diabetes, but the benefit: risk remains favorable, which suggests that statins should be continued in patients with newly diagnosed diabetes.[29,30] Based on data from the Cholesterol Treatment Trialists' Collaboration[7] and a report by Collins and colleagues,[23] it is estimated that statin therapy in 10,000 patients for 5 years, with an LDL-C reduction of 2 mmol/L (77 mg/dL), would result in 100 new cases of diabetes, but also prevent major vascular events in 1000 patients with CVD, and 500 patients with no history of CVD.

Long-term trials of statins, and meta-analyses of these trials show that those who develop diabetes, commonly have risk factors for diabetes,[31,32] although the absolute risk is low, approximately 0.2% per year.[5] The risk is higher with high-intensity statin therapy.[30]

Box 3
Statin intolerance

- Symptoms usually not caused by the statin cause the patient to discontinue the statin.

- About half of the symptoms are muscle-related, such as muscle pain and/or weakness without significant elevation of the muscle enzyme CK.

- Most double-blind RCTs show no difference between placebo and statin groups in the percent of participants with muscle symptoms.

- In double-blind RCTs of patients with statin intolerance due to muscle symptoms, muscle symptoms are similar on active drug and placebo. This shows that the intolerance depends on the patient knowing what they are taking.

- Patients with statin intolerance should be encouraged to take a statin, either the same statin at a lower dose, or a different statin. This is successful in most patients.

In JUPITER, physician-reported diabetes was significantly higher in the rosuvastatin 20 mg group compared with placebo: 270 versus 216; $P = .01.$[33] Of 17,603 participants, 65% had at least one risk factor for diabetes at baseline: metabolic syndrome, impaired fasting glucose, BMI 30 kg/m^2 or greater, or hemoglobin A1C above 6.0%.[31] In this subgroup, allocation to rosuvastatin significantly increased newly diagnosed diabetes (hazard ratio [HR] 1.28; 95% confidence interval [CI], 1.07–1.54; $P = .01$); however, CVD events were significantly reduced (HR 0.61; 95% CI, 0.47–0.79; $P = .00001$). Further analysis found that rosuvastatin 20 mg accelerated the time to diagnosis of diabetes by 5.4 weeks.[31]

SPARCL found a significant reduction in cardiovascular events and total stroke in patients with a history of stroke or transient ischemic attack (TIA) randomized to atorvastatin 80 mg in comparison to placebo.[34] Diabetes was diagnosed in 8.7% of patients in the atorvastatin group, compared with 6.1% in the placebo group.[32] In the SPARCL, TNT, and IDEAL trials of atorvastatin 80 mg, factors associated with new diabetes were elevated fasting glucose, and components of the metabolic syndrome: higher TG, higher BMI, and hypertension (**Box 4**).[32]

Statins may reduce glycemic control in people with diabetes, although the effect is small. Pooled studies found a 0.12% increase in HbA1C.[35] Two RCTs reported statistically significant increases in HbA1C: 0.1% at 4 years in CARDS[36,37] and 0.3% at 4 months in AFFORD.[38] However, in the Heart Protection Study, small increases in HbA1C (0.15% and 0.12%) in the simvastatin 40 mg and placebo groups, respectively, did not significantly differ.[39]

The mechanism underlying new-onset diabetes in statin-treated patients is not understood, but has been hypothesized to be related to the LDL-C lowering effect of the drug. Some studies of reduced function genetic variants for HMG-CoA reductase, PCSK9, and Niemann-Pick D1-Like-1 found a reduction in LDL-C and CVD events and increased prevalence of diabetes mellitus.[40–42] However, one study of a different PCSK9 genetic variant did not find an association with LDL-C and diabetes.[43]

Liver

Statins may cause asymptomatic dose-related elevations in hepatic transaminases, without increases in bilirubin, or changes in albumin or prothrombin time. Clinical trials have documented transaminase elevation greater than 3 times ULN, with a similar repeat measurement, in 1% of patients taking the highest statin doses.[11] Elevations in alanine aminotransferase (ALT) usually exceed elevations in aspartate aminotransferase (AST).[44,45] If AST exceeds ALT, another etiology, such as muscle injury or alcohol, could be the cause. Monitoring of hepatic transaminases does not prevent liver disease, and routine monitoring is no longer recommended by the FDA.[46]

Box 4
Clinical points about statins and diabetes

- New diabetes in patients taking statins is more common in people with risk factors for diabetes.
- Incidence in clinical trials is 0.2% per year, depending on the population.
- CVD benefit of statin therapy outweighs the risk of diabetes.
- It is important to continue statin therapy.
- Manage diabetes with lifestyle, and as needed medication (such as metformin).

Severe liver injury related to statin therapy is rare, and not detected in clinical trials. A Swedish registry study reported statin-related liver injury in 1 in 100,000 patients over a 22-year period (1998–2010).[47] The US FDA adverse event reporting system (2000–2009) contained very few reports of serious liver injury, death, or liver transplantation, and no cases were highly likely or definitively caused by a statin[46] A meta-analysis of 9 studies of patients with hepatocellular carcinoma found that statin use was associated with a lower rate of recurrence after liver surgery[48] Studies of patients with nonalcoholic fatty liver disease or hepatitis C have found that statins did not increase liver disease progression.[49–52]

Hemorrhagic Stroke

RCTs of statins in people with and without a history of stroke have shown a decrease in total stroke, largely due to ischemic stroke. RCTs of patients without a history of stroke (a primary prevention stroke population) have not found increased hemorrhagic stroke with statin therapy[53] or with high- versus low-intensity statin therapy.[54] In SPARCL, the only RCT in patients with prior stroke or TIA, and without CVD, total stroke was reduced in participants allocated to atorvastatin 80 mg compared with placebo; however, hemorrhagic stroke was increased (HR 1.66; 95% CI, 1.08–2.55) and was higher with age, and in those with a history of hemorrhagic stroke as the entry event.[34,55] Recurrent stroke was reduced in those with ischemic stroke at study entry, but not reduced in those with hemorrhagic stroke at entry, and was not related to achieved LDL-C levels.

The American Heart Association (AHA) Scientific Statement, "Statin Safety and Associated Adverse Events", concluded that statins may cause a small increase in hemorrhagic stroke in people with a history of stroke; however, the beneficial effects of statins on overall stroke and other vascular events usually outweigh the risk of hemorrhagic stroke.[5]

Other Adverse Events

Other adverse events have been attributed to statins, although there is no evidence supporting a causal effect.[5] These include cancer, cataracts, cognitive dysfunction or memory disturbances, hypogonadism, kidney disease or progression, erectile dysfunction (all studied in RCTs), and fatigue, peripheral neuropathy, tendonitis, and tendon rupture.

Drug Interactions

Statins are subject to numerous drug interactions usually due to medications that inhibit CYP 3A4, or inhibit the hepatic drug membrane transporters OAT1B1 or P-glycoprotein (**Table 3**).[14,56] Inhibitors of CYP 3A4 can raise the plasma levels of statins metabolized by CYP3A4 (simvastatin, lovastatin, and to a lesser extent atorvastatin), and increase the risk of serious muscle adverse effects (myopathy with increased CK > 10× ULN).

Pregnancy and Breastfeeding

Statins had been contraindicated in pregnancy because of teratogenic effects observed in the original animal studies of lovastatin, which used very high doses that caused maternal toxicity in rats. Available observational data in pregnant individuals do not show a serious hazard. In July 2021, the US FDA issued a Drug Safety Communication, requesting revision of all statin labels, removing the contraindication in pregnancy, and recommending that practitioners discontinue statins in most pregnant individuals, but consider continuing statins in those with a high risk of

Table 3
Statins, pharmacokinetic parameters and principal drug interactions

	Lova	Simva	Atorva	Prava	Fluva	Rosuva	Pitava
Half life	2 h	2 h	14 h	2 h	3 h	19 h	12 h
Substrate of CYP3A4 or CYP2C9	CYP3A4	CYP3A4	CYP3A4	No	CYP2C9	CYP2C9	CYP2C9
Maximal dose recommended							
Antiarrhythmics			None	None	None	None	None
Amiodarone	40 mg	20 mg					
Dronedarone	20 mg	10 mg					
Antifungal azoles				None		None	None
Fluconazole	....	....	Consider B/R.		20 mg BID		
Itraconazole	Avoid	Avoid	Caution		....		
Ketoconazole	Avoid	Avoid	Consider B/R.		....		
Posaconazole	Avoid	Avoid	Consider B/R.		....		
Voriconazole	Avoid	Avoid	Consider B/R.		....		
Calcium channel blockers			None	None	None	None	None
Amlodipine	....	20 mg					
Diltiazem	20 mg	10 mg					
Verapamil	20 mg	10 mg					

						None	
Macrolide antibiotics							
Clarithromycin	Avoid	Avoid	20 mg	40 mg	20 mg	1 mg	....
Erythromycin	Avoid	Avoid	Consider B/R	Caution	....	1 mg	
Telithromycin	Avoid	Avoid	Consider B/R.	Caution	....	1 mg	
Immunosuppressants							
Cyclosporine	Avoid	Avoid	Avoid	20 mg	20 mg	5 mg	Avoid
Tacrolimus	Avoid	Avoid	10 mg	20 mg	40 mg	5 mg	Avoid
Everolimus	Avoid	Avoid	10 mg	20 mg	40 mg	5 mg	Avoid
Sirolimus	Avoid	Avoid	10 mg	20 mg	40 mg	5 mg	Avoid
Other							
Gemfibrozil	Avoid	Avoid	Avoid	Avoid	Avoid	Avoid	Avoid
Nefazodone	Avoid	Avoid	....	....	....	....	....
Danazol	20 mg	Avoid	....	....	....	....	....
Ranolazine	Caution	20 mg	....	....	....	....	....
Colchicine	Caution	Caution	Caution	Caution	Caution	Caution.	Caution
HIV protease inhibitors, hepatitis C protease inhibitors	Numerous interactions, see Prescribing information						

Abbreviations: Atorva, atorvastatin; Fluva, fluvastatin; Lova, lovastatin; Pitava, pitavastatin; Prava, pravastatin; Rosuva, rosuvastatin; Simva, simvastatin. The dose indicates the maximal statin dose recommended.

B/R benefit/risk; .... Not discussed in the prescribing information.

Data from Refs.[5,56]

Table 4
Adverse effects of nonstatin medications[a]

Medication	Drug Class or Mechanism of Action	Principal Drug Interactions	Contraindications	Warnings	Nonserious Adverse Events
Ezetimibe	Cholesterol and phytosterol absorption inhibitor	Cyclosporine, gemfibrozil	Contraindicated if active liver disease if used with a statin	Potential for myopathy	Diarrhea, arthralgia, extremity pain, URI, sinusitis
Monoclonal antibodies to PCSK9, Evolocumab Alirocumab	PCSK 9 inhibition	None known	History of hypersensitivity reaction	Hypersensitivity reactions (pruritus, rash, urticaria)	Injection site reactions, nasopharyngitis, URI
Bile acid sequestrant, colesevelam	Bile acid sequestrant	Concomitant administration may decrease levels of phenytoin, thyroid hormone, warfarin, oral contraceptives with ethinyl estradiol and norethindrone, olmesartan, medoxomil, sulfonylureas	Serum TG > 500 mg/dL, history of hypertriglyceridemic pancreatitis, history of bowel obstruction	Vitamin K or fat-soluble vitamin deficiencies; may harm patients with phenylketonuria	Constipation, dyspepsia, nausea
Bempedoic acid	Citrate lyase inhibitor	Doses of simvastatin > 20 mg, doses of pravastatin > 40 mg	None	Elevations in uric acid, tendon rupture	Hyperuricemia, elevated hepatic transaminases, anemia, URI, muscle spasms, back pain, abdominal pain or discomfort, bronchitis, extremity pain

Gemfibrozil	Fibrate, mechanism not known	Coumarin, statins, repaglinide, colchicine, bile acid–binding resins, drugs metabolized by CYP 2 C 8,[b] substrates of OAT 1B1 (all statins, ezetimibe, atrasentan, bosentan, glyburide, irinotecan, rifampin, valsartan, olmesartan)	Hepatic or severe renal dysfunction, gallbladder disease, severe hypoglycemia in combination with repaglinide, hypersensitivity	Cholecystitis, cholelithiasis, cataracts, increased risk of rhabdomyolysis when taken with a statin, severe anemia, leukopenia, thrombocytopenia, risk of worsened renal function if creatinine > 2.0 mg/dL	Elevated LFTs (SGOT, ALT, bilirubin, alkaline phosphatase), dyspepsia, abdominal pain, acute appendicitis, atrial fibrillation
Fenofibrate	Peroxisome proliferator-activated receptor (PPAR) alpha agonist	Coumarin anticoagulants, immunosuppressants, bile acid resins	Severe renal disease, active liver disease, gallbladder disease, nursing mothers, hypersensitivity	Hepatotoxicity, myopathy/rhabdomyolysis when taken with a statin,[c] increased serum creatinine, cholelithiasis, bleeding potential with coumarin anticoagulants, hypersensitivity reactions including anaphylaxis and angioedema, small increase in risk of pulmonary embolus	Abnormal LFTs, increased AST, ALT, increased CPK, rhinitis

(continued on next page)

Table 4
(continued)

Medication	Drug Class or Mechanism of Action	Principal Drug Interactions	Contraindications	Warnings	Nonserious Adverse Events
Icosapent ethyl, omega-3 acid ethyl esters, omega-3 carboxylic acid	Omega-3 fatty acid	Antiplatelet and anticoagulant, increased risk of bleeding	Hypersensitivity to drug or its components	Use cautiously in patients with sensitivity to fish or shellfish, increased risk of atrial fibrillation or flutter, monitor ALT, AST if hepatic dysfunction	Diarrhea, nausea, dyspepsia, abdominal pain; for icosapent ethyl musculoskeletal pain, peripheral edema, gout in clinical trials

[a] Each class of medication includes at least one medication in that class. Inclisiran, lomitapide and niacin are not included in this table.

[b] Drugs metabolized by CYP2C8 are dabrafenib, enzalutamide, loperamide, montelukast, paclitaxel, pioglitazone, and rosiglitazone.

[c] In using concomitantly with a statin, the risk of myopathy with gemfibrozil is greater than the risk with fenofibrate.

Data from Merck and Co., Inc. ZETIA (Ezetimibe tablets) U.S. Prescribing Information January 2012; Amgen Inc. REPATHA (evolocumab) injection. U.S. Prescribing Information Sept. 2021; Sanofi-Aventis U.S. LLC. Praluent (alirocumab) injection. U.S. Prescribing Information Sept. 2021; Daiichi Sankyo Inc. WELCHOL (colesevelam) tablets. U.S. Prescribing Information. October 2021; Pharmacia and Upjohn Company. Division of Pfizer Inc.; Esperion Therapeutics. NEXLETOL (bempedoic acid). U.S. Product Information Feb 2020; Parke-Davis, Division of Pfizer Inc. LOPID (gemfibrozil). U.S. Prescribing Information Dec 2020; Abb Vie Inc. TRICOR (fenofibrate tablet). U.S. Prescribing Information. March 2021; Amarin Pharma Inc. VASCEPA (icosapent ethyl) capsules. U.S. Prescribing Information Dec 2019; GlaxoSmithKline. LOVAZA (omega-3-acid ethyl esters capsules). U.S. Prescribing Information Sept 2020; AstraZeneca Pharmaceuticals LP. EPANOVA (omega-3-carboxylic acids) capsules. U.S. Prescribing Information March 2017.

cardiovascular events.[57] The FDA communication advises practitioners to reassure patients who have taken statins during early pregnancy that this is unlikely to be harmful. The communication also advises practitioners to recommend discontinuation of statins in patients who wish to breastfeed; however, for patients who must take statins because of cardiovascular risk, breastfeeding is not recommended as statins may be secreted into breast milk.

NONSTATIN MEDICATIONS FOR DYSLIPIDEMIA

This section summarizes the main adverse effects of nonstatin medications. **Table 4** lists contraindications, warnings, and drug interactions. For additional information, please see the Prescribing Information.

Ezetimibe

Ezetimibe has a good safety profile and is well tolerated.

Skeletal muscle

Ezetimibe is unlikely to cause myopathy. In the 6-year RCT IMPROVE-IT, which compared ezetimibe 10 mg/simvastatin 40 mg to simvastatin 40 mg alone in 18,144 patients with acute coronary syndrome, prespecified muscle adverse events, including myopathy and rhabdomyolysis, were similar in each group.[2] Nevertheless, cases of myopathy have been reported to the FDA in patients taking ezetimibe alone or in combination with a statin.

Liver

IMPROVE-IT found no difference between study groups in prespecified liver or gallbladder adverse events.[2] Nevertheless, the prescribing information cautions against using ezetimibe in patients with moderate or severe liver disease.

Diabetes mellitus

A systematic review and meta-analysis of 16 clinical trials, including 5 trials that were placebo-controlled, suggests that ezetimibe does not reduce glycemic control, or cause new-onset diabetes either when used alone or in combination with a statin.[58] Most of these trials were short-term: 16 weeks or less.

Cancer

Although an increased risk of cancer was suggested by data from the SEAS trial, subsequent analysis of data from SEAS, SHARP, and IMPROVE-IT found no overall increase in cancer.[59–61]

Drug interactions

Ezetimibe interacts with cyclosporine, causing increased plasma levels of both drugs (see **Table 4**). Ezetimibe may be used with fenofibrate but not with other fibrates because of the potential for increased cholesterol excretion into the bile and cholelithiasis.

Pregnancy

There are no adequate studies of ezetimibe in pregnant women. The FDA recommends that ezetimibe be used in pregnant women only if the potential benefit to the mother justifies the potential risk to the fetus.

Monoclonal Antibodies to PCSK9 (Proprotein Convertase Subtilisin/Kexin Type 9)

Evolocumab[62] and alitrocumab[63] were approved in the United States in 2015. The RCTs FOURIER and ODYSSEY OUTCOMES in participants with CVD taking a statin demonstrated significant reduction in ASCVD events in the PCSK9 inhibitor group.[3,4]

Adverse effects

The most common adverse effects of monoclonal antibodies to PCSK9 are pain, itching, swelling or erythema at the injection site, and rare hypersensitivity reactions, including angioedema (see **Table 4**). Early clinical trial data suggested potential adverse effects on cognition; however, EBBINHAUS, a study of 1204 patients, a subgroup of the FOURIER trial, showed no significant differences in cognitive function between those randomized to evolocumab or placebo for a median duration of 19 months.[64]

PCSK-9 inhibitors, in combination with statins and/or other medications that lower LDL-C, can cause a marked reduction in LDL-C to levels below 20 mg/dL. As discussed in Jonathan Tobert's article, "LDL Cholesterol - How Low Can We Go?," in this issue, there is no evidence to date showing that such low LDL-C concentrations are harmful.[65,66]

Diabetes

Similar rates of new diabetes in the PCSK-9 inhibitor and placebo groups of FOURIER[67] (8.1% vs 7.7%, respectively) and ODYSSEY OUTCOMES[68] (9.6% vs 10.1%, respectively) were reported. The median duration of each trial was 2.2 years and 2.8 years, respectively.

To date, no signal of a risk of newly diagnosed diabetes has been detected in the PCSK-9 inhibitor class of medications. For statins, diabetes was not known to be an adverse effect until multiple long-term trials of 2 to 5 years duration were completed. This occurred more than 20 years after the approval of lovastatin in 1987. Indeed, genetic studies have found that loss-of-function PCSK9 variants that cause lower LDL-C levels are associated with a 19% to 29% higher risk of diabetes, HR 1.29 (1.11–1.50)[69] and HR 1.19 (1.02–1.38).[42] However, it is not known whether this increase in diabetes risk, which develops over a lifetime, correlates with treatment with PCSK9 inhibitors beginning in adulthood.[70]

Drug interactions

There are no known drug interactions.

Pregnancy

Other monoclonal antibodies cross the placenta in the second and third trimesters, but are unlikely to do so in the first trimester. There are insufficient data on evolocumab and alirocumab in pregnant women to provide accurate information on risk. Potential benefits and risks to the pregnant woman, and the fetus, should be considered before prescribing these medications.

Inclisiran

Inclisiran, a small interfering RNA molecule that reduces translation of PCSK9 in the hepatocyte,[71] was approved in the United Kingdom and European Union in December 2020 for use alone or in combination with a statin or other lipid-lowering therapies, as an adjunct to diet, in adults with primary hypercholesterolemia and mixed dyslipidemia.[71] Inclisiran was approved in the United States in December 2021 as an adjunct to diet and maximally tolerated statin therapy for the treatment of adults with heterozygous FH or with clinical ASCVD, who require additional LDL-C reduction. Inclisiran, at a dose of 284 mg, is administered subcutaneously initially, 3 months after the first injection, and then every 6 months. Dose adjustment is not needed for individuals with mild, moderate, or severe renal impairment, or with mild to moderate hepatic impairment. However, no data are available for patients with end-stage renal disease or severe hepatic disease. Reduction in LDL-C is about 50%.[72]

Adverse effects

A patient-level meta-analysis of 3 RCTs (ORION-9,10,11) in 3660 participants taking maximally tolerated statin therapy, randomized to inclisiran for a duration of 18 months, found significantly more injection site pain and reactions, and bronchitis (4.3% vs 2.7%) in the inclisiran group compared with placebo.[73] The study groups did not differ in liver function tests (LFTs), CK, and platelet counts. The Summary of Product Characteristics (SPC) for Inclisiran in the EU cautions against use in people with severe renal or hepatic impairment, although no data in these populations are available.[71] Additional data are needed to address the long-term safety of inclisiran. A cardiovascular outcomes trial is ongoing.

Drug interactions

Drug interactions are not expected because inclisiran is not a substrate or inhibitor of CYP450 enzymes or common transporters. Studies showed no meaningful interactions with rosuvastatin or atorvastatin.[71]

Bile Acid Sequestrants

Bile acid sequestrants (BAS) used in the United States to reduce cholesterol include colestipol,[74] cholestyramine,[75] and colesevelam.[76] Colesevelam is also indicated for the treatment of type 2 diabetes.

Gastrointestinal adverse effects

BAS are not absorbed. The most common side effect is constipation, which is usually mild and transient, but can lead to bowel obstruction (see **Table 4**). Less common gastrointestinal (GI) adverse effects are abdominal pain, bloating, flatulence, indigestion, diarrhea, nausea, and vomiting. Transient elevations of AST, ALT, and alkaline phosphatase may occur.

Increased TGs

BAS may increase TG levels and should not be prescribed for people with TG above 500 mg/dL.[77]

Drug interactions

BAS may decrease absorption of fat-soluble vitamins and some medications.[76] If vitamin K deficiency occurs, bleeding will be increased. Absorption of certain medications listed in **Table 4** may be reduced. These medications should be given 4 hours before the ingestion of a BAS. INR should be monitored in patients on warfarin or other anticoagulants.

Pregnancy and breastfeeding

Although animal studies did not show fetal harm, there are no adequate, well-controlled studies of BAS in pregnant women or nursing women. The effect on the absorption of fat-soluble vitamins has not been studied. BAS should only be used during pregnancy if clearly needed. Excretion into human milk is unlikely because BAS are not systemically absorbed.

Bempedoic Acid

Bempedoic acid is an adenosine triphosphate-citrate lyase (ACL) inhibitor, indicated as adjunct to diet and maximally tolerated statin therapy for LDL-C reduction in adults with heterozygous FH or ASCVD.[78] Bempedoic acid lowers LDL-C by 18% to 20%. A cardiovascular outcomes trial is ongoing.

Hyperuricemia, gout

Bempedoic acid may increase plasma uric acid (see **Table 4**) through an unknown mechanism. In the 52-week CLEAR Harmony trial, in 1487 patients with heterozygous FH and/or ASCVD, gout developed in 1.2% of patients allocated to bempedoic acid and 0.3% of patients allocated to placebo ($P = .03$).[79] Uric acid increased from baseline by 0.73 mg/dL in the bempedoic acid group and decreased by 0.06 mg/dL in the placebo group. The risk for gout is greater in patients with prior gout (11.2% bempedoic acid vs 1.7% placebo).[78] The prescribing information recommends monitoring patients for signs and symptoms of gout, evaluation of uric acid as clinically indicated, and treatment with urate-lowering drugs as needed (**Box 5**).

Musculoskeletal system

In CLEAR Harmony, muscle pain, spasm, or weakness were reported in more patients allocated to bempedoic acid compared with placebo (13.1% vs 10.1%, HR 1.30 [95% CI, 1.01, 1.67]). Elevations in CK above 5 times ULN were 0.5% for bempedoic acid versus 0.1% for placebo.[79] These differences require further exploration.

The US Prescribing Information reports a small increase in tendon rupture in patients taking bempedoic acid compared with placebo (0.5% vs 0.0%, respectively) and recommends discontinuation of bempedoic acid if tendinitis or tendon rupture occurs.

Diabetes

New-onset diabetes was less frequent in the bempedoic acid group versus the placebo group (3.3% vs 5.4%; $P = .02$) in CLEAR Harmony.[79] Additional long-term trials are needed to assess the risk of diabetes.

Other adverse effects

Asymptomatic transient elevations in hepatic transaminases greater than 3-fold ULN occurred in a clinical trial (incidence 0.5% vs 0.1% placebo). In several clinical trials, bempedoic acid was associated with increased creatinine by 0.5 mg/dL (2.2% bempedoic acid vs 1.1% placebo) and a doubling of blood urea nitrogen (3.8% bempedoic acid vs 1.5% placebo).[78] Decreases in hemoglobin of 2 or more g/dL, decrease in leukocyte count, and increase in platelet count have been observed. Most of these patients were asymptomatic.

Drug interactions

Bempedoic acid increases the plasma concentrations of simvastatin and pravastatin. Doses of simvastatin above 20 mg, and of pravastatin above 40 mg are not recommended.

Box 5
Bempedoic acid

- Inhibitor of ATP citrate lyase, an enzyme in the cholesterol synthesis pathway
- Adjunct to statin therapy
- CVD outcomes trial pending
- Increases uric acid: approximately 1%
- Muscle symptoms: approximately 3%
- Precipitates gout: in approximately 10% of people with a history of gout

Pregnancy

Bempedoic acid has not been evaluated in pregnant women and should be discontinued when pregnancy is discovered. Bempedoic acid has not been evaluated in breastfeeding women or in breast milk, and should be avoided.

Fibrates

Gemfibrozil

Gallstones. Patients taking gemfibrozil have an increased risk of cholelithiasis and cholecystitis (see **Table 4**). In a substudy of 450 participants in the Helsinki Heart Study, the rate of gallstones in the gemfibrozil group was 7.5% compared with 4.9% in the placebo group.[80]

Muscle adverse effects. Rhabdomyolysis, when gemfibrozil is given with a statin, is the most serious safety concern and the main reason why gemfibrozil has been largely displaced by fenofibrate. The probable mechanism is inhibition of the organic anion transporter OATB1B1, reducing statin elimination in the bile.

Common adverse effects. Common adverse effects are GI (dyspepsia and abdominal pain) and worsening renal function in people with creatinine above 2.0 mg/dL.

Drug interactions. The use of gemfibrozil with a statin or with colchicine can cause myopathy/rhabdomyolysis (see **Table 4**). The increase in rhabdomyolysis and death from rhabdomyolysis associated with cerivastatin (subsequently withdrawn from the market) occurred when the full dose (0.8 mg/day) was taken or when cerivastatin was taken with gemfibrozil.[81]

The dose of warfarin should be reduced when given with gemfibrozil. As gemfibrozil inhibits CYP2C8, it may increase exposure to drugs metabolized by CYP2C8 (see **Table 4**). Gemfibrozil inhibits the OATP1B1 transporter and may increase exposure to drugs that are substrates of OATP1B1 (see **Table 4**). The doses of these drugs should be reduced. The combination of gemfibrozil and repaglinide is contraindicated because of the risk of severe hypoglycemia.

Fenofibrate

Muscle, LFTs, creatinine. In comparison to gemfibrozil, the use of fenofibrate with a statin carries a much lower risk of myopathy/rhabdomyolysis.[82,83] Fenofibrate may increase LFTs (3%–7% of patients) and plasma creatinine (see **Table 4**). Monitoring of LFTs and creatinine is recommended.

Serious adverse events. Serious adverse events include cholelithiasis and potentially a small increased risk of pulmonary embolism, demonstrated in the FIELD trial.[84]

Drug interactions. Cyclosporine and tacrolimus may impair kidney function, and therefore should not be taken with fenofibrate, which is excreted through the kidney.[85] A BAS may reduce absorption of fenofibrate. Therefore, fenofibrate should be taken at least 1 hour before or 4 to 6 hours after the BAS. Myopathy has been reported when fenofibrate has been taken in combination with colchicine. Adjustment of the dose of a coumarin anticoagulant is recommended to maintain the prothrombin time/INR at the desired level to prevent bleeding.

Pregnancy. Limited data are available in pregnant women. Fenofibrate should be taken by pregnant women only when the potential benefit to the mother outweighs the potential harm to the fetus.

Omega-3 Fatty Acids

Omega-3 fatty acids available by prescription in the United States are icosapent ethyl,[86] which consists of pure eicosapentaenoic acid (EPA) ethyl ester, as well as omega-3-acid ethyl esters,[87] and omega-3 carboxylic acid,[88] which are combinations of EPA and DHA (docosahexaenoic acid). The main tolerability concerns are GI (diarrhea, nausea, abdominal pain, and dyspepsia). Serious adverse effects are atrial fibrillation or flutter, and bleeding, especially in patients taking anticoagulants or antiplatelet drugs.

Atrial fibrillation

The STRENGTH trial compared 4 gm omega-3-carboxylic acid to a corn oil placebo in high-risk subjects taking statins for a median duration of 3.5 years.[89] The primary composite endpoint of cardiovascular events in the omega-3-carboxylic acid and placebo groups did not differ. Atrial fibrillation occurred in 2.2% of participants in the omega-3 fatty acid group, compared with 1.3% of those allocated corn oil, relative risk (RR) 1.69 ($P < .001$). REDUCE-IT compared a pure EPA omega-3-fatty acid, icosapent ethyl, to mineral oil, in statin-treated patients, and found a marked reduction in CVD in the icosapentethyl group. Serious adverse events in the icosapent ethyl group and the mineral oil placebo group, were hospitalization for atrial fibrillation or flutter (3.1% vs 2.1% $P = .004$), atrial fibrillation (5.3% vs 3.9%, $P = .003$), and serious bleeding events (2.7% vs 2.1%, $P = .06$).[90]

Drug interactions

In people taking anticoagulants or antiplatelet drugs, bleeding may be prolonged.

Pregnancy

No severe birth defects have been identified. Omega-3 fatty acids should be considered only if the benefit to the mother exceeds the risk to the mother and fetus. Omega-3 fatty acids are secreted into breast milk.

Lomitapide

Lomitapide, an inhibitor of microsomal transfer protein, is only available through a restricted program for the treatment of patients with homozygous FH (prevalence of 1 in 1,000,000) in combination with a statin or LDL apheresis.[91] LDL-C reduction is about 50% with 40 mg daily.[92]

Liver and GI adverse effects

Lomitapide can cause hepatic steatosis, associated with an increase in liver fat from 1% to 8% in one clinical trial.[92] GI adverse reactions are common and may affect the absorption of other medications.[91]

Pregnancy

Lomitapide should not be taken during pregnancy, which is rare in people with homozygous FH, or during nursing.

Drug interactions

Strong and moderate CYP 3A4 inhibitors are contraindicated. Doses of simvastatin and lovastatin must be decreased to avoid high plasma levels of these statins which increase the risk of myopathy. Lomitapide also increases plasma levels of warfarin.

Niacin

Niacin lowers total cholesterol, LDL-C, and TG, and increases high-density lipoprotein cholesterol. Common adverse effects are pruritus and flushing. The negative impact of niacin on glucose control (increasing plasma glucose, worsening glucose control in diabetes, and causing diabetes)[93,94] and the serious adverse events of infection, GI bleeding, myopathy, and rare hepatoxicity seen in 2 RCTs (AIM High[95] and HPS-2 THRIVE[96]) have raised serious questions about its use for lipid management.[97] It has taken 50 years for the discovery of all these adverse effects. In Europe, prescription niacin is no longer available.

SUMMARY

The statin class of medications has been used for more than 30 years, and serious adverse effects are rare. Myopathy/rhabdomyolysis (0.1% and 0.01% of patients) can be detected by measuring CK in a patient with muscle symptoms, and is reversible. Myalgia with normal CK is rarely caused by the statin, but rather by expectations of harm, the nocebo effect. New diabetes, which was detected after 20 years of marketed use, may occur in patients with risk factors for diabetes. However, the benefit: risk is favorable because of the substantial reduction in cardiovascular risk when patients with diabetes take a statin. Ezetimibe is well tolerated as are the PCSK9 inhibitors evolocumab and alirocumab. Bempedoic acid increases uric acid in about 1% of patients and precipitates gout in 10% of patients with a history of gout. Bile acid sequestrants have GI adverse effects, which interfere with tolerability in some patients, but the cost is much lower in comparison with PCSK9 inhibitors and bempedoic acid. Icosapent ethyl, which is the only omega-3 fatty acid approved for reduction in CVD morbidity, has GI adverse effects, and may cause atrial fibrillation. All omega-3 fatty acids are approved for the treatment of hypertriglyceridemia when TG exceeds 500 mg/dL. Also approved to lower TG are gemfibrozil and fenofibrate; however, fenofibrate is the preferred medication because gemfibrozil carries a very high risk of myopathy/rhabdomyolysis when added to statin therapy.

Using a combination of a statin and a PCSK9 inhibitor and possibly ezetimibe too, very low levels of LDL-C, below 10 to 20 mg/dL, may be achieved. Analysis of data from clinical trials of evolocumab[65] and alirocumab[66] shows that very low LDL-C does not pose a safety concern. This is discussed in the article, *LDL-C: How Low Can We Go.*

CLINICS CARE POINTS

- Continue statin therapy in patients with new-onset diabetes mellitus because the benefit exceeds the risk.

- Prevent statin intolerance by carefully explaining to patients 1) the low risk of muscle injury, which can easily be detected with a blood test (CK), and 2) middle age and elderly people commonly have muscle aches and pains.

- When a combination of a statin and a fibrate is needed to reduce TG, use fenofibrate rather than gemfibrozil, because gemfibrozil has a much greater risk of myopathy/rhabdomyolysis.

- In patients taking bempedoic acid, evaluate uric acid levels periodically, especially in patients with a history of gout.

- When treating patients with omega-3 fatty acids, check for signs of atrial fibrillation and bleeding.

REFERENCES

1. Cholesterol Treatment Trialists' (CTT) Collaboration. Efficacy and safety of more intensive lowering of LDL cholesterol: a meta-analysis of data from 170,000 participants in 26 randomised trials. Lancet 2010;376:1670–81.

2. Cannon CP, Blazing MA, Giugliano RP, et al. Ezetimibe added to statin therapy after acute coronary syndromes. N Engl J Med 2015;372(25):2387–97.

3. Schwartz GG, Steg PG, Szarek M, et al. Alirocumab and Cardiovascular Outcomes after Acute Coronary Syndrome. N Engl J Med 2018;379(22):2097–107.

4. Sabatine MS, Giugliano RP, Keech AC, et al. Evolocumab and Clinical Outcomes in Patients with Cardiovascular Disease. N Engl J Med 2017;376(18):1713–22.

5. Newman CB, Preiss D, Tobert JA, et al. on behalf of the American Heart Association Clinical Lipidology, Lipoprotein, Metabolism and Thrombosis Committee, a Joint Committee of the Council on Atherosclerosis, Thrombosis and Vascular Biology and Council on Lifestyle and Cardiometabolic Health; Council on Cardiovascular Disease in the Young; Council on Clinical Cardiology; and Stroke Council. Statin safety and associated adverse events: a scientific statement from the American Heart Association. Arterioscler Thromb Vasc Biol 2018;38:e38–81.

6. Cholesterol Treatment Trialists Collaboration, Fulcher J, O'Connell R, et al. Efficacy and safety of LDL-lowering therapy among men and women: meta-analysis of individual data from 174,000 participants in 27 randomised trials. Lancet 2015; 385(9976):1397–405.

7. Cholesterol Treatment Trialists Collaboration, Baigent C, Blackwell L, et al. Efficacy and safety of more intensive lowering of LDL cholesterol: a meta-analysis of data from 170,000 participants in 26 randomised trials. Lancet 2010; 376(9753):1670–81.

8. Cholesterol Treatment Trialists Collaboration. Efficacy and safety of statin therapy in older people: a meta-analysis of individual participant data from 28 randomised controlled trials. Lancet 2019;393(10170):407–15.

9. Carlsson L, Lind L, Larsson A. Reference values for 27 clinical chemistry tests in 70-year-old males and females. Gerontology 2010;56(3):259–65.

10. Newman C, Tsai J, Szarek M, et al. Comparative safety of atorvastatin 80 mg versus 10 mg derived from analysis of 49 completed trials in 14,236 patients. Am J Cardiol 2006;97(1):61–7.

11. LaRosa JC, Grundy SM, Waters DD, et al. Intensive lipid lowering with atorvastatin in patients with stable coronary disease. N Engl J Med 2005;352(14):1425–35.

12. Link E, Parish S, Armitage J, et al. SLCO1B1 variants and statin-induced myopathy–a genomewide study. N Engl J Med 2008;359(8):789–99.

13. Neuvonen PJ, Niemi M, Backman JT. Drug interactions with lipid-lowering drugs: Mechanisms and clinical relevance. Clin Pharmacol Ther 2006;80(6):565–81.

14. Kellick KA, Bottorff M, Toth PP. The National Lipid Association's Safety Task Force. A clinician's guide to statin drug-drug interactions. J Clin Lipidol 2014;8(3 Suppl): S30–46.

15. Panel on Antiretroviral Guidelines for Adults and Adolescents. Guidelines for the Use of Antiretroviral Agents in Adults and Adolescents with HIV. Department of Health and Human Services. Jan 2022. Available at: https://clinicalinfo.hiv.gov/sites/default/files/guidelines/documents/ AdultandAdolescentGL.pdf. Accessed Feb 27, 2022.

16. Gong Y, Haque S, Chowdhury P, et al. Pharmacokinetics and pharmacodynamics of cytochrome P450 inhibitors for HIV treatment. Expert Opin Drug Metab Toxicol 2019;15(5):417–27.

17. Newman CB, Tobert JA. Statin-Related Myopathy and Rhabdomyolysis. Endocr Metab Med Emergencies 2018;760–74.

18. Nazir S, Lohani S, Tachamo N, et al. Statin-Associated Autoimmune Myopathy: A Systematic Review of 100 Cases. J Clin Rheumatol 2017;23(3):149–54.

19. Newman CB, Tobert JA. Statin intolerance: Reconciling clinical trials and clinical experience. JAMA 2015;313(10):1011–2.
20. Tobert JA, Newman CB. Statin tolerability: In defence of placebo-controlled trials. Eur J Prev Cardiol 2016;23(8):891–6.
21. Tobert JA, Newman CB. The nocebo effect in the context of statin intolerance. J Clin Lipidol 2016;10(4):739–47.
22. Colloca L, Barsky AJ. Placebo and Nocebo Effects. N Engl J Med 2020;382(6): 554–61.
23. Collins R, Reith C, Emberson J, et al. Interpretation of the evidence for the efficacy and safety of statin therapy. Lancet 2016;388(10059):2532–61.
24. Moriarty PM, Thompson PD, Cannon CP, et al. Efficacy and safety of alirocumab vs ezetimibe in statin-intolerant patients, with a statin rechallenge arm: The ODYSSEY ALTERNATIVE randomized trial. J Clin Lipidol 2015;9(6):758–69.
25. Nissen SE, Stroes E, Dent-Acosta RE, et al. Efficacy and tolerability of evolocumab vs ezetimibe in patients with muscle-related statin intolerance: The GAUSS-3 randomized clinical trial. JAMA 2016;315(15):1580–90.
26. Joy TR, Monjed A, Zou GY, et al. N-of-1 (single-patient) trials for statin-related myalgia. Ann Intern Med 2014;160:301–10.
27. Wood FA, Howard JP, Finegold JA, et al. N-of-1 Trial of a Statin, Placebo, or No Treatment to Assess Side Effects. N Engl J Med 2020;383(22):2182–4.
28. Herrett E, Williamson E, Brack K, et al. Statin treatment and muscle symptoms: series of randomised, placebo controlled n-of-1 trials. BMJ 2021;372:n135.
29. Sattar N, Preiss D, Murray HM, et al. Statins and risk of incident diabetes: a collaborative meta-analysis of randomised statin trials. Lancet 2010;375:735–42.
30. Preiss D, Seshasai SR, Welsh P, et al. Risk of incident diabetes with intensive-dose compared with moderate-dose statin therapy: A meta-analysis. JAMA 2011;305(24):2556–64.
31. Ridker PM, Pradhan A, MacFadyen JG, et al. Cardiovascular benefits and diabetes risks of statin therapy in primary prevention: an analysis from the JUPITER trial. Lancet 2012;380(9841):565–71.
32. Waters DD, Ho JE, DeMicco DA, et al. Predictors of new-onset diabetes in patients treated with atorvastatin: results from 3 large randomized clinical trials. J Am Coll Cardiol 2011;57(14):1535–45.
33. Ridker PM, Danielson E, Fonseca FA, et al. Rosuvastatin to prevent vascular events in men and women with elevated C-reactive protein. N Engl J Med 2008;359(21):2195–207.
34. The Stroke Prevention by Aggressive Reduction in Cholesterol Levels (SPARCL) Investigators. High-dose atorvastatin after stroke or transient ischemic attack. N Engl J Med 2006;355:549–59.
35. Erqou S, Lee CC, Adler AI. Statins and glycaemic control in individuals with diabetes: a systematic review and meta-analysis. Diabetologia 2014;57(12): 2444–52.
36. Colhoun HM, Betteridge DJ, Durrington PN, et al. Primary prevention of cardiovascular disease with atorvastatin in type 2 diabetes in the Collaborative Atorvastatin Diabetes Study (CARDS): multicentre randomised placebo-controlled trial. Lancet 2004;364(9435):685–96.
37. Newman CB, Szarek M, Colhoun HM, et al. The safety and tolerability of atorvastatin 10 mg in the Collaborative Atorvastatin Diabetes Study (CARDS). Diab Vasc Dis Res 2008;5:177–83.

38. Holman RR, Paul S, Farmer A, et al. Atorvastatin in Factorial with Omega-3 EE90 Risk Reduction in Diabetes (AFORRD): a randomised controlled trial. Diabetologia 2009;52(1):50–9.

39. Collins R, Armitage J, Parish S, et al. MRC/BHF Heart Protection Study of cholesterol-lowering with simvastatin in 5963 people with diabetes: a randomised placebo-controlled trial. Lancet 2003;361(9374):2005–16.

40. Besseling J, Kastelein JP, Defesche JC, et al. Association between familial hypercholesterolemia and prevalence of type 2 diabetes mellitus. JAMA 2015;313(10): 1029–36.

41. Ference BA, Robinson JG, Brook RD, et al. Variation in PCSK9 and HMGCR and Risk of Cardiovascular Disease and Diabetes. N Engl J Med 2016;375(22): 2144–53.

42. Lotta LA, Sharp SJ, Burgess S, et al. Association Between Low-Density Lipoprotein Cholesterol-Lowering Genetic Variants and Risk of Type 2 Diabetes: A Meta-analysis. JAMA 2016;316(13):1383–91.

43. Bonnefond A, Yengo L, Le May C, et al. The loss-of-function PCSK9 p.R46L genetic variant does not alter glucose homeostasis. Diabetologia 2015;58(9): 2051–5.

44. Tobert JA. Efficacy and long-term adverse effect pattern of lovastatin. Am J Cardiol 1988;62(15):28j–34j.

45. Dujovne CA, Chremos AN, Pool JL, et al. Expanded clinical evaluation of lovastatin (EXCEL) study results: IV. Additional perspectives on the tolerability of lovastatin. Am J Med 1991;91(1b):25s–30s.

46. FDA Drug Safety Communication: Important safety label changes to cholesterol-lowering statin drugs. 2012. Available at: https://www.fda.gov/drugs/drug-safety-and-availability/fda-drug-safety-communication-important-safety-label-changes-cholesterol-lowering-statin-drugs. Accessed March 1, 2022.

47. Björnsson E, Jacobsen EI, Kalaitzakis E. Hepatotoxicity associated with statins: Reports of idiosyncratic liver injury post-marketing. J Hepatol 2012;56(2):374–80.

48. Khajeh E, Moghadam AD, Eslami P, et al. Statin use is associated with the reduction in hepatocellular carcinoma recurrence after liver surgery. BMC Cancer 2022;22(1):91. https://doi.org/10.1186/s12885-022-09192-1.

49. Lewis JH, Mortensen ME, Zweig S, et al. Efficacy and safety of high-dose pravastatin in hypercholesterolemic patients with well-compensated chronic liver disease: Results of a prospective, randomized, double-blind, placebo-controlled, multicenter trial. Hepatology 2007;46(5):1453–63.

50. Kargiotis K, Athyros VG, Giouleme O, et al. Resolution of non-alcoholic steatohepatitis by rosuvastatin monotherapy in patients with metabolic syndrome. World J Gastroenterol 2015;21(25):7860–8.

51. Atsukawa M, Tsubota A, Kondo C, et al. Combination of fluvastatin with pegylated interferon/ribavirin therapy reduces viral relapse in chronic hepatitis C infected with HCV genotype 1b. J Gastroenterol Hepatol 2013;28(1):51–6.

52. Selic Kurincic T, Lesnicar G, Poljak M, et al. Impact of added fluvastatin to standard-of-care treatment on sustained virological response in naive chronic hepatitis C Patients infected with genotypes 1 and 3. Intervirology 2014;57(1): 23–30.

53. Amarenco P, Labreuche J. Lipid management in the prevention of stroke: review and updated meta-analysis of statins for stroke prevention. Lancet Neurol 2009;8: 453–63.

54. Waters DD, LaRosa JC, Barter P, et al. Effects of high-dose atorvastatin on cere-
    brovascular events in patients with stable coronary disease in the TNT (Treating
    to New Targets) study. J Am Coll Cardiol 2006;48(9):1793–9.

55. Goldstein LB, Amarenco P, Szarek M, et al. Secondary analysis of hemorrhagic
    stroke in the Stroke Prevention by Aggressive Reduction in Cholesterol Levels
    (SPARCL) Study. Neurology 2008;70:2364–70.

56. Wiggins BS, Saseen JJ, Page RL, et al. Recommendations for Management of
    Clinically Significant Drug-Drug Interactions With Statins and Select Agents
    Used in Patients With Cardiovascular Disease: A Scientific Statement From the
    American Heart Association. Circulation 2016;134(21):e468–95.

57. FDA Drug Safety Communication. 7-20-2021. FDA requests removal of strongest
    warning against cholesterol-lowering statins during pregnancy; still advises most
    pregnant patients should stop taking statins. Available at: https://www.fda.gov/
    media/150774/download. Accessed October 18 2021.

58. Wu H, Shang H, Wu J. Effect of ezetimibe on glycemic control: a systematic re-
    view and meta-analysis of randomized controlled trials. Endocrine 2018;60(2):
    229–39.

59. Peto R, Emberson J, Landray M, et al. Analyses of cancer data from three ezeti-
    mibe trials. N Engl J Med 2008;359(13):1357–66.

60. Baigent C, Landray MJ, Reith C, et al. The effects of lowering LDL cholesterol with
    simvastatin plus ezetimibe in patients with chronic kidney disease (Study of Heart
    and Renal Protection): a randomised placebo-controlled trial. Lancet 2011;
    377(9784):2181–92.

61. Giugliano RP, Gencer B, Wiviott SD, et al. Prospective evaluation of malignancy in
    17,708 patients randomized to ezetimibe versus placebo: Analysis from
    IMPROVE-IT. J Am Cardiol CardioOnc 2020;2(3):385–96.

62. Amgen Inc.REPATHA (evolocumab) injection. U.S. Prescribing Information Sept.
    2021.

63. Sanofi-Aventis U.S. LLC. Praluent (alirocumab) injection. U.S. Prescribing Infor-
    mation Sept. 2021.

64. Giugliano RP, Mach F, Zavitz K, et al. Cognitive Function in a Randomized Trial of
    Evolocumab. N Engl J Med 2017;377(7):633–43.

65. Giugliano RP, Pedersen TR, Park JG, et al. Clinical efficacy and safety of
    achieving very low LDL-cholesterol concentrations with the PCSK9 inhibitor evo-
    locumab: a prespecified secondary analysis of the FOURIER trial. Lancet 2017;
    390(10106):1962–71.

66. Schwartz GG, Gabriel Steg P, Bhatt DL, et al. Clinical Efficacy and Safety of
    Alirocumab After Acute Coronary Syndrome According to Achieved Level
    of Low-Density Lipoprotein Cholesterol: A Propensity Score-Matched Analysis
    of the ODYSSEY OUTCOMES Trial. Circulation 2021;143(11):1109–22.

67. Sabatine MS, Leiter LA, Wiviott SD, et al. Cardiovascular safety and efficacy of
    the PCSK9 inhibitor evolocumab in patients with and without diabetes and the ef-
    fect of evolocumab on glycaemia and risk of new-onset diabetes: a prespecified
    analysis of the FOURIER randomised controlled trial. Lancet Diabetes Endocrinol
    2017;5(12):941–50.

68. Ray KK, Colhoun HM, Szarek M, et al. Effects of alirocumab on cardiovascular
    and metabolic outcomes after acute coronary syndrome in patients with or
    without diabetes: a prespecified analysis of the ODYSSEY OUTCOMES rando-
    mised controlled trial. Lancet Diabetes Endocrinol 2019;7(8):618–28.

69. Schmidt AF, Swerdlow DI, Holmes MV, et al. PCSK9 genetic variants and risk of type 2 diabetes: a mendelian randomisation study. Lancet Diabetes Endocrinol 2017;5(2):97–105.
70. Lee J, Hegele RA. PCSK9 inhibition and diabetes: turning to Mendel for clues. Lancet Diabetes Endocrinol 2017;5(2):78–9.
71. Novartis Europharm Limited. Leqvio 284 mg solution for injection (Inclisiran). Summary of Product Characteristics. 2020. Available at: https://www.ema.europa.eu/en/documents/product-information/leqvio-epar-product-information_en.pdf. Accessed October 25 2021.
72. Ray KK, Wright RS, Kallend D, et al. Two Phase 3 Trials of Inclisiran in Patients with Elevated LDL Cholesterol. N Engl J Med 2020;382(16):1507–19.
73. Wright RS, Ray KK, Raal FJ, et al. Pooled Patient-Level Analysis of Inclisiran Trials in Patients With Familial Hypercholesterolemia or Atherosclerosis. J Am Coll Cardiol 2021;77(9):1182–93.
74. Pharmacia and Upjohn Company. Division of Pfizer Inc. Colestid (colestipol hydrochloride tablets). U.S. Prescribing Information May 2017.
75. Riaz S, John S. Cholestyramine Resin. StatPearls. Treasure Island (FL)2021.
76. Daiichi Sankyo Inc. WELCHOL (colesevelam) tables. U.S. Prescribing Information. October 2021.
77. Newman CB, Blaha MJ, Boord JB, et al. Lipid Management in Patients with Endocrine Disorders: An Endocrine Society Clinical Practice Guideline. J Clin Endocrinol Metab 2020;105(12).
78. Esperion Therapeutics. NEXLETOL ('mpedoic acid). U.S. Product Information Feb 2020.
79. Ray KK, Bays HE, Catapano AL, et al. Safety and Efficacy of Bempedoic Acid to Reduce LDL Cholesterol. N Engl J Med 2019;380(11):1022–32.
80. Parke-Davis, Division of Pfizer Inc. LOPID (gemfibrozil). U.S. Prescribing Information Dec 2020.
81. Furberg CD, Pitt B. Withdrawal of cerivastatin from the world market. Curr Control Trials Cardiovasc Med 2001;2(5):205–7.
82. Ginsberg HN, Elam MB, et al, ACCORD Study Group. Effects of combination lipid therapy in type 2 diabetes mellitus. N Engl J Med 2010;362(17):1563–74.
83. Jones PH, Davidson MH. Reporting rate of rhabdomyolysis with fenofibrate + statin versus gemfibrozil + any statin. Am J Cardiol 2005;95(1):120–2.
84. Keech A, Simes RJ, Barter P, et al. Effects of long-term fenofibrate therapy on cardiovascular events in 9795 people with type 2 diabetes mellitus (the FIELD study): randomised controlled trial. Lancet 2005;366(9500):1849–61.
85. Abb Vie Inc. TRICOR (fenofibrate tablet). U.S. Prescribing Information. March 2021.
86. Amarin Pharma Inc. VASCEPA (icosapent ethyl) capsules. U.S. Prescribing Information Dec 2019.
87. GlaxoSmithKline. LOVAZA (omega-3-acid ethyl esters capsules). U.S. Prescribing Information Sept 2020.
88. AstraZeneca Pharmaceuticals LP. EPANOVA (omega-3-carboxylic acids) capsules. U.S. Prescribing Information March 2017.
89. Nicholls SJ, Lincoff AM, Garcia M, et al. Effect of High-Dose Omega-3 Fatty Acids vs Corn Oil on Major Adverse Cardiovascular Events in Patients at High Cardiovascular Risk: The STRENGTH Randomized Clinical Trial. JAMA 2020;324(22):2268–80.
90. Bhatt DL, Steg PG, Miller M, et al. Cardiovascular Risk Reduction with Icosapent Ethyl for Hypertriglyceridemia. N Engl J Med 2019;380(1):11–22.

91. AMRYT Pharma. JUXTAPID (lomitapide) prescribing information. Dec 2019.
92. Cuchel M, Meagher EA, du Toit Theron H, et al. Efficacy and safety of a micro-somal triglyceride transfer protein inhibitor in patients with homozygous familial hypercholesterolaemia: a single-arm, open-label, phase 3 study. Lancet 2013; 381(9860):40–6.
93. Elam MB, Hunninghake DB, Davis KB, et al. Effect of niacin on lipid and lipopro-tein levels and glycemic control in patients with diabetes and peripheral arterial disease: the ADMIT study: A randomized trial. Arterial Disease Multiple Interven-tion Trial. JAMA 2000;284(10):1263–70.
94. Goldie C, Taylor AJ, Nguyen P, et al. Niacin therapy and the risk of new-onset dia-betes: a meta-analysis of randomised controlled trials. Heart 2016;102(3): 198–203.
95. Anderson TJ, Boden WE, Desvigne-Nickens P, et al. Safety profile of extended-release niacin in the AIM-HIGH trial. N Engl J Med 2014;371(3):288–90.
96. Landray MJ, Haynes R, Hopewell JC, et al. Effects of extended-release niacin with laropiprant in high-risk patients. N Engl J Med 2014;371(3):203–12.
97. Lloyd-Jones D3. Niacin and HDL cholesterol–time to face facts. N Engl J Med 2014;371(3):271–3.

LDL Cholesterol—How Low Can We Go?

Jonathan A. Tobert, MD, PhD

KEYWORDS

- LDL cholesterol • Hypocholesterolemia • Guidelines • Safety
- Cardiovascular risk reduction

KEY POINTS

- Most if not all mammalian nucleated cells can produce cholesterol, so LDL particles are needed only to recycle it.
- Normal human newborns have very low LDL cholesterol, showing that it is physiologic.
- Randomized controlled trials have shown that lowering LDL cholesterol below 70 mg/dL reduces the risk of atherosclerotic vascular events with minimal adverse effects.
- There is no known threshold below which lowering LDL cholesterol is harmful.
- Reducing LDL cholesterol below 40 mg/dL is often feasible with combination therapy and can be considered in patients who have had 2 or more major vascular events, but below 25 mg/dL further reduction may provide little if any further benefit.

INTRODUCTION

Forty years ago, 300 mg/dL was generally considered the upper limit of normal for total plasma cholesterol in Western countries. In that era, the risks associated with high concentrations of plasma and low-density lipoprotein cholesterol (LDL-C) were only beginning to be appreciated and were vigorously debated, so the normal range was based on population statistics, not biology. In 1984, an NIH Consensus Conference concluded that lowering elevated LDL-C with diet and drugs would reduce the risk of coronary heart disease (CHD). Efforts to educate physicians and the public about the importance of treating hypercholesterolemia followed. However, the effectiveness of diet and the available drugs was limited. The 1987 introduction of lovastatin, the first statin, was a radical advance. Lovastatin is generally well tolerated and could produce a 40% mean reduction in LDL-C at its maximal dose, and subsequently atorvastatin and rosuvastatin expanded that to about 55%. The cholesterol absorption inhibitor ezetimibe, introduced in 2001, lowers LDL-C by a further 20% when added to a statin. From 2015 onwards, adding a PCSK9 inhibitor to high-intensity statin treatment

Nuffield Department of Population Health, University of Oxford, Richard Doll Building, Old Road Campus, Oxford OX3 7LF, UK
E-mail address: jonathan.tobert@cantab.net

Endocrinol Metab Clin N Am 51 (2022) 681–690
https://doi.org/10.1016/j.ecl.2022.01.005
0889-8529/22/© 2022 Elsevier Inc. All rights reserved.

Abbreviation	
LDL	low-density lipoprotein

(atorvastatin or rosuvastatin at maximal or near-maximal doses) with or without ezetimibe made possible the reduction of LDL-C to well below 1 mmol/L (38.7 mg/dL) in many patients.

Doubts about the value of lowering LDL-C, and the safety of doing so, were largely quenched in 1994 with the publication of the Scandinavian Simvastatin Survival Study (4S), in which a 30% reduction in total mortality (P = .0003) was demonstrated.[1] The 25 years that followed saw a steady stream of large-scale randomized controlled trials (RCTs) of statins and other lipid-modifying agents,[2] including those mentioned earlier, which collectively showed that the reduction in the risk of myocardial infarction and ischemic stroke, and other atherosclerotic events, was proportional to the absolute reduction in LDL-C, with a reduction of 1 mmol/L (~40 mg/dL) producing an average reduction in risk of 22%.[2] The PCSK9 monoclonal antibodies alirocumab and evolocumab, introduced in 2015, lower LDL-C by about 50% when added to a statin. This has created a new question: is there any level of LDL-C below which reducing it does not produce any worthwhile cardiovascular risk reduction and/or creates an unacceptable increase in adverse effects[3,4]?

In cardiovascular outcome trials with both alirocumab[5] and evolocumab[6] compared to placebo on a background of statin therapy, the mean on-treatment value of LDL-C was around 40 mg/dL (~1 mmol/L). Neither study raised any safety concerns. Indeed, current European guidelines[7] suggest 1 mmol/L (~40 mg/dL) as the target of treatment in patients who have suffered 2 or more major atherosclerotic events.

CHOLESTEROL TRANSPORT

Very low-density lipoprotein (VLDL) is synthesized in the liver and released into the circulation to transport triglycerides and fat-soluble vitamins to tissues. VLDL particles also contain liver-derived esterified cholesterol, which stabilizes them. Lipoprotein lipase liberates fatty acids from triglycerides in VLDL and chylomicrons, thus converting VLDL into remnant lipoproteins and subsequently LDL. Cholesterol is required for the formation of cell membranes and bile acids, and for steroidogenesis, but nucleated mammalian cells can synthesize cholesterol from acetate.[8] Intricate control mechanisms enable cells to synthesize cholesterol when it is depleted.[8,9] But circulating LDL can penetrate the vascular endothelium, which may lead to atherosclerotic lesions and eventually serious outcomes, including myocardial infarction and ischemic stroke. A high concentration of LDL particles is the primary cause of atherosclerosis.

LDL is what remains after most of the triglyceride in VLDL particles has been lipolyzed. Thus, LDL is essentially a byproduct. Removal of LDL from the circulation is accomplished predominantly by the LDL receptors on the surface of hepatocytes, which bind the apolipoprotein B component of LDL. LDL is then taken up mostly into the liver but also peripheral tissues, and the apolipoprotein B it contains is catabolized, while the cholesterol is either recycled into VLDL, used for steroidogenesis and to produce bile acids, or incorporated into cell membranes. Some cholesterol is excreted in the bile, and enterohepatic recirculation returns most intestinal cholesterol to the liver via chylomicrons. Dietary cholesterol is superfluous, as indicated by the health of vegans. A simplified diagram of these pathways is shown in **Fig. 1**, reproduced from Feingold,[10] and Kenneth R Feingold's article, "Lipid and Lipoprotein

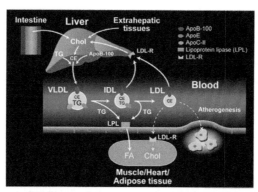

Fig. 1. A simplified diagram of cholesterol transport. (*From* Feingold KR. Introduction to Lipids and Lipoproteins. [Updated 2021 Jan 19]. In: Feingold KR, Anawalt B, Boyce A, et al., editors. Endotext [Internet]. South Dartmouth (MA): MDText.com, Inc.; 2000-. https://www.ncbi.nlm.nih.gov/books/NBK305896/. 2021).

Metabolism," in this issue provides in-depth information beyond the scope of this article, as do Goldstein and Brown,[8] who led much of the effort to work out these pathways. In this article, very low LDL-C is somewhat arbitrarily defined as a concentration less than 40 mg/dL (1 mmol/L). The conversion factor is 38.7, approximated to 40 in the case of 1 mmol/L. When this article cites the work of authors who use the SI system, SI values are provided with traditional units in parentheses.

Cholesterol is an essential component of mammalian cell membranes, and nucleated cells have the capacity to synthesize it.[8] Because LDL has no essential function other than recycling cholesterol back to the liver,[8,9] very low LDL-C—defined here as less than 40 mg/dL (approximately 1 mmol/L)—should be compatible with health, as long as the other components of the lipidome are within normal limits. This should be true regardless of whether very low LDL-C is the result of normal physiology, or mutations that are associated with these very low levels, or is reduced to very low levels by drug treatment. We shall examine in turn each of these 3 components of the hypothesis that very low LDL-C is not harmful.

LOW CHOLESTEROL STATES
Neonatal Human Physiology

It has long been known that LDL-C concentrations are much lower in neonates than in young children or adults. For example, Khoury and colleagues[11] reported mean LDL-C in 122 cord blood samples of 23 mg/dL with a standard deviation of 10 mg/dL, indicating that about one-third of the newborns had LDL-C at or below 13 mg/dL (0.34 mmol/L). Plasma triglycerides and apolipoprotein B were also much lower than in children or adults. This very low level of LDL-C is compatible with the rapid growth of the near-term fetus because, as previously mentioned, mammalian nucleated cells are capable of cholesterol biosynthesis; in particular, the large quantities of cholesterol required for fetal cerebral development are produced within the brain. VLDL production appears to be minimal in the intrauterine environment, in which nutrients are supplied via the placenta and not the gastrointestinal system, so that few LDL particles are formed. Concentrations of LDL-C, triglycerides, and apolipoprotein B rise rapidly in the days following birth,[11] when the infant must process breast milk and later solid food.

Mutations

Mutations of the LDL receptor have been a key resource in the elucidation of the mechanisms that control circulating levels of LDL. Homozygosity for loss of function LDL receptor mutations prevents receptor-mediated uptake of LDL into hepatocytes and other cells, leading to LDL-C concentrations of 500 mg/dL or higher. This condition, homozygous familial hypercholesterolemia (FH), is found in approximately one in a million individuals, whereas heterozygous FH occurs in about one in 300 and typically leads to untreated LDL-C levels of 250 mg/dL or higher. If untreated, patients with homozygous FH frequently succumb as children or adolescents due to myocardial infarctions and other atherosclerotic events, whereas in untreated heterozygous FH, these events typically occur in midlife. The lethality of homozygous FH in children, who have no other risk factors for atherosclerosis, was strong evidence for the pathogenicity of LDL-C and the physiologic requirement for pathways to control it. Elucidation of the LDL receptor control mechanisms[12] led to the award of the 1985 Nobel Prize in Physiology or Medicine to Michael Brown and Joseph Goldstein.

Mutations that are associated with low LDL-C concentrations have been useful but have not led to such clear-cut results. Familial hypobetalipoproteinemia[13] generally results from mutant alleles coding for apolipoprotein B that disrupt the production of VLDL, the precursor of LDL-C. Plasma concentrations of LDL-C fall to around 30 mg/dL. Although most patients with heterozygous mutant alleles are generally healthy, they are at risk of fatty liver, chronic diarrhea, steatorrhea, and deficiency of fat-soluble vitamins.[14] However, all apolipoprotein B containing lipoproteins are depleted, not just LDL, so the relevance of familial hypobetalipoproteinemia to the question at hand is limited.

Heterozygous genetic variants that cause loss of function of PCSK9 have a frequency of 2% to 3% in the United States and are associated with moderate reductions of LDL-C, not large enough to bring LDL-C down to very low levels.[15] Nevertheless, these variants have a disproportionately large beneficial effect on the risk of CHD, presumably because the LDL-C reduction is lifelong, in contrast to a few years in cardiovascular outcome trials. Reports of individuals homozygous for PCSK9 loss of function mutations are minimal. Details of one subject with undetectable circulating PCSK9 were published in 2006.[16] Genetic analysis indicated that she was a compound heterozygote with 2 loss-of-function PCSK9 mutant alleles. At that time, she was an apparently healthy, fertile, college-educated African-American woman who worked as an aerobics instructor. Liver and renal function tests were normal. Her LDL-C was 14 mg/dL, whereas HDL-cholesterol and triglycerides were well within the normal range. Another subject with very low LDL-C, 0.4 mmol/L (15 mg/dL), and homozygosity for the C679X loss-of-function variant was found in a study of 653 women attending antenatal clinics in Zimbabwe[17]; further details have not been published. Identifying and where possible studying more subjects who are homozygotes or compound heterozygotes for loss-of-function variants would be of great interest; but if such individuals are not only very rare but also typically healthy, and have a very low rate of CHD and other atherosclerotic events later in life,[15] they are unlikely to come to the attention of geneticists or lipid specialists.

Studies of PCSK9 human genetics, therefore, suggest that this enzyme is not essential for health. The apparent normality of PCSK9-knockout mice is consistent with this conclusion.[18] The implication is that the very low levels of LDL-C that follow from the absence of PCSK9 are compatible with health, at least in a well-nourished population under contemporary conditions. Possibly under earlier evolutionary conditions there might have been a greater need for PCSK9, which serves as an additional regulator of cholesterol homeostasis.

Drug Treatment

As with all drugs, the adverse effects of lipid-lowering drugs are dose-related, but there is no evidence that these are augmented at low achieved LDL-C concentrations. For example, cerivastatin was removed from the market in 2001 because of a much higher frequency of rhabdomyolysis compared with other statins,[19] particularly when taken with concomitant gemfibrozil. But cerivastatin was a moderate efficacy statin, reducing LDL-C by only about 40% on average at the maximal 0.8 mg dose, and target LDL-C levels were less aggressive than today. In contrast, the most commonly used statin, atorvastatin, reduces LDL-C by about 55% at its maximal dose and it rarely causes rhabdomyolysis.

Statins are the bedrock of lipid-lowering therapy. The most effective statins, atorvastatin and rosuvastatin, produce a mean reduction in LDL-C of about 55%, which is not usually sufficient to lower LDL-C much below 70 mg/dL when used as monotherapy. However, the addition of monoclonal antibodies against PCSK9, alirocumab or evolocumab, or the small interfering RNA inclisiran,[20] that blocks PCSK9 transcription, will often reduce LDL-C below 40 mg/dL. The adverse effects of statins and the safety of the LDL-C reductions produced have been a subject of intense interest for many years. However, the currently marketed statins have a history going back to 1987 and an excellent safety profile,[21] as discussed in Connie B. Newman's article, "Safety of Statins and Non-Statins for Treatment of Dyslipidemia," in this issue. The well-established adverse effects of statins are serious muscle injury, including rhabdomyolysis, with an incidence less than 0.1%, and a 0.2% risk of newly diagnosed diabetes.[22] Both of these adverse effects appear to be caused by statins directly, as opposed to indirectly via the lipid-lowering they produce; the main evidence for this is that PCSK9 inhibitors lower LDL-C at least as much as statins and, to date at least, do not appear to cause rhabdomyolysis or newly diagnosed diabetes.[23,24]

Unexplained muscle symptoms without significant elevation of creatine kinase are commonly reported by statin-treated patients and are a barrier to therapy, but in RCTs, the incidence of these symptoms is consistently very similar in the statin and placebo groups (see Connie B. Newman's article, "Safety of Statins and Non-Statins for Treatment of Dyslipidemia," in this issue). Furthermore, several studies have shown that statin intolerance due to muscle symptoms is not reproducible under double-blind conditions.[21,22,25,26] Consequently these symptoms are mostly attributed to the nocebo effect.

The safety of lipid-lowering agents is discussed in detail in Connie B. Newman's article, "Safety of Statins and Non-Statins for Treatment of Dyslipidemia," in this issue. Here we consider only adverse effects arising from treatment that produces very low concentrations of LDL-C. The ODYSSEY-Outcomes protocol specified blinded replacement of active alirocumab with placebo if LDL-C fell below 15 mg/dL on 2 occasions.[5] This occurred in 730 patients, who had a median duration on active treatment of 6.8 months. There was no excess of neurocognitive disorders or new-onset diabetes in patients who achieved LDL-C levels less than 15 mg/dL, and there were no cases of hemorrhagic stroke. In FOURIER,[24] comparing evolocumab versus placebo, 1335 (5%) patients allocated to evolocumab had an on-treatment LDL-C concentration of less than $0 \cdot 4$ mmol/L (15 mg/dL) and 504 (2%) less than $0 \cdot 26$ mmol/L (10 mg/dL). No safety signal was detected in either of these groups.

Inclisiran is a recently approved double-stranded small interfering RNA (siRNA) that suppresses hepatic PCSK9 translation. It reduces the concentration of circulating

PCSK9 by 80% to 90%, which leads to LDL reductions of about 50%, similar to that achieved by the PCSK9 monoclonal antibodies.[20] This siRNA is given subcutaneously at 6-month intervals, with an extra dose at month 3. It too has an excellent safety profile,[27] although ORION-4, a cardiovascular outcome study, is still in progress, so treatment duration in RCTs is still relatively short, less than 2 years. In a pooled analysis of phase 3 studies with inclisiran that included 3660 participants,[27] 52% of patients randomized achieved LDL-C values below 50 mg/dL and 14% below 25 mg/dL. No safety signal emerged, except for injection site reactions and a slightly higher incidence of bronchitis in the inclisiran group (4.3% vs 2.7%).

Overall, experience to date indicates that bringing LDL-C down to below 40 mg/dL involves little if any additional risk compared with less aggressive targets. Longer follow-up of patients with these low and ultralow concentrations of LDL-C may be informative, but as of 2021, there is no good evidence of a threshold below which new adverse effects emerge.

This is encouraging, but possibly not the last word. Two decades passed before statins were found to increase the risk of new-onset diabetes, for example, and the mechanism of the hallmark adverse effect of statins, myopathy/rhabdomyolysis, is still unclear. The biology of PCSK9 is complex and an active field of research.[9] Experience with PCSK9 inhibitors has not raised any major concerns, but these agents have been available for prescription for less than 5 years, compared with nearly 35 years for statins. There is even less experience with inclisiran.

UTILITY OF REDUCING LDL-C BELOW 40 MG/dL

Having arrived at the conclusion that there is no detectable hazard arising from very low LDL-C concentrations, the next question to consider is whether reducing LDL-C to below 40 mg/dL confers additional cardiovascular benefit, with the caveat that measurement of low (<100 mg/dL) concentrations of LDL-C by the traditional Friedewald equation is subject to clinically important inaccuracies (see Lucero and colleagues' article, "Lipoprotein Assessment in the 21st Century," in this issue). In particular, when plasma triglyceride concentration exceeds 150 mg/dL, the relative contribution of VLDL-C to the estimate of low LDL-C is appreciable and underestimation of LDL-C results.[28] Various methods, particularly the Martin/Hopkins equation[29] and the Sampson-NIH equation,[30] can be used to increase the accuracy of LDL-C estimation by adjustments to the relationship of VLDL-C to triglycerides. Alternatively, LDL-C can be measured directly by various chemical methods, but the methods are proprietary and may not be well validated. A further source of error is the inclusion of cholesterol in lipoprotein(a) when measuring LDL-C. In a patient with low LDL-C and high lipoprotein(a), this can lead to substantial overestimation of LDL-C. Lucero and colleagues' article, "Lipoprotein Assessment in the 21st Century," in this issue provides a full discussion of these analytical issues.

More than 30 large-scale cardiovascular outcome trials have provided data on cardiovascular risk reduction and LDL-C reduction, with statins in most cases but also PCSK9 inhibitors, the cholesterol absorption inhibitor ezetimibe, and CETP inhibitors. The 2010 meta-analysis by the Cholesterol Treatment Trialists Collaboration (CTTC)[2] was confined to statins and included a subgroup with baseline LDL-C less than 2 mmol/L (77 mg/dL). The overall number of patients with major vascular events was 24,323 and the overall reduction in major vascular events was 22% per 1 mmol/L LDL-C lowering, with very similar reductions in all the subgroups determined by baseline LDL-C, all the way down to the subgroup with the lowest LDL-C, less than 2 mmol/L (77 mg/dL). In this subgroup, the risk reduction was also 22% per 1 mmol/L

LDL-C lowering, but with a much wider confidence interval, because the subgroup included only 1922 participants with endpoint events, 8% of the total.

Subgroup analyses[23,24,31] addressing the utility and safety of on-treatment very low LDL-C concentrations are available from various cardiovascular outcome trials. Whenever an RCT population is divided into subgroups defined by postrandomization characteristics (as opposed to baseline values), the rigor of randomization is lost and bias may well be introduced, requiring careful application of statistical techniques to minimize it. Therefore, interpretation should be cautious. One such study is a prespecified analysis of ODYSSEY Outcomes,[23] the cardiovascular outcome trial for alirocumab in patients with acute coronary syndrome. The authors considered and listed numerous possible sources of bias and used propensity scoring to match the placebo control groups to the groups allocated to active treatment. Sensitivity analyses were used for confirmation.

The subgroups were 3 prespecified strata of LDL-C in patients allocated to active treatment, measured at 4 months after randomization: less than 25 (n = 3357), 25 to 50 (n = 3692), or greater than 50 mg/dL (n = 2197). LDL-C was calculated using the Friedewald equation unless the calculated value was less than 15 mg/dL or the concurrent triglyceride level was greater than 400 mg/dL, in which case LDL-C was measured directly by preparative ultracentrifugation and β-quantitation. The primary endpoint, major vascular events, was a composite of nonfatal myocardial infarction, ischemic stroke, or hospitalization for unstable angina.

The treatment benefit of alirocumab was similar in patients in the lowest and middle strata, and less in the upper stratum, in which adherence to study medication was relatively poor. The respective primary endpoint hazard ratios were 0.74, 0.74, and 0.87. This suggests that lowering LDL-C to 25 to 50 mg/dL is optimal in patients with atherosclerotic vascular disease and that further reduction of LDL-C in a patient with a level of about 25 mg/dL may be unproductive, no matter how high their cardiovascular risk. This is consistent with current guidelines. However, a large prespecified 2017 subgroup analysis of FOURIER,[24] also based on on-treatment values of LDL-C, reported no detectable utility threshold with evolocumab all the way down to 0.2 mmol/L (8 mg/dL). Both FOURIER and ODYSSEY Outcomes compared PCSK9 monoclonal antibodies, evolocumab or alirocumab, respectively, versus placebo in patients on statin therapy. The statistical methodology of the FOURIER subgroup analysis,[24] including adjustment for covariates, was different from that used in the subgroup analysis of ODYSSEY Outcomes. This might account for its different conclusions; indeed, the authors of a 2021 reanalysis[32] of the FOURIER subgroup results acknowledged the possibility of confounding in the original subgroup analysis.[24] Using statistical methodology that preserved randomization, they found that lowering LDL-C to ≤40 mg/dL proportionally reduced cardiovascular risk, but they did not claim evidence for benefit of reducing LDL-C to any particular value below 40 mg/dL. Thus, the results of FOURIER and ODYSSEY Outcomes are no longer inconsistent.

DISCUSSION

ODYSSEY Outcomes demonstrate a possible threshold of 25 mg/dL below which further lowering of LDL-C does not further reduce the risk of major atherosclerotic vascular events. This is consistent with FOURIER and is plausible, as we cannot assume that the CTTC meta-analysis[2] 22% reduction in cardiovascular risk per 1 mmol/L reduction of LDL-C holds down to very low levels. Even if it does hold, lowering LDL-C by 50% from 25 mg/dL would provide an absolute reduction of only 12.5 mg/dL (0.32 mmol/L) and an expected risk reduction of only 7%. A patient whose

LDL-C is 25 mg/dL is probably already taking a high-intensity statin and a PCSK9 inhibitor. To obtain a yet further 50% reduction might require the addition of inclisiran or some other equally effective but not yet developed agent. Interventions targeting risk factors other than LDL-C, such as lipoprotein(a), seem a more promising avenue for reducing residual risk. A small interfering RNA that produces a 90% reduction in lipoprotein(a) concentration is currently being tested in a large-scale cardiovascular outcome trial (NCT04023552).[33] Trial completion is scheduled for 2024.

There is no evidence for a threshold below which lowering LDL-C leads to adverse effects, nor does the biology of LDL lead to any expectation of a threshold. Nevertheless, evidence for rare but serious adverse effects could emerge in long-term studies when large numbers of patients are treated down to around 25 mg/dL or below. If that happens, experience with statins indicates that interpretation should be cautious. At various times concerns arose that statins might increase the risk of cataracts, breast cancer, or neurocognitive adverse effects. None of these concerns survived critical scrutiny and the acquisition of more data.[21,22]

To put the question that titles this article into perspective, residual uncertainty about reducing LDL-C below 25 mg/dL is far less of a barrier to treatment than the reluctance of many patients, even those at high risk with LDL-C far above 25 mg/dL, to take a statin, as discussed in Connie B. Newman's article, "Safety of Statins and Non-Statins for Treatment of Dyslipidemia," in this issue.

SUMMARY

The cardiovascular benefit and safety of reducing LDL-C to about 40 mg/dL (1 mmol/L) has been demonstrated in large-scale RCTs. The current therapeutic armamentarium makes further reduction of LDL-C achievable in some high-risk patients, but clinicians should be aware that the benefit of further reduction of LDL-C to below 25 mg/dL has not been established. If there is a hazard related to reducing LDL-C to very low levels, as of 2021 it has not been detected.

CLINICAL PEARLS

- In patients who have had 2 or more atherosclerotic events or are otherwise at very high risk, consider treatment to lower LDL cholesterol below 40 mg/dL.
- There is no evidence for any threshold below which further lowering of LDL cholesterol is harmful, but below 25 mg/dL, the reduction of cardiovascular risk is likely to be small if not nonexistent.

DISCLOSURE

The author has nothing to disclose.

REFERENCES

1. Scandinavian Simvastatin Survival Study Group. Randomised trial of cholesterol lowering in 4444 patients with coronary heart disease: the Scandinavian Simvastatin Survival Study (4S). Lancet 1994;344:1383–9.
2. Cholesterol Treatment Trialists' (CTT) Collaboration. Efficacy and safety of more intensive lowering of LDL cholesterol: a meta-analysis of data from 170,000 participants in 26 randomised trials. Lancet 2010;376:1670–81.
3. Olsson AG, Angelin B, Assmann G, et al. Can LDL cholesterol be too low? Possible risks of extremely low levels. J Intern Med 2017;281(6):534–53.

4. Gotto AM Jr. Low-density lipoprotein cholesterol and cardiovascular risk reduction: how low is low enough without causing harm? JAMA Cardiol 2018;3(9): 802–3.

5. Schwartz GG, Steg PG, Szarek M, et al. Alirocumab and cardiovascular outcomes after acute coronary syndrome. N Engl J Med 2018;379(22):2097–107.

6. Sabatine MS, Giugliano RP, Keech AC, et al. Evolocumab and clinical outcomes in patients with cardiovascular disease. N Engl J Med 2017;376(18):1713–22.

7. Mach F, Baigent C, Catapano AL, et al. 2019 ESC/EAS Guidelines for the management of dyslipidaemias: lipid modification to reduce cardiovascular risk: The Task Force for the management of dyslipidaemias of the European Society of Cardiology (ESC) and European Atherosclerosis Society (EAS). Eur Heart J 2019;41(1):111–88.

8. Goldstein JL, Brown MS. A century of cholesterol and coronaries: from plaques to genes to statins. Cell 2015;161(1):161–72.

9. Shapiro MD, Tavori H, Fazio S. PCSK9. Circ Res 2018;122(10):1420–38.

10. Feingold KR. Introduction to Lipids and Lipoproteins. [Updated 2021 Jan 19]. In: Feingold KR, Anawalt B, Boyce A, et al, editors. Endotext [Internet]. South Dartmouth (MA): MDText.com, Inc.; 2000. Available from: https://www.ncbi.nlm.nih.gov/books/NBK305896/.

11. Khoury J, Henriksen T, Christophersen B, et al. Effect of a cholesterol-lowering diet on maternal, cord, and neonatal lipids, and pregnancy outcome: a randomized clinical trial. Am J Obstet Gynecol 2005;193(4):1292–301.

12. Brown MS, Goldstein JL. A receptor-mediated pathway for cholesterol homeostasis. Science 1986;232(4746):34–47.

13. Jakubowski B, Shao Y, McNeal C, et al. Monogenic and polygenic causes of low and extremely low LDL-C levels in patients referred to specialty lipid clinics: Genetics of low LDL-C. J Clin Lipidol 2021;15(5):658–64.

14. Rimbert A, Vanhoye X, Coulibaly D, et al. Phenotypic differences between polygenic and monogenic hypobetalipoproteinemia. Arterioscler Thromb Vasc Biol 2021;41(1):e63–71.

15. Cohen JC, Boerwinkle E, Mosley TH Jr, et al. Sequence variations in PCSK9, low LDL, and protection against coronary heart disease. N Engl J Med 2006;354(12): 1264–72.

16. Zhao Z, Tuakli-Wosornu Y, Lagace TA, et al. Molecular characterization of loss-of-function mutations in PCSK9 and identification of a compound heterozygote. Am J Hum Genet 2006;79(3):514–23.

17. Hooper AJ, Marais AD, Tanyanyiwa DM, et al. The C679X mutation in PCSK9 is present and lowers blood cholesterol in a Southern African population. Atherosclerosis 2007;193(2):445–8.

18. Rashid S, Curtis DE, Garuti R, et al. Decreased plasma cholesterol and hypersensitivity to statins in mice lacking PCSK9. Proc Natl Acad Sci U S A 2005;102(15): 5374–9.

19. Tobert JA. Lovastatin and beyond: the history of the HMG-CoA reductase inhibitors. Nat Rev Drug Discov 2003;2(7):517–26.

20. Ray KK, Landmesser U, Leiter LA, et al. Inclisiran in patients at high cardiovascular risk with elevated LDL cholesterol. N Engl J Med 2017;376(15):1430–40.

21. Collins R, Reith C, Emberson J, et al. Interpretation of the evidence for the efficacy and safety of statin therapy. Lancet 2016;388(10059):2532–61.

22. Newman CB, Preiss D, Tobert JA, et al. Statin safety and associated adverse events: a scientific statement from the american heart association. Arterioscler Thromb Vasc Biol 2019;39(2):e38–81.

23. Schwartz GG, Gabriel Steg P, Bhatt DL, et al. Clinical efficacy and safety of alir-ocumab after acute coronary syndrome according to achieved level of low-density lipoprotein cholesterol: a propensity score-matched analysis of the OD-YSSEY OUTCOMES trial. Circulation 2021;143(11):1109–22.
24. Giugliano RP, Pedersen TR, Park JG, et al. Clinical efficacy and safety of achieving very low LDL-cholesterol concentrations with the PCSK9 inhibitor evo-locumab: a prespecified secondary analysis of the FOURIER trial. Lancet 2017; 390(10106):1962–71.
25. Herrett E, Williamson E, Brack K, et al. Statin treatment and muscle symptoms: series of randomised, placebo controlled n-of-1 trials. BMJ 2021;372:n135.
26. Wood FA, Howard JP, Finegold JA, et al. N-of-1 trial of a statin, placebo, or no treatment to assess side effects. N Engl J Med 2020;383(22):2182–4.
27. Wright RS, Ray KK, Raal FJ, et al. Pooled patient-level analysis of inclisiran trials in patients with familial hypercholesterolemia or atherosclerosis. J Am Coll Cardiol 2021;77(9):1182–93.
28. Martin SS, Blaha MJ, Elshazly MB, et al. Friedewald-estimated versus directly measured low-density lipoprotein cholesterol and treatment implications. J Am Coll Cardiol 2013;62(8):732–9.
29. Martin SS, Blaha MJ, Elshazly MB, et al. Comparison of a novel method vs the Friedewald equation for estimating low-density lipoprotein cholesterol levels from the standard lipid profile. JAMA 2013;310(19):2061–8.
30. Sampson M, Ling C, Sun Q, et al. A New equation for calculation of low-density lipoprotein cholesterol in patients with normolipidemia and/or hypertriglyceride-mia. JAMA Cardiol 2020;5(5):540–8.
31. Everett BM, Mora S, Glynn RJ, et al. Safety profile of subjects treated to very low low-density lipoprotein cholesterol levels (<30 mg/dl) with rosuvastatin 20 mg daily (from JUPITER). Am J Cardiol 2014;114(11):1682–9.
32. Marston NA, Giugliano RP, Park JG, et al. Cardiovascular benefit of lowering low-density lipoprotein cholesterol below 40 mg/dL. Circulation 2021;144(21):1732–4.
33. Plakogiannis R, Sorbera M, Fischetti B, et al. The role of antisense therapies tar-geting lipoprotein(a). J Cardiovasc Pharmacol 2021;78(1):e5–11.

Moving?

Make sure your subscription moves with you!

To notify us of your new address, find your **Clinics Account Number** (located on your mailing label above your name), and contact customer service at:

Email: journalscustomerservice-usa@elsevier.com

800-654-2452 (subscribers in the U.S. & Canada)
314-447-8871 (subscribers outside of the U.S. & Canada)

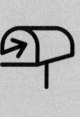

Fax number: 314-447-8029

Elsevier Health Sciences Division
Subscription Customer Service
3251 Riverport Lane
Maryland Heights, MO 63043

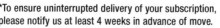

ELSEVIER

Printed and bound by CPI Group (UK) Ltd, Croydon, CR0 4YY

08/05/2025

01864723-0005